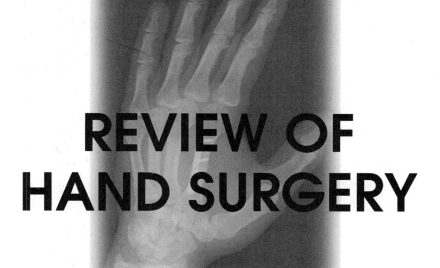

REVIEW OF HAND SURGERY

Pedro K. Beredjiklian, MD
Assistant Professor,
Department of Orthopaedic Surgery
University of Pennsylvania School of Medicine
Philadelphia, Pennsylvania

David J. Bozentka, MD
Associate Professor,
Department of Orthopaedic Surgery
University of Pennsylvania School of Medicine
Chief, Hand Surgery Section
Hospital of the University of Pennsylvania
Philadelphia, Pennsylvania

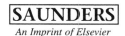

SAUNDERS
An Imprint of Elsevier

SAUNDERS
An Imprint of Elsevier

The Curtis Center
Independence Square West
Philadelphia, PA 19106-3399

REVIEW OF HAND SURGERY   ISBN 0-7216-0188-X
Copyright © 2004, Elsevier Inc. All rights reserved.

Permissions may be sought directly from Elsevier Inc. Rights Department in Philadelphia, USA: phone: (+1) 215 238 7869, fax: (+1) 215 238 2239, email: healthpermissions@elsevier.com. You may also complete your request on-line via the Elsevier Inc. homepage (http://www.elsevier.com), by selecting "Customer Support" and then "Obtaining Permissions."

Notice

Orthopaedics is an ever-changing field. Standard safety precautions must be followed, but as new research and clinical experience broaden our knowledge, changes in treatment and drug therapy may become necessary or appropriate. Readers are advised to check the most current product information provided by the manufacturer of each drug to be administered to verify the recommended dose, the method and duration of administration, and contraindications. It is the responsibility of the treating physician, relying on experience and knowledge of the patient, to determine dosages and the best treatment for each individual patient. Neither the Publisher nor the editors assume any liability for any injury and/or damage to persons or property arising from this publication.

The Publisher

Library of Congress Cataloging-in-Publication Data

Review of hand surgery / [edited by] Pedro K. Beredjiklian, David J. Bozentka.—1st ed.
    p. ; cm.
  ISBN 0-7216-0188-X
    1. Hand—Surgery. I. Beredjiklian, Pedro K. II. Bozentka, David J.
  [DNLM: 1. Hand—surgery. WE 830 R454 2004]
  RD559.R485 2004
  617.5′75059—dc21

                                                                    2003050659

Acquisitions Editor: Daniel Pepper
Developmental Editor: Heather Krehling
Project Manager: Linda Lewis Grigg

CE/MVY

Printed in the United States of America.

Last digit is the print number: 9   8   7   6   5   4   3

DEDICATION

To our families, for their endless support and encouragement.

CONTRIBUTORS

Mark E. Baratz, MD
Professor of Orthopaedic Surgery,
Department of Orthopaedic Surgery,
Drexel University College of Medicine,
Philadelphia; Vice Chairman and Director,
Division of Hand and Upper Extremity Surgery,
Department of Orthopaedic Surgery,
Allegheny General Hospital,
Pittsburgh, Pennsylvania
VASCULAR DISORDERS OF THE HAND AND
UPPER EXTREMITY

Pedro K. Beredjiklian, MD
Assistant Professor, Department of Orthopaedic Surgery,
University of Pennsylvania School of Medicine,
Philadelphia, Pennsylvania
REHABILITATION

Philip E. Blazar, MD
Assistant Clinical Professor of Orthopaedic
Surgery, Department of Orthopaedics,
Harvard Medical School; Orthopaedic Surgeon,
Brigham and Women's Hospital,
Boston, Massachusetts
DISLOCATIONS/INSTABILITY

David J. Bozentka, MD
Associate Professor, Department of Orthopaedic
Surgery, University of Pennsylvania School of Medicine;
Chief, Hand Surgery Section, Hospital of the University
of Pennsylvania, Philadelphia, Pennsylvania
REHABILITATION

Kent H. Chou, MD
Attending, Department of Orthopaedic Surgery,
University of Pittsburgh Medical Center,
Pittsburgh, Pennsylvania
FRACTURES OF THE HAND, WRIST, AND
FOREARM AXIS

Aaron Daluiski, MD
Instructor, Department of Orthopaedic Surgery,
Weill Medical College of Cornell University;
Assistant Attending, Hand Service, and Assistant
Scientist, Research Division, Hospital for Special
Surgery, New York, New York
TENDON

Rakesh Donthineni-Rao, MD
Assistant Professor, Department of Orthopaedics,
University of California Davis School of Medicine;
Chief, Orthopaedic Oncology, University of California
Davis Medical Center, Sacramento, California
TUMORS

Richard D. Goldner, MD
Associate Professor, Department of Surgery,
Division of Orthopaedic Surgery, Duke University
School of Medicine, Durham, North Carolina
MICROVASCULAR HAND SURGERY

Ranjan Gupta, MD
Assistant Professor—Hand and Upper
Extremity Surgery, Department of Surgery,
University of California, Irvine, School of Medicine,
Irvine, California
NERVE

Thomas R. Hunt III, MD
Head, Section of Hand Surgery, and Director,
Occupational Hand Therapy,
Department of Orthopaedic Surgery,
Cleveland Clinic, Cleveland, Ohio
INFECTION

Mark A. Katz, MD
Clinical Instructor, Department of Orthopaedic
Surgery, Presbyterian Medical Center of the
University of Pennsylvania Health System,
Philadelphia, Pennsylvania; Director,
The Princeton Hand Center,
Lawrenceville, New Jersey
MICROVASCULAR HAND SURGERY

Scott H. Kozin, MD
Associate Professor, Department of Orthopaedic
Surgery, Temple University School of Medicine;
Hand Surgeon, Shriners Hospital for Children,
Philadelphia, Pennsylvania
PEDIATRIC HAND SURGERY

Y. Leo Leung, MD*
Resident, Department of Orthopaedic Surgery,
Hospital of the University of Pennsylvania,
Philadelphia, Pennsylvania
REHABILITATION

L. Scott Levin, MD
Professor, Department of Plastic and Orthopaedic
Surgery, Duke University School of Medicine;
Chief, Division of Plastic, Reconstructive,
Maxillofacial and Oral Surgery,
Duke University Medical Center, Durham,
North Carolina
MICROVASCULAR HAND SURGERY

*Deceased.

Alexander M. Marcus, MD
Orthopedic Associates of Central Jersey,
Edison, New Jersey
INFECTION

Bruce A. Monaghan, MD
Chief, Division of Orthopaedic Surgery, and
Vice Chairman, Department of Surgery,
Underwood Memorial Hospital,
Woodbury, New Jersey
ANATOMY

Sanjiv H. Naidu, MD, PhD
Associate Professor,
Department of Orthopaedic Surgery,
Pennsylvania State University College of Medicine,
Hershey, Pennsylvania
ARTHRITIS

Nikolaos G. Papadimitriou, MD, PhD
Research Fellow, Department of Orthopaedic Surgery,
Division of Hand and Upper Extremity Surgery,
University of Pittsburgh School of Medicine,
Pittsburgh, Pennsylvania
FRACTURES OF THE HAND, WRIST, AND
FOREARM AXIS

Tamara D. Rozental, MD
Instructor, Department of Orthopaedic Surgery,
University of Pennsylvania School of Medicine,
Philadelphia, Pennsylvania
SKIN AND SOFT TISSUE DEFECTS

Ioannis Sarris, MD, PhD
Professor, Department of Orthopaedics,
Athens University School of Medicine,
Athens, Greece; Fellow, Department of
Orthopaedics, Allegheny General Hospital,
Pittsburgh, Pennsylvania
FRACTURES OF THE HAND, WRIST, AND
FOREARM AXIS

Christopher C. Schmidt, MD
Director, Microvascular Reconstruction of the Upper
Limb, Department of Orthopaedic Surgery,
Allegheny General Hospital,
Pittsburgh, Pennsylvania
VASCULAR DISORDERS OF THE HAND AND
UPPER EXTREMITY

Dean G. Sotereanos, MD
Professor, Department of Orthopaedics,
Drexel University College of Medicine;
Vice Chairman, Department of Orthopaedics,
Allegheny General Hospital,
Pittsburgh, Pennsylvania
FRACTURES OF THE HAND, WRIST, AND
FOREARM AXIS

David R. Steinberg, MD
Associate Professor, Department of Orthopaedic
Surgery, University of Pennsylvania School of Medicine;
Director, Hand and Upper Extremity Fellowship,
Hospital of the University of Pennsylvania,
Philadelphia, Pennsylvania
SKIN AND SOFT TISSUE DEFECTS

Virak Tan, MD
Assistant Professor, Department of Orthopaedic
Surgery, UMDNJ–New Jersey Medical School,
Newark; Attending Surgeon, Department of
Orthopaedic Surgery, Overlook Hospital,
Summit, New Jersey
TENDON

John D. Temple, MD
Resident in Orthopaedics, Penn State Orthopaedics,
Milton S. Hershey Medical Center,
Hershey, Pennsylvania
ARTHRITIS

James R. Urbaniak, MD
Virginia Flowers Baker Professor of Orthopaedic
Surgery and Vice Chairman, Department of Surgery,
Duke University School of Medicine,
Durham, North Carolina
MICROVASCULAR HAND SURGERY

Jonathan A. Uroskie, MD
Orthopaedic Surgeon,
Sports Medicine North,
Lynnfield, Massachusetts
VASCULAR DISORDERS OF THE HAND AND
UPPER EXTREMITY

FOREWORD

The upper extremity in general and the hand in particular received a quantum boost in recognition as a distinct entity during World War II. Norman Kirk, the Surgeon General, recognized that surgeons were not adequately trained to care for the complicated upper extremity injuries that the war produced. Operative treatment was deficient as were proper postoperative care and hand therapy, all requisites for regaining hand function. Dr. Kirk appointed Sterling Brunnell to organize nine centers managed by nine surgeons for the treatment of hand injuries in World War II. This group became the core who established the American Society for Surgery of the Hand. Comprehensive books about hand surgery have been published, including those by Brunnell, Flynn, Tubiano, and Green.

In 1989, hand surgery became the first specialty to have separated itself from other root surgical fields by creating an examination, the certificate for added qualifications of the hand (CAQ). It is a privilege to contribute a Foreword for this excellent and badly needed book. It organizes material in subjects that have been covered in previous examinations. These include the orthopaedic in-training examination (OITE), boards, and the CAQ examination. The text will be of enormous value to medical students, residents, fellows, hand therapists, and emergency room surgeons as a study guide, and it will be a ready source of reference for practicing Hand Surgeons. Drs. Beredjiklian and Bozentka have gathered a group of colleagues, all of whom are acknowledged experts in their particular field. The resultant work has a delightful evenness of style that is unusual in a multiauthored book, and this is the work of the editors.

F. William Bora, Jr.

PREFACE

This text is designed to be a comprehensive review of disorders related to hand and upper extremity surgery. We believe that this work will fill a void in the available body of textbooks dedicated to this field by providing the reader with a complete yet easy-to-access source of information. We have integrated information involving a wide range of topics in hand surgery to create an all-inclusive guide for study. Chapters dealing in areas including pediatric hand surgery, microvascular surgery, and the treatment of bony and soft tissue injuries complement one another and serve to broaden the scope of the text.

We hope the book will serve as a ready source of reference for Hand Surgeons and physical and occupational therapists involved in the care of patients with hand and wrist disorders. In addition, we expect that this text will be invaluable to surgeons in training as an outline for study. Hand surgery fellows, orthopaedic and plastic surgery residents, and medical students will find *Review of Hand Surgery* a helpful asset for test preparation such as the boards, the certificate for added qualifications of the hand (CAQ), and in-training residency examinations.

We would like to thank the chapter authors for their dedication to the field. We are also indebted to Richard Lampert for his guidance throughout the editorial process and to Fran Reilly for her tireless work on this project.

Pedro K. Beredjiklian
David J. Bozentka

CONTENTS

*Deceased.

1

✧ Bruce A. Monaghan, MD

ANATOMY

Introduction

Osteology

1. Bone can be classified as either cortical (compact) or cancellous (spongy).
2. Endochondral bone formation is a process whereby bone is formed from a cartilaginous model. This can occur by embryonic long bone formation, longitudinal growth through a physis, and fracture healing. Intramembranous ossification occurs without a cartilage model and can be seen in flat bone formation (i.e., clavicle) or with distraction osteogenesis.
3. Appositional bone growth also does not require a cartilaginous model and occurs when bones grow in width with periosteal new bone formation.

Arthrology

1. Joints are specialized structures that mechanically coordinate motion between bones.
2. In addition to bone structures, diarthrodial joints are composed of ligaments, joint capsule, synovium, and articular cartilage. Ligaments are supporting structures. The joint capsule separates the joint from surrounding structures. The synovium is a layer of the capsule that is involved in joint nutrition and lubrication.
3. Synovial fluid, produced by type B synoviocytes, is composed of hyaluronic acid, proteinases, collagenases, prostaglandins, and lubricin, a glycoprotein involved in lubrication.
4. Articular cartilage functions to decrease friction and to transfer load transmission. It is aneural and avascular, receiving its nutrition from the synovial fluid through diffusion.
5. Joints are classified by their freedom of motion (Table 1-1).
   a. Synarthroses typically have no motion at maturity (i.e., skull suture lines).
   b. Amphiarthrodial joints have limited motion and possess an articular disk between the articular or hyaline cartilage (i.e., symphysis pubis, sternoclavicular).
   c. Diarthrodial joints are specialized structures that efficiently coordinate motion. These joints are classified according to mobility and anatomy.

Nerves (see Chapter 5)

1. Most peripheral nerves originate from the ventral rami of spinal nerves. Efferent fibers carry motor signals from the central nervous system to muscles. Afferent fibers typically carry sensory information back to the central nervous system (Fig. 1-1).
2. Peripheral nerves consist of numerous axons (surrounded by the endoneurium), which are organized into fascicles that are bound by the perineurium, a layer of connective tissue.
   a. The fascicles of the peripheral nerves are surrounded by a loose connective tissue layer (epineurium) (Fig. 1-2).
   b. Nerve fibers are characterized by function and other characteristics (Table 1-2).
   c. Peripheral nerves have several sensory end organs in skin.
      i. Meissner corpuscles are disklike, approximately 3 μm thick and 30 μm in diameter. They are activated by touch (moving two-point).
      ii. Pacinian corpuscles are larger (100 to 500 μm × 2 mm) and respond to pressure and vibration.
      iii. Ruffini corpuscles are activated by cold and heat.
      iv. Merkel's disks are activated by continuous touch (static two-point discrimination).
      v. Naked A-delta fibers—sharp pain.
      vi. Naked C fibers—burning pain.

✧ Table 1-1		
TYPES OF JOINTS		
Planes of Freedom	**Anatomic Description**	**Example**
Uniaxial	Ginglymus (hinge)	Interphalangeal
	Trochoid (pivot)	Distal radioulnar
Biaxial	Condyloid	Metacarpophalangeal
	Ellipsoid	Radiocarpal
	Saddle	Thumb carpometacarpal
Polyaxial	Spheroid (ball-and-socket)	Glenohumeral
Plane	Gliding	Scapholunate

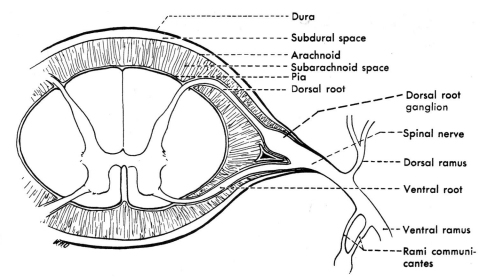

Figure 1-1 ❖ Spinal nerves. *(From Jenkins DB: Hollinshead's Functional Anatomy of the Limbs and Back, 6th ed. Philadelphia, WB Saunders, 1991.)*

Tendon (see Chapter 2)

1. Tendon is composite tissue that consists primarily of type I collagen (86% of dry weight) in a matrix of proteoglycans and a sparse density of fibroblasts.
2. Each collagen molecule is a triple left-handed helix of three polypeptide chains. The collagen molecules are arranged longitudinally and quarter staggered in microfibrils. Tendon fibrils are incorporated into tendon fascicles in a matrix of proteoglycans, glycoproteins, and water.
3. Fascicles are bound within the endotenon, a loose connective tissue that supports a blood supply, lymphatic drainage, and a nerve supply as well as allows longitudinal motion between individual fibrils.

4. The epitenon is a highly cellular, fibrous outer layer that is continuous with endotenon and contains most of the capillaries and blood supply.

Ligament

1. Ligaments, dense connective tissue with structure similar to tendons, serve to connect bones or to support viscera.
2. Collagen type I composes about 70% of the dry weight of ligament (less than of tendon), but there is more ground substance. In addition, the collagen is less organized than in tendon, forming more of a weaving pattern.
3. Most of the blood supply to ligaments originates from the origin and insertion sites.

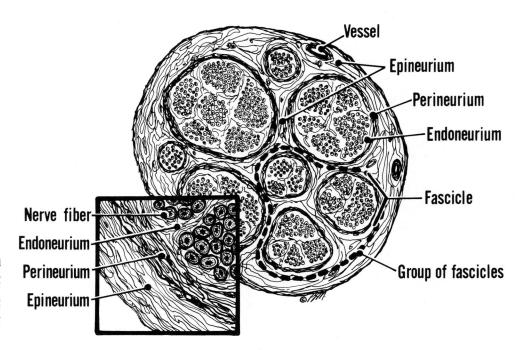

Figure 1-2 ❖ Cross-sectional anatomy of a peripheral nerve. *(From Brushart TM: Nerve repair and grafting. In Green DP, Hotchkiss RN, Pederson WC, eds: Operative Hand Surgery, 4th ed. New York, Churchill Livingstone, 1999.)*

◆ Table 1-2

TYPES OF NERVE FIBERS

Type	Size (μm)	Myelination	Speed	Examples
A	10–20	Heavy	Fast	Touch
B	<3	Intermediate	Medium	Autonomic
C	<1.3	None	Slow	Pain

Hand

Osteology (Fig. 1-3)

PHALANGES

1. There are 14 phalanges (5 proximal, 4 middle, and 5 distal).
2. Primary ossification occurs in the shaft in the 8th to 9th week of development for the distal phalanges, the 10th week for the middle phalanges, and the 11th week or later for the proximal phalanges. Secondary ossification centers appear in the proximal phalanges first (2 to 3 years). All phalangeal growth plates fuse by 15 to 16 years in girls and 17 to 18 years in boys.
3. The base of each phalanx has smooth facets to articulate with the more proximal metacarpal or phalangeal head.
4. The heads of the proximal and middle phalanges are pulley shaped to form the hinge joints of the interphalangeal joints.
5. The volar surface of the distal phalanx has a roughened surface that attaches to the pulp of the fingertip with multiple vertical septa of dense connective tissue.

METACARPALS

1. There are five metacarpals in the hand. They are long bones with a base, shaft, neck, and head.

The primary ossification center in the shaft appears at 8 weeks of age, and the secondary ossification (physis) appears at 3 years. Because the thumb metacarpal is similar to a proximal phalanx, its secondary ossification is located at the base.

2. The collateral recesses appear along the radial and ulnar aspects of the metacarpal head as an origin of the proper collateral ligaments.
3. The metacarpal shaft is concave longitudinally on the volar surface. This concavity makes the dorsal surface the tension side of the bone.
4. Whereas the medial four metacarpals are tightly bound side by side, the thumb metacarpal is rotated 90 degrees with respect to the others to facilitate prehension.

Arthrology

INTERPHALANGEAL JOINTS (FIG. 1-4)

1. The proximal interphalangeal (PIP) and distal interphalangeal (DIP) joints are uniaxial hinge joints.
2. The DIP joints experience the greatest amount of longitudinal stress of any joints in the hand.
3. The major soft tissue constraints are the capsule and extensor tendons dorsally, the collateral ligaments laterally, and the volar plate volarly.
4. The primary stability of the joint is conferred by articular congruity, the collateral ligaments, and the volar plate.
   a. The collateral ligaments arise from fossae on the lateral aspect of the phalangeal heads and insert into the volar third of the phalangeal base (proper collateral ligament) and the volar plate (accessory collateral ligament).

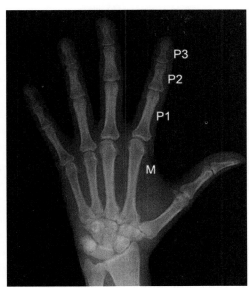

Figure 1-3 ◆ Posteroanterior radiograph of the hand. P3, distal phalanx; P2, middle phalanx; P1, proximal phalanx; M, metacarpal.

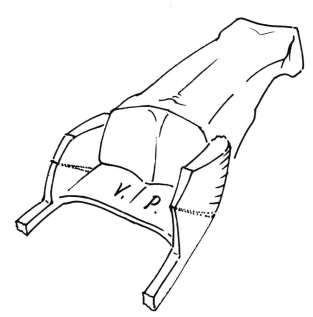

Figure 1-4 ◆ Schematic of an interphalangeal joint without the more proximal phalanx revealing the volar plate (V.P.) and the collateral ligaments. *(From Glickel S, Barron OA, Eaton RG: Dislocations and ligament injuries in the digits. In Green DP, Hotchkiss RN, Pederson WC, eds: Operative Hand Surgery, 4th ed. New York, Churchill Livingstone, 1999.)*

b. The collateral ligaments are the primary restraints to radial and ulnar deviation of the joint.

c. Checkrein ligaments are fibrous connections between the proximal aspect of the volar plate and the volar bone ridges of the proximal phalanx in the PIP joint. These are implicated in flexion contractures of the PIP joint (Fig. 1-5).

5. The palmodigital crease corresponds to the midshaft of the proximal phalanx. The distal palmar crease corresponds to the metacarpophalangeal joint.

METACARPOPHALANGEAL JOINTS

1. The metacarpophalangeal (MP) joints of the medial digits are condyloid joints, allowing flexion-extension, abduction-adduction, and some rotation.

2. They are less susceptible to injury because of their protected position and the additional soft tissue stability conferred by the surrounding extensor, flexor, and intrinsic tendons and the transverse intermetacarpal ligaments.

3. The volar plate, which is thicker distally than proximally, is continuous with the deep transverse intermetacarpal ligament.

4. The metacarpal head is wider on its volar surface than on its dorsal surface, allowing more bone contact and stability with increasing flexion.

5. On the sagittal plane, the distance from the center of rotation of the metacarpal head to the articular surface of the MP joint is smallest at the most distal aspect and greatest at the most volar aspect of the metacarpal head (Fig. 1-6).

a. This creates a "cam" effect as the MP joint is taken from extension into flexion.

b. As a result, the collateral ligaments are lax in extension and taut in flexion.

c. For this reason, the MP joints should be immobilized in flexion (intrinsic plus position). If the joints are immobilized in extension, the collateral ligaments can contract, preventing flexion of the joint and leading to an extension contracture.

d. In addition, maintaining the MP joints in extension leads to an imbalance of the extrinsic muscles. Tension on the finger flexors leads to a flexion deformity of the PIP joints.

Thumb MP Joint

1. The thumb MP joint combines the features of a ginglymus and condyloid joint.

2. The range of motion is variable between individuals because of differences in metacarpal head radius of curvature.

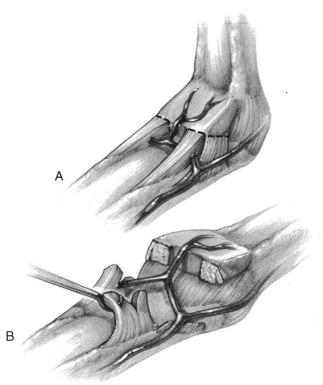

Figure 1-5 ◆ Checkrein pathologic bands. **A,** The checkreins attach proximally to the assembly line and distally to the volar plate on both the radial and ulnar sides. The transverse communicating vessels traverse the collagen band approximately 2 mm proximal to the volar plate. **B,** Complete excision of the checkreins often requires resection dorsal as well as volar to the transverse communicating vessels. These vessels should be preserved. *(From Watson HK, Weinzweig J: Stiff joints. In Green DP, Hotchkiss RN, Pederson WC, eds: Operative Hand Surgery, 4th ed. New York, Churchill Livingstone, 1999.)*

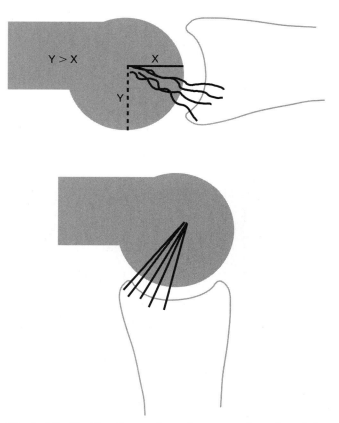

Figure 1-6 ◆ The distance from the center of rotation of the metacarpal head to the articular surface of the MP joint is greatest at the most volar aspect of the joint (Y) and smallest at the most distal aspect of the head (X). For this reason, in full extension, the collateral ligaments are relaxed in extension but become taut with MP joint flexion.

3. Bone congruity is much less a determinant of stability than are soft tissues (volar plate, collateral ligaments).
4. There are no checkrein ligaments, but the accessory collateral ligaments insert into the sesamoids as well as the volar plate.
5. The adductor aponeurosis lies directly over the ulnar collateral ligament. Interposition of the aponeurosis between torn ulnar collateral ligament and base of the proximal phalanx can occur, resulting in a Stener lesion (see Chapter 7).

Nerve (Fig. 1-7)

MEDIAN NERVE

1. The median nerve enters the hand through the carpal tunnel along with the flexor tendons.

2. The nerve supplies sensation to the volar aspect of the thumb and index and long fingers and the radial half of the ring finger. It innervates the index and long finger lumbrical muscles and the majority of the thenar muscles including the abductor pollicis brevis, the opponens pollicis, and the superficial head of the flexor pollicis brevis.

3. As it enters the palm of the hand, the median nerve branches into the motor branch to the thenar muscles and the sensory common digital nerves.
   a. The point of origin of the motor branch is variable with respect to the overlying transverse carpal ligament (46% extraligamentous, 31% subligamentous, and 23% transligamentous).
   b. Studies have shown that the transligamentous median nerve may be more infrequent (7%) (Fig. 1-7B).

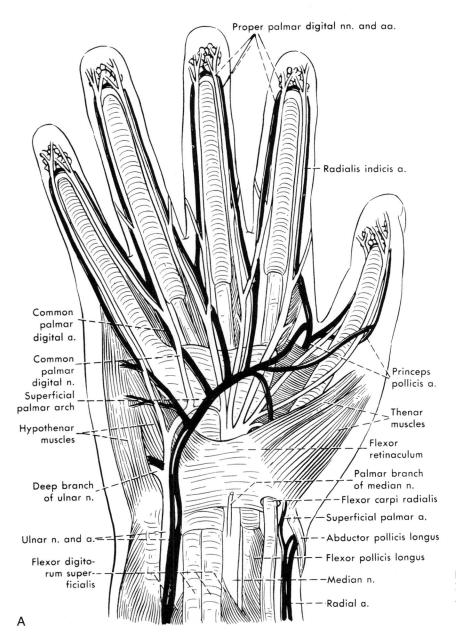

Proper palmar digital nn. and aa.

Radialis indicis a.

Common palmar digital a.

Common palmar digital n.

Superficial palmar arch

Hypothenar muscles

Deep branch of ulnar n.

Ulnar n. and a.

Flexor digitorum superficialis

Princeps pollicis a.

Thenar muscles

Flexor retinaculum

Palmar branch of median n.

Flexor carpi radialis

Superficial palmar a.

Abductor pollicis longus

Flexor pollicis longus

Median n.

Radial a.

A

Figure 1-7 ◈ **A,** Nerves and vessels of the hand. *(A from Jenkins DB: Hollinshead's Functional Anatomy of the Limbs and Back, 6th ed. Philadelphia, WB Saunders, 1991.)*

(Continued)

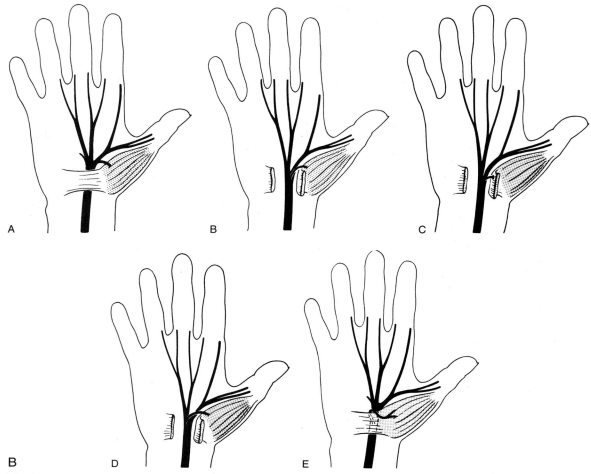

Figure 1-7 ◆ cont'd **B,** Variations of the motor branch of the median nerve in the carpal tunnel. The motor branch may be extraligamentous (**A,** 46% to 90%), subligamentous (**B,** 31%), or transligamentous (**C,** 23%). Less commonly, the motor branch may lie ulnar to the median nerve in the carpal tunnel (**D**) or lie on top of the transverse carpal ligament (**E**). *(**B** from Green DP, Hotchkiss RN, Pederson WC, eds: Operative Hand Surgery, 4th ed. New York, Churchill Livingstone, 1999.)*

4. The palmar cutaneous nerve branch of the median nerve supplies sensation to the thenar skin and originates from the radial aspect of the median nerve variably 0 to 5 cm proximal to the wrist flexor crease.

5. High median nerve division and bifid median nerve are associated with aberrant muscles or a persistent median artery.

ULNAR NERVE

1. The ulnar nerve enters the hand through Guyon's canal.

2. Guyon's canal is formed by the volar carpal ligament volarly, the transverse carpal ligament dorsally, the hook of the hamate laterally, and the pisiform medially (Fig. 1-8).

3. The nerve supplies sensation to the small finger and ulnar half of the ring finger. It innervates the intrinsic muscles of the hand with the exception of the median-innervated thenar muscles and the radial two lumbricals.

4. The nerve branches into a superficial branch and deep branch. The superficial component has branches to the palmaris brevis muscle and sensory branches to the small and ring fingers. The deep branch supplies branches to the deep intrinsics.
   a. The deep branch of the ulnar nerve pierces between the abductor digiti minimi and the flexor digiti minimi brevis.

5. The dorsal sensory branch of the ulnar nerve originates approximately 7 cm proximal to the wrist crease and provides sensation to the dorsal aspect of the ulnar hand and the ring finger proximal to the PIP joints.

RADIAL NERVE

1. The dorsal sensory radial nerve supplies the dorsal aspect of the radial hand, the dorsum of the thumb, and the dorsal aspect of the radial fingers proximal to the PIP joints. The lateral antebrachial cutaneous nerve, the terminal branch of the musculocutaneous nerve, also supplies sensory branches to the radial aspect of the wrist overlapping the region of the dorsal radial sensory nerve.

2. The radial nerve does not innervate any of the intrinsic muscles of the hand.

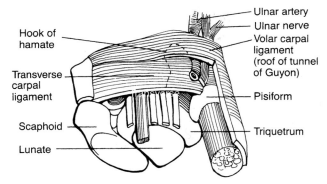

Hook of hamate

Transverse carpal ligament

Scaphoid

Lunate

Ulnar artery

Ulnar nerve

Volar carpal ligament (roof of tunnel of Guyon)

Pisiform

Triquetrum

Figure 1-8 ◈ The carpal tunnel is formed by the transverse carpal ligament volarly and the carpal bones on the floor and sides. Guyon's canal is formed by the volar carpal ligament (roof), the hamate (lateral wall), and the pisiform (medial wall). *(From Beim GM, Warner JP: Clinical and radiographic evaluation of the acromioclavicular joint. Oper Tech Sports Med 5:68, 1997.)*

COMMON AND PROPER DIGITAL NERVES

1. Common digital nerves are branches from the median and ulnar nerves. Proper digital nerves arise from the common digital nerves.
   a. The proper ulnar digital nerve to the small finger arises from the ulnar nerve.
   b. The fourth common digital nerve originates from contributions of the ulnar and median nerves. This nerve then divides distally into the radial digital nerve to the small finger and the ulnar nerve to the ring finger.
   c. The rest of the common digital nerves originate from the median nerve.
2. The digital nerves lie dorsal to the digital arteries in the palm. At the level of the digital web, the position changes and the digital nerves lie volar to the digital arteries.
3. The dorsal branches of the digital nerves supply the skin distal to the PIP joint in the index, middle, and ring fingers and the entire dorsum of the small finger.
4. Cleland's and Grayson's ligaments are fascial bands that maintain the position of the digital skin on flexion and extension of the finger.
   a. They originate from the flexor tendon sheath and travel dorsal (Cleland's [C—ceiling]) and volar (Grayson's [G—ground]) to the digital neurovascular bundles.
   b. They insert on the digital fascia.
   c. Cleland's ligaments are not involved in Dupuytren's contracture (see Chapter 10).
5. Distal to the DIP joint, the digital nerves trifurcate into branches supplying the finger pulp, fingertip, and the dorsal nail fold.

Artery (Fig. 1-7)

See Chapter 4.
1. The hand is most commonly vascularized by a dual supply from the radial and ulnar arteries.
2. The superficial palmar arch is a continuation of the ulnar artery and is most commonly the dominant blood supply to the hand (88%).

3. The deep palmar arch is a continuation of the radial artery and is the dominant blood supply to the hand in 12% of cases.
4. The superficial arch is more variable than the deep arch.
   a. It is coapted by the radial artery in 35% of cases, by the deep arch in 30% of cases, and by the median artery in 5% of cases. It is incomplete in 21% of cases.
5. The deep arch is incomplete in 3% of cases.
6. In a majority of hands, blood supply to the digits is derived from both the deep and superficial arches (86% to 98%).
7. The blood supply to the thumb is variable. The most common pattern is from the princeps pollicis artery (first palmar metacarpal artery) which divides into the proper digital arteries.
8. The first and second dorsal metacarpal arteries supply the skin over the proximal phalanx of the index and middle fingers. They are the vascular pedicles of the first and second dorsal metacarpal artery flaps (see Chapter 3).
9. The dorsal branch of the radial artery enters the hand between the two heads of the first dorsal interosseous muscle.

Extensor Tendons (Fig. 1-9)

EXTENSOR MECHANISM

1. Digital extension occurs through a coordinated effort of the radially innervated extrinsic extensor tendons and the median- and ulnar-innervated intrinsic system.
2. There are independent extrinsic tendons for index and small finger extension, the extensor indicis proprius (EIP) and the extensor digiti minimi (EDM). These tendons lay ulnar to the common extensor tendons on the dorsum of the hand before inserting into the dorsal expansion with the extensor digitorum communis (EDC) tendon.
3. Juncturae tendinum interconnect the common digital extensors on the dorsum of the hand and can allow MP joint extension in the setting of a complete single EDC laceration. They prevent independent finger extension.
   a. The juncturae are most constant between the middle and ring fingers.
   b. EIP is typically not involved, whereas EDM typically has juncturae.
   c. Three types have been described:
      i. Filamentous bands, more common in the radial digits.
      ii. Thicker, well-defined bands.
      iii. Tendon slips, R or Y shaped, more common in the ulnar digits.
4. The EDC to the small finger is absent in up to 50% of cadaver specimens. If absent, the tendon is replaced by juncturae from the ring finger.
5. Distal to the MP joint, the EDC divides into three parts.
   a. The central part (central slip) continues on to insert on the base of the dorsum of the

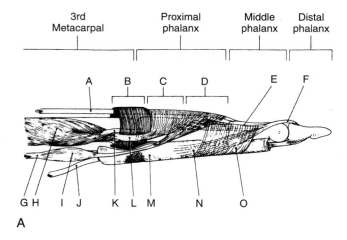

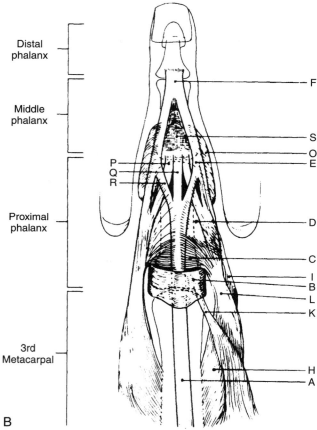

Figure 1-9 ◈ **A,** Diagrammatic representation (radial view, left middle finger) of the muscles, tendons, and fascia that directly influence the motion of the finger. **B,** Dorsal aspect of the left middle finger. A, common extensor tendon; B, sagittal band; C, transverse fibers of the interossei; D, oblique fibers of the interossei; E, lateral conjoined tendon; F, terminal tendon; G, flexor digitorum profundus tendon; H, interosseus muscle (second dorsal), deep head; I, lumbrical muscle; J, flexor digitorum superficialis tendon; K, medial tendon, superficial head of second dorsal interosseus; L, lateral tendon of deep head of second dorsal interosseus muscle; M, fibrous flexor pulley; N, oblique retinacular ligament; O, transverse retinacular ligament; P, medial interosseus band; Q, central slip of the common extensor; R, lateral slip of the common extensor; S, triangular ligament. *(From Smith RJ: Balance and kinetics of the fingers under normal and pathological conditions. Clin Orthop 104:92-111, 1974.)*

middle phalanx. Before insertion onto the phalanx, the central slip is joined by contributions from the interosseous muscles. The primary role of the central slip is extension of the PIP joint.

b. The two lateral slips of the EDC join the deep head of the interosseous and lumbrical muscles to become the conjoined lateral band. The two lateral bands become conjoined over the middle phalanx and go on to insert on the base of the dorsum of the distal phalanx as the terminal tendon. The primary role of the terminal tendon is extension of the DIP joint.

The extensor mechanism is complemented by retinacular elements that help stabilize the tendons and aid in digital motion. There are several components to the digital extensor aponeurosis.

Sagittal Bands
The extensor tendon at the level of the MP joint is held centrally by sagittal bands.

1. The sagittal bands arise from the volar plate and intermetacarpal ligaments volarly and attach to the extensor tendon dorsally.
2. The sagittal bands are also named the "shroud" ligament because it covers or wraps the MP joint.
3. Disruption of the sagittal bands can lead to extensor tendon subluxation into the space between metacarpal heads ("intermetacarpal valleys").
   a. If the extensor tendon subluxates, there will be incomplete extension of the affected MP joint and the digit will assume a deviated position because of the eccentric line of pull of the tendon.
   b. Attritional lengthening of the radial sagittal bands can develop in patients with rheumatoid arthritis because of proliferative synovitis at the MP joint. Insufficiency of the radial sagittal bands leads to ulnar subluxation of the extensor tendon. This subluxation leads to the characteristic rheumatoid hand deformity of MP joint flexion and ulnar deviation of the digits (see Chapter 9).
   c. Sagittal bands can also rupture acutely, often as a result of a traumatic injury to an extended finger. The most commonly injured sagittal band is the radial sagittal band of the long finger (see Chapter 2).
   d. Initiation of extension in the fully flexed finger occurs via the action of the EDC on the sagittal bands (Fig. 1-10).

Transverse and Oblique Fibers
These fibers are located distal to the sagittal bands.

1. The oblique fibers originate from the interossei and lumbrical muscles.
2. In contrast to the sagittal bands, the transverse fibers facilitate flexion of the MP joint (Fig. 1-10).

Transverse Retinacular Ligament
1. The transverse retinacular ligament originates from the flexor tendon sheath and inserts onto the lateral border of the conjoined lateral bands.
2. It functions to prevent dorsal subluxation of the lateral bands.

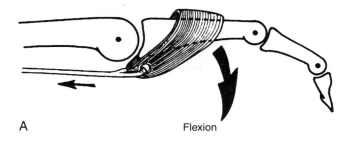

A   Flexion

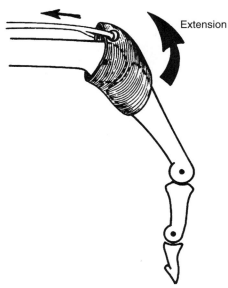

Extension

B

Figure 1-10 ◈ The transverse fibers of the interosseous tendons overlie the midshaft of the proximal phalanx. They serve to flex the proximal phalanx as diagrammed in **A**. The sagittal bands of the common extensor tendon insert volarly into the volar plate (and part of the periosteum of the proximal phalanx). They act to extend the proximal phalanx as seen in **B**. Thus, the sagittal bands and the transverse fibers of the interosseous tendons have completely opposite functions, although they lie adjacent to each other. *(From Smith RJ: Balance and kinetics of the fingers under normal and pathological conditions. Clin Orthop 104:92-111, 1974.)*

3. In cases of chronic boutonnière deformity, the ligament contracts, potentiating the volar subluxation of the lateral bands and the resultant flexion deformity of the PIP joint.
4. In cases of chronic swan-neck deformity, the ligament becomes attenuated, potentiating the dorsal subluxation of the lateral bands and the resultant extension deformity of the PIP joint.

Oblique Retinacular Ligament
1. The oblique retinacular ligament originates from the flexor tendon sheath and inserts onto the terminal tendon of the extensor mechanism.
2. It functions to extend the DIP joint through its attachment to the terminal tendon when the PIP joint is extended (tenodesis effect).

3. It maintains DIP extension in patients treated with a terminal tendon tenotomy for chronic boutonnière deformity (Fowler's distal tenotomy).
4. It can be reconstructed in patients with chronic swan-neck or mallet deformity.

Triangular Ligament
1. The triangular ligament joins the two lateral bands before their joining to become the terminal tendon.
2. It functions to prevent volar subluxation of the lateral bands.

Flexor Tendons

1. The medial four digits have two flexor tendons that originate from forearm muscles.
2. Unlike the extensor mechanism, in which the extension of the digital joints is linked, flexion of the PIP and DIP joints is effected by two independent muscle groups.
   a. The flexor digitorum superficialis (FDS) tendon is responsible for flexion of the PIP joint by its attachment on the middle phalanx.
      i. The FDS tendon divides into two slips along the proximal phalanx to allow passage of the profundus tendon.
      ii. The superficial flexor tendon slips rejoin dorsally at Camper's chiasma (named because of the crossing fibers) before inserting into the middle 3/5 of the volar shaft of the middle phalanx.
   b. The flexor digitorum profundus (FDP) is responsible for flexion of the DIP joint by its attachment on the volar base of the distal phalanx.
      i. The FDP tendons of the long, ring, and small fingers originate from a common muscle and cannot flex each digit independently. The FDP tendon of the index finger has an independent muscle origin.
      ii. Because of this common origin, limiting the excursion of one tendon will limit the excursion of the tendons of the other digits (quadriga effect; see Chapter 2).
   c. The thumb has only one extrinsic flexor, the flexor pollicis longus (FPL), which inserts into the distal phalanx of the thumb.
      i. It is the most radial tendon in the carpal tunnel.
3. Up to 9 cm of digital tendon excursion may be needed for composite wrist and digital flexion; only 2.5 cm may be required for digital flexion with the wrist in neutral.
4. Passive range of motion generates forces of 2 to 4 N in digital flexor tendons. Flexion with moderate resistance can generate 17 N of force. Thumb to index fingertip pinch can generate 120 N of force.

TENDON SHEATH

The flexor tendons travel through fibro-osseous sheaths in the digits (Fig. 1-11).
1. The tendon sheaths are composed of fibrous pulleys that provide structural stability to the sheath.

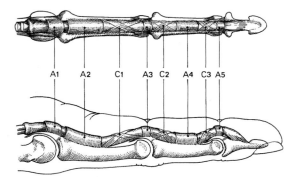

Figure 1-11 ◆ Annular pulleys. *(From Lisfranc R: Flexor tendon lesions in rheumatoid arthritis. In Tubiana R, ed: The Hand, vol V. Philadelphia, WB Saunders, 1999.)*

  a. There are five annular pulleys and three cruciate pulleys for the four fingers.
    i. The odd-numbered annular pulleys arise from the volar plates of the MP, PIP, and DIP joints.
    ii. The even-numbered annular pulleys, A2 and A4, arise from the periosteum of the proximal and middle phalanges, respectively.
    iii. The A2 and A4 pulleys are most important biomechanically because they prevent tendon bowstringing. If injury leads to bowstringing, they should be repaired or reconstructed.
    iv. The cruciate pulleys are located over joints. The orientation of the fibers allows them to collapse, which prevents "crimping" of the tendon sheath with digital flexion.
  b. The fingers have a palmar aponeurosis pulley, which is a condensation of palmar fascia proximal to the A1 pulley. This pulley becomes mechanically important if other pulleys are injured or nonfunctional.
  c. The thumb has two annular pulleys (A1 and A2 overlying the MP and interphalangeal joints, respectively) and one oblique pulley. The oblique pulley is centered on the proximal phalanx and is in continuity with the adductor pollicis insertion. The oblique pulley of the thumb is the most important pulley of the thumb in preventing bowstringing.
2. The primary function of the digital sheath is to maintain the tendons close to the phalanges. By maintenance of the tendons close to the axes of rotation of the joints, the angular rotation of the joint is maximized as a function of tendon excursion. If bowstringing occurs, joint rotation is decreased, and digital contractures may develop.
3. The sheaths are lined by visceral and parietal synovial layers, which provide nutrition and a smooth gliding surface for the flexor tendons.
  a. Synovial cells within the sheath produce synovial fluid, which contains nutrients and provides lubrication for the flexor tendons.

  b. The nutrients can enter the tendon through diffusion or a process called imbibition, whereby the synovial fluid is driven mechanically into the tendon parenchyma with digital motion.
  c. The flexor tendons in the hand also have direct vascular supply through vincula.
    i. Vincula are folds of mesotenon on the dorsal surface of the flexor tendons carrying nutrient vessels from the digital arteries. There are short (breve) and long (longum) vincula for each tendon (Fig. 1-12).
    ii. Other minor contributors to the blood supply of the tendons include muscle branches at the musculotendinous junction and periosteal branches at the site of bone insertion.
  d. The sheaths of the index, long, and ring fingers start at the level of the metacarpal necks with the palmar aponeurosis pulleys and end at the point of insertion of the FDP into the distal phalanx (Fig. 1-13).
  e. The sheath of the thumb flexor (FPL) extends proximal to the wrist joint to the level of the pronator quadratus muscle.
  f. The sheath of the small finger also extends proximal to the wrist joint.
    i. It incorporates the rest of the digital flexors at the level of the carpal tunnel.

Fascial Spaces (Fig. 1-14)

See Chapter 11.

MIDPALMAR SPACE

1. The midpalmar space is bounded volarly by the palmar aponeurosis and the flexor tendons of the long, ring, and small fingers.

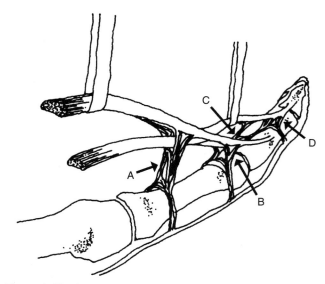

Figure 1-12 ◆ The direct vascular supply to the flexor tendons in the digits comes from vincula. Each tendon is supplied by two *vincula.* A, vinculum longum superficialis; B, vinculum breve superficialis; C, vinculum longum profundus; D, vinculum breve profundus. *(From Beredjiklian PK: Biologic aspects of flexor tendon healing. J Bone Joint Surg Am 85:539-550, 2003.)*

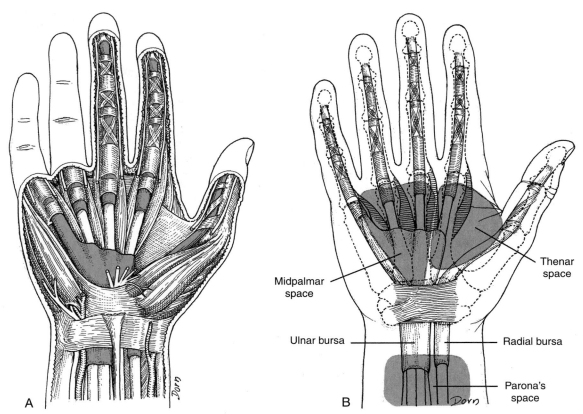

Figure 1-13 ◈ Coronal sections of the hand and distal forearm showing the flexor tendon sheaths, spaces, and bursae. *(From Drukker S, Masson J, Grossman JAI: Common bacterial infections. In Tubiana R, ed: The Hand, vol V. Philadelphia, WB Saunders, 1999.)*

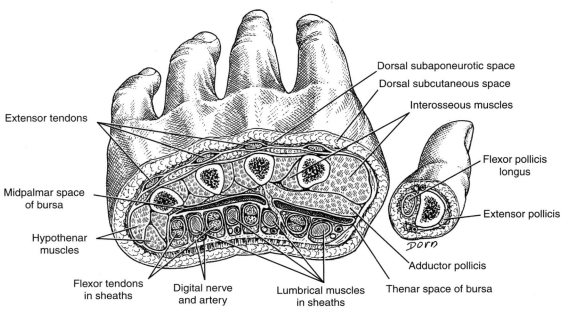

Figure 1-14 ◈ Cross-sectional anatomy of the palm revealing the thenar, midpalmar, hypothenar, and dorsal subaponeurotic spaces and the tendon sheaths. *(From Drukker S, Masson J, Grossman JAI: Common bacterial infections. In Tubiana R, ed: The Hand, vol V. Philadelphia, WB Saunders, 1999.)*

2. It is bounded dorsally by the fascia of the volar interossei and the metacarpals of the long and ring fingers.
3. It is limited radially by the midpalmar (oblique) septum and ulnarly by the hypothenar septum.
4. It may have attritional connections to the radial and ulnar bursa.

Thenar Space

1. The thenar space is bordered volarly by the index flexor tendon.
2. It is bounded dorsally by the adductor pollicis muscle.
3. It is bounded ulnarly by the oblique septum. The radial border is the adductor insertion and thenar muscle fascia.

Hypothenar Space

1. The hypothenar space is bounded radially by the hypothenar septum.
2. It is bordered dorsally and ulnarly by the fascia of the hypothenar musculature.

Interdigital Web Space

1. The interdigital web space is bounded volarly by palmar fascia, dorsally by the dorsal fascia and skin, and radially and ulnarly by the extensor mechanism and the MP joint capsule.
2. Infection in this space is termed a collar-button abscess.

Parona's Space

1. Parona's space is bordered dorsally by the pronator quadratus muscle and volarly by the digital flexors.
2. It is bordered on the radial side by the radial bursa (FPL sheath) and ulnarly by the flexor carpi ulnaris (FCU) muscle.
3. This space can become infected by extension from the radial or ulnar bursa and can provide a conduit for development of a horseshoe abscess.

Dorsal Subaponeurotic Space

1. The dorsal subaponeurotic space is bordered by the extensor tendons dorsally and the interosseous muscles and metacarpals volarly.

Nail

See Chapter 3.

Palmar Fascia (Fig. 1-15)

See Chapter 10.
1. The palmar fascia is a fine reticular system of ligaments that provides channels and restraint for the flexor tendons and anchor points for the skin.
2. The elements of the palmar fascia are shown in Figure 1-15.

Intrinsic Muscles (Table 1-3)

1. The intrinsic muscle system (lumbricals and interossei) acts volar to the flexion axis of rotation of the MP joints (thus, the intrinsic muscles are

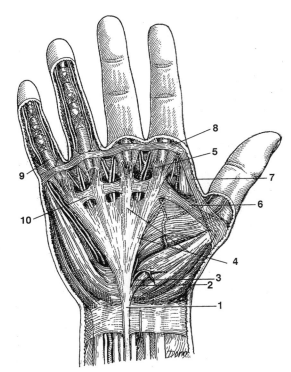

Figure 1-15 ◆ The superficial palmar fascia: 1, palmaris longus tendon; 2, tendon for the superficial fascicle of the abductor pollicis brevis; 3, palmar cutaneous branch of the median nerve; 4, pretendinous bands; 5, fibers of the pretendinous bands inserted into the dermis; 6, proximal commissural ligament of the first web space; 7, distal commissural ligament of the first web space; 8, natatory ligament; 9, fibrous flexor tendon sheath; 10, transverse superficial ligament. *(From Mawhinney I, et al: Dupuytren's disease. In Tubiana R, ed: The Hand, vol V. Philadelphia, WB Saunders, 1999.)*

flexors of the MP joints) and dorsal to the axis of rotation of the PIP and DIP joints (thus, the intrinsic muscles are extensors of the PIP and DIP joints).
2. The intrinsic muscles join the extrinsic finger extensors just proximal to the PIP joints.

Interossei

There are four dorsal and three volar interossei. The dorsal muscles abduct (Dorsal ABduct—DAB) and the volar muscles adduct (Palmar ADduct—PAD) the digits. Abduction and adduction of the digits are stated relative to the long finger axis.

Dorsal Interossei

1. The first, second, and fourth dorsal interossei have two distinct muscle bellies.
2. The superficial belly of each originates from the adjacent metacarpal shaft and inserts onto the base of the respective proximal phalanx.
3. It is this component that provides primary abduction and weak flexion of the MP joint. Because there are no insertions into the dorsal aponeurosis, they have no effect on the middle or distal phalanx.
4. The deep bellies of the first, second, and fourth dorsal interossei originate from the radial side of the index and middle and the ulnar side of the ring metacarpal. They insert onto the dorsal

◈ **Table 1-3**

MUSCLES OF THE HAND AND WRIST

Muscle	Origin	Insertion	Action	Innervation
Thenar muscles				
Abductor pollicis brevis (APB)	Scaphoid, trapezoid	Base of proximal phalanx, radial side	Abduct thumb	Median
Opponens pollicis	Trapezium	Thumb metacarpal	Abduct, flex, med. rotation	Median
Flexor pollicis brevis (FPB)	Trapezium, capitate	Base of proximal phalanx, radial side	Flex MCP	Median, ulnar
Adductor pollicis	Capitate, 2nd/3rd metacarpals	Base of proximal phalanx, ulnar side	Adduct thumb	Ulnar
Hypothenar muscles				
Palmaris brevis (PB)	TCL, palmar aponeurosis	Ulnar palm	Retract skin	Ulnar
Abductor digiti minimi (ADM)	Pisiform	Base of proximal phalanx, ulnar side	Abduct small finger	Ulnar
Flexor digiti minimi brevis (FDMB)	Hamate, TCL	Base of proximal phalanx, ulnar side	Flex MCP	Ulnar
Opponens digiti minimi (ODM)	Hamate, TCL	Small finger metacarpal	Abduct, flex, lat. rotation	Ulnar
Intrinsic muscles				
Lumbricals	Flexor digitorum profundus (FDP)	Lateral bands (radial)	Extend PIP	Median, ulnar
Dorsal interosseous (DIO)	Adjacent metacarpals	Proximal phalanx base/extensor apparatus	Abduct, flex MCP	Ulnar
Volar interosseous (VIO)	Adjacent metacarpals	Proximal phalanx base/extensor apparatus	Adduct, flex MCP	Ulnar

From Miller MD, Gomez BA: Anatomy. In Miller MD, ed: Miller's Review of Orthopaedics, 3rd ed. Philadelphia, WB Saunders, 2000, p 545.

---

extensor hood through the lateral tendon or lateral band.

5. The third dorsal interosseous has a single muscle belly that inserts onto the dorsal hood of the middle finger. The deep head flexes and weakly abducts the MP joint while extending the PIP and DIP joints through the lateral bands.

Volar Interossei

The three volar interossei arise from the metacarpal shafts and insert onto the dorsal hood on the ulnar side of the index and the radial sides of the ring and small fingers. They cause adduction through their insertion onto the dorsal aponeurosis.

LUMBRICALS

The first and second lumbricals arise from the index and long profundus tendons; the third and fourth arise from the ring and small profundus tendons, respectively. The lumbricals contribute fibers to the extensor hood at the level of the proximal phalanx. They are flexors of the MP joints and "relax their own antagonist" (contraction of the lumbrical relaxes the profundus tendon, facilitating DIP joint extension) and extensors of the interphalangeal joints.

INTEROSSEOUS TENDONS

At the metacarpal neck level, the interosseous tendons are a confluence from the neighboring dorsal and palmar interossei muscles.

1. The interossei lie dorsal to the deep transverse metacarpal ligament, and the lumbrical lies volar to it.

2. The intrinsic tendons from the lumbricals (radial to the metacarpal head) and the interossei join the extensor tendon at the proximal and middle aspect of the proximal phalanx.

ANOMALOUS EXTENSOR MUSCLES OF THE HAND

1. Although common and largely asymptomatic, these may cause dorsal wrist pain because the muscle belly is contained within the extensor retinaculum. The EIP can pass beyond the extensor retinaculum in 4% of cadavers.

2. The extensor digitorum brevis manus muscle is present in 1% to 9% of cadavers and is bilateral in 30%. Its origin is variable (most commonly the dorsal radiocarpal ligament), but its insertion is similar to that of the EIP.

3. The extensor medii proprius (0.8% to 10.4% incidence) originates from the ulna and inserts into the dorsal aponeurosis of the middle finger.

4. The extensor indicis et medius communis is like an EIP to the index and middle finger with its muscle belly within the extensor retinaculum.

Wrist

Osteology (Figs. 1-16 and 1-17)

DISTAL RADIUS

1. The radial shaft flares distally into a metaphyseal region to articulate with the distal ulna and the proximal carpal row.

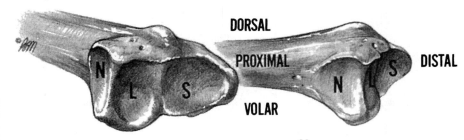

Figure 1-16 ◆ The distal radius is viewed from the ulnar aspect of the carpus on the left and from directly ulnar on the right. Note the confluence of the lunate facet and the sigmoid notch (ulnar facet). *(From Bowers WH: The distal radioulnar joint. In Green DP, Hotchkiss RN, Pederson WC, eds: Operative Hand Surgery, 4th ed. New York, Churchill Livingstone, 1999.)*

2. Lister's tubercle is a dorsal prominence that redirects the extensor pollicis longus tendon and is a landmark in dorsal surgical approaches to the wrist and in arthroscopy (1 cm proximal to the 3-4 portal). Lister's tubercle is also 1 cm proximal to the scapholunate joint.
3. The distal articular surface is composed of two fossae, which are concave in the dorsal-palmar and medial-lateral planes.
   a. The smaller lunate fossa is ovoid. The scaphoid fossa is more triangular.
4. The distal articular surface is tilted with 22 degrees of radial inclination and 11 degrees of palmar tilt. The average radial height (longitudinal distance from the tip of the radial styloid to the most ulnar aspect of the distal radius) is 11 mm (see Chapter 6).
5. The sigmoid notch articulates with the ulnar seat at the distal radioulnar joint (DRUJ). Although the notch is classically described as concave, there can be variability. The arc of curvature of the notch covered with articular cartilage averages 60 degrees.
6. The distal radius physis appears at 2 years of age and fuses at 17 to 20 years.
7. Blood supply
   a. The intraosseous blood supply of the distal radius has numerous implications for local vascularized bone grafts about the carpus.

   b. The distal radius is supplied by the radial, ulnar, anterior interosseous, and posterior interosseous arteries.
   c. Branches of these arteries are identified by location relative to the extensor compartments.
      i. The 1,2 intercompartmental suprareti-nacular artery (branch of the radial artery) and the fourth and fifth extensor compartment arteries (branches of the posterior interosseous artery) are the most commonly employed pedicles for vascularized bone grafts (see Chapter 4).

DISTAL ULNA

1. The distal ulna is the articular extension of the ulnar shaft into the carpus and DRUJ.
2. It is composed of the ulnar head (faces the undersurface of the triangular fibrocartilage complex), seat (articulates with the sigmoid notch), styloid, and fovea.
3. The arc of curvature of the ulnar seat is 105 degrees.
4. The distal ulna physis appears at 5 years of age and fuses at 20 years.

CARPAL BONES (Fig. 1-18)

1. There are eight carpal bones (scaphoid, lunate, triquetrum, pisiform, hamate, capitate, trapezoid, and trapezium) that are arranged in two rows

Figure 1-17 ◆ The radioulnar articulation in neutral or zero rotation as viewed from the dorsum and from end on. Note that the arc of the notch circumscribes a circle of greater diameter than that of the ulnar head. *(From Bowers WH: The distal radioulnar joint. In Green DP, Hotchkiss RN, Pederson WC, eds: Operative Hand Surgery, 4th ed. New York, Churchill Livingstone, 1999.)*

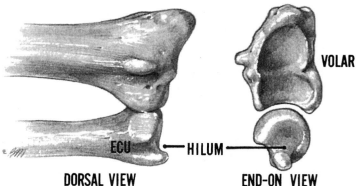

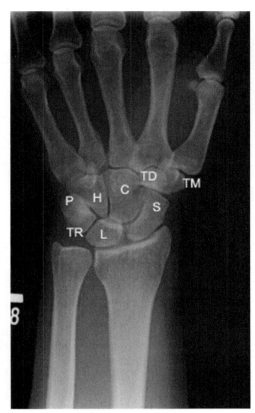

Figure 1-18 ◈ Posteroanterior radiograph of the wrist. S, scaphoid; L, lunate; TR, triquetrum; P, pisiform; H, hamate; C, capitate; TD, trapezoid; TM, trapezium.

◈ **Table 1-4**

APPEARANCE OF OSSIFICATION OF CARPAL BONES

Capitate	1st months of life
Hamate	1st year
Triquetrum	2nd-3rd year
Lunate	4th year
Scaphoid	4th-6th year
Trapezium	4th-6th year
Trapezoid	4th-6th year
Pisiform	8th-10th year

10. The lunate has been classified morphologically into two types (Fig. 1-19).
    a. The type I lunate occurs in about 30% of patients; it does not articulate with the hamate and is associated with a low incidence of proximal pole of hamate arthrosis (2%).
    b. A type II lunate has a medial facet that articulates with the proximal hamate; it occurs about 70% of the time and can be associated with proximal pole of hamate arthrosis (44%).

CARPAL BLOOD SUPPLY

1. The extraosseous blood supply to the carpus is provided by dorsal and palmar transverse arches (three dorsal and three palmar) formed by branches of the radial, anterior interosseous, and ulnar arteries.
2. Scaphoid (Fig. 1-20)
    a. The main blood supply to the scaphoid is dorsal (70% to 80%) through the radial artery entering at its dorsal ridge at the scaphoid waist.
    b. For this reason, the blood supply to the proximal pole of the scaphoid is retrograde and can lead to avascular necrosis with injury.

between the metacarpal bases distally and the distal radius and ulna (with the intervening triangular fibrocartilage complex) proximally.
2. Whereas the proximal and distal surfaces are articular, the dorsal and volar surfaces are primarily points of ligament attachment and vascular supply.
3. The scaphoid occupies a position in both the proximal and distal rows.
4. The pisiform is a sesamoid bone within the tendon of the FCU that articulates with the volar surface of the triquetrum.
5. The hamulus, or hook of the hamate, serves as an attachment point for the flexor retinaculum, the hypothenar muscles, and the pisohamate fascia (Guyon's canal).
6. Although ossification is variable, the capitate usually appears first and sequential bones ossify in a counterclockwise direction (right hand viewed with the palm up) (Table 1-4).
7. In a skeletally immature individual, incomplete ossification of the scaphoid may mimic scapholunate dissociation.
8. The os styloideum is an accessory ossicle at the tip of the radial styloid.
9. A lunatotriquetral coalition is the most common bone coalition in the carpus.

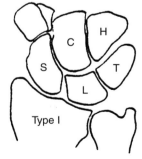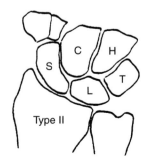

Figure 1-19 ◈ *Left,* Diagram illustrating a type I lunate with the proximal subchondral line of the capitate lined up with the proximal subchondral line of the hamate (CH line), the distal subchondral line of the lunate lined up with the distal subchondral line of the triquetrum (LT line), and the medial subchondral line of the capitate lined up with the medial subchondral line of the lunate (CL line). *Right,* A type II lunate, in which the CH, the LT, and the CL lines do not line up. S, scaphoid; C, capitate; H, hamate; L, lunate; T, triquetrum. *(From Viegas SF, Wagner K, Patterson R, Peterson P: Medial [hamate] facet of the lunate. J Hand Surg Am 15:564–571, 1990.)*

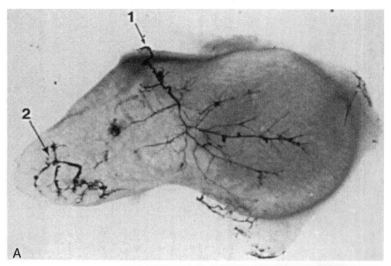

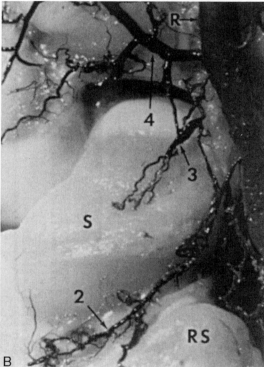

Figure 1-20 ◆ **A**, Photograph of a cleared specimen showing the internal vascularity of the scaphoid. (The vessels in the dorsal and volar scapholunate ligaments do not penetrate the bone.) 1, dorsal scaphoid branch of the radial artery; 2, volar scaphoid branch. **B**, Close-up view of the dorsoradial aspect of the wrist demonstrating nutrient vessels entering the dorsal ridge of the scaphoid. RS, radial styloid; S, scaphoid; R, radial artery; 2, dorsal radiocarpal arch; 3, branch to the dorsal ridge of the scaphoid; 4, dorsal intercarpal arch. (*A from Gelberman RH, Menon J: The vascularity of the scaphoid bone. J Hand Surg Am 5:508–513, 1990. B from Gelberman RH, Panagis JS, Taleisnik J, et al: The arterial anatomy of the human carpus. Part I: The extraosseous vascularity. J Hand Surg Am 8:367–375, 1983.*)

c. The volar blood supply (20% to 30%) also arises from the radial artery and enters the bone at the scaphoid tubercle.
3. Lunate
a. The lunate receives its blood supply from both dorsal and volar (80% of the time) or volar alone (20%). There are three patterns of intraosseous blood supply in the lunate (Fig. 1-21).

Arthrology

RADIOCARPAL JOINT

The radiocarpal joint is an ellipsoid biaxial joint that allows flexion, extension, radial deviation, and ulnar deviation through a complex combination of muscle contraction, intrinsic and extrinsic ligament constraints, and intra-articular motion.

INTERCARPAL JOINT

The distal carpal row (trapezium, trapezoid, capitate, and hamate) articulates with the distal aspect of the scaphoid, lunate, and triquetrum.

DISTAL RADIOULNAR JOINT

The DRUJ is a trochoid or pivot joint. The bone components include the sigmoid notch of the distal radius and the ulnar head and seat. The triangular fibrocartilage complex also confers the primary stability of the joint. There is a mismatch in the radii of curvature of

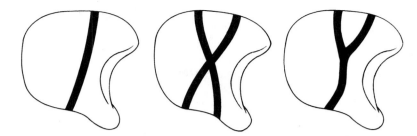

Figure 1-21 ◆ Schematic representation of I, X, and Y intraosseous vascular patterns. *(From Gelberman RH, Bauman RD, Menon J, Akeson WH: The vascularity of the lunate bone and Kienböck's disease. J Hand Surg Am 5:272–278, 1980.)*

the articular surfaces of the radius and ulna, which leads to a combination rolling, sliding, and gliding in pronation-supination.

THUMB CARPOMETACARPAL (BASAL) JOINT

1. The thumb metacarpal base is a saddle or double ginglymus joint between the two facets of the thumb metacarpal base and the trapezium.
2. It is specifically designed to maximize mobility to place the thumb ray at any point in space and stability to allow firm grip and pinch with the medial four digits.
3. The radiovolar ligament (Kaplan's beak, volar oblique, anterior oblique, or deep ulnar ligament) is the primary stabilizer of the joint. Laxity of this ligament is thought to be of importance in the pathogenesis of basilar joint arthritis.
4. Other stabilizers of this joint include the intermetacarpal, posterior oblique, ulnar collateral, and dorsoradial ligaments.

INDEX THROUGH SMALL CARPOMETACARPAL JOINTS

1. The second and third carpometacarpal joints are the central axis of the hand and have almost no mobility. These joints are stabilized by dorsal (strongest), palmar, and interosseous carpometacarpal ligaments.
2. The carpal boss is a bone protuberance on the dorsal aspect of the second or third carpometacarpal joint where the second and third metacarpals articulate with the trapezoid and capitate, respectively. The carpal boss may represent a partial bone coalition in this region.
3. The fourth and fifth carpometacarpal joints have approximately 30 degrees of flexion and extension. This mobility is important in power grip.

Extensor Tendons (Fig. 1-22)

1. Six distinct synovial sheaths firmly fix thumb, digital, and wrist extensor tendons to the dorsal distal radius.

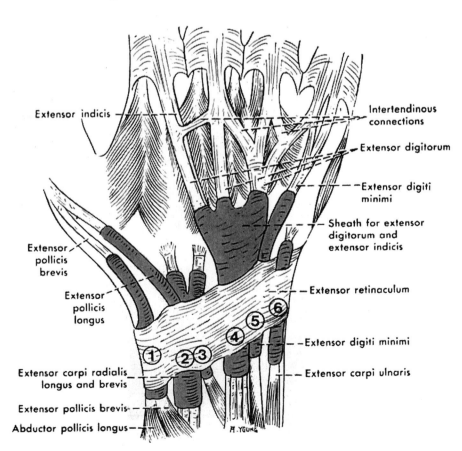

Extensor indicis — Intertendinous connections — Extensor digitorum — Extensor digiti minimi — Sheath for extensor digitorum and extensor indicis — Extensor pollicis brevis — Extensor pollicis longus — Extensor retinaculum — Extensor digiti minimi — Extensor carpi radialis longus and brevis — Extensor carpi ulnaris — Extensor pollicis brevis — Abductor pollicis longus

Figure 1-22 ◆ Extensor compartments of the wrist, 1 to 6. *(From Jenkins DB: Hollinshead's Functional Anatomy of the Limbs and Back, 6th ed. Philadelphia, WB Saunders, 1991.)*

2. The anatomic snuffbox lies over the dorsal scaphoid waist; its borders are the extensor pollicis longus (EPL) tendon dorsally, the abductor pollicis longus (APL) and extensor pollicis brevis (EPB) volarly, and the radial styloid proximally. The scaphoid represents the floor of the snuffbox.

COMPARTMENTS

1. The first dorsal compartment contains the APL and EPB tendons.
   a. The first dorsal compartment can have variable anatomy but most commonly has two slips of the APL tendon and one EPB tendon.
   b. A septum can separate the EPB and APL tendon (24% to 34% of cadavers) and may be implicated in the pathogenesis of de Quervain's stenosing tenosynovitis.
2. The second dorsal compartment contains the two radial wrist extensors, the extensor carpi radialis brevis (ECRB, inserts on the base of the long finger metacarpal) and the extensor carpi radialis longus (ECRL, inserts on the base of the index finger metacarpal).
3. The third dorsal compartment contains the EPL tendon.
4. The fourth dorsal compartment contains the four EDC tendons and the EIP.
   a. The posterior interosseous artery and nerve are located on the floor of the fourth compartment on the radial aspect.
5. The fifth dorsal compartment contains the EDM.
6. The sixth dorsal compartment contains the extensor carpi ulnaris (ECU) tendon.

Ligament

A series of extrinsic ligaments (connect carpal bones to forearm bones) and intrinsic ligaments (connect carpal bones) bind the bones of the wrist.

EXTRINSIC LIGAMENTS

Dorsal Radiocarpal Ligaments (Fig. 1-23)
1. The dorsal radiocarpal ligament originates from the dorsal rim of the lunate fossa of the distal radius and inserts into the dorsal triquetrum.
   a. It must be ruptured to produce a static volar intercalated segment instability.
   b. It can be divided into the radioscaphoid and radiotriquetral ligaments.
2. The dorsal intercarpal ligament originates from the dorsal triquetrum and inserts largely onto the dorsal ridge of the scaphoid and to a lesser extent onto the trapezium and trapezoid.
3. It is thought that the dorsal radiocarpal and dorsal intercarpal ligaments stabilize the proximal pole of the scaphoid and prevent its dorsal subluxation.

Palmar Radiocarpal Ligaments (Figs. 1-24 and 1-25)
The palmar radiocarpal and ulnocarpal ligaments are visible during wrist arthroscopy.
1. The radioscaphocapitate is the most radial ligament (Fig. 1-26); it is the radial component of the

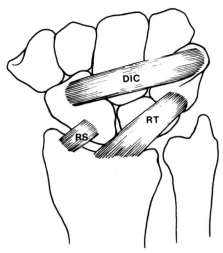

Figure 1-23 ❖ Dorsal wrist ligaments. DIC, dorsal intercarpal ligament; RS, radioscaphoid ligament; RT, radiotriquetral ligament (dorsal radiocarpal ligament). *(From Weber ER: Physiologic bases of wrist function. In Lichtman DM, Alexander AH, eds: The Wrist and Its Disorders. Philadelphia, WB Saunders, 1997.)*

arcuate complex. An aggressive radial styloidectomy may compromise the site of origin of the radioscaphocapitate ligament. The radioscaphocapitate ligament is transected in a volar approach to the scaphoid.
2. The long radiolunate ligament originates from the palmar scaphoid fossa of the radius and passes deep to the proximal pole of the scaphoid before inserting in the palmar radial aspect of the lunate.

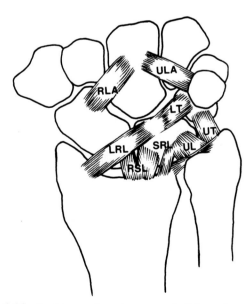

Figure 1-24 ❖ Ligaments: palmar aspect of the wrist—extrinsic. LRL, long radiolunate ligament; LT, lunotriquetral ligament; RLA, radial arm of the arcuate ligament; RSL, radioscapholunate ligament; SRL, short radiolunate ligament; UL, ulnolunate ligament; ULA, ulnar arm of the arcuate ligament; UT, ulnotriquetral ligament. *(From Weber ER: Physiologic bases of wrist function. In Lichtman DM, Alexander AH, eds: The Wrist and Its Disorders. Philadelphia, WB Saunders, 1997.)*

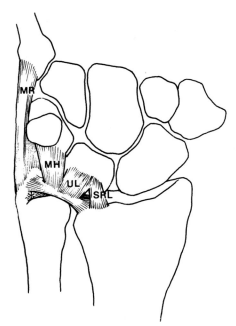

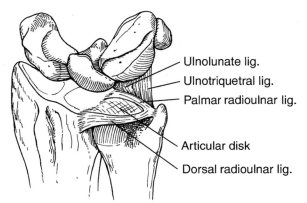

Figure 1-27 ◈ Schematic of the triangular fibrocartilage complex revealing the radioulnar ligaments and the triangular fibrocartilage. *(From Loftus JB, Palmer AK: Disorders of the DRUJ and TFCC. In Lichtman DM, Alexander AH, eds: The Wrist and Its Disorders. Philadelphia, WB Saunders, 1997.)*

Figure 1-25 ◈ Palmar view: ligaments of the ulnar side of the carpus. MH, meniscus homologue; MR, meniscus reflection; SRL, short radiolunate ligament; UL, ulnolunate ligament. *(From Weber ER: Physiologic bases of wrist function. In Lichtman DM, Alexander AH, eds: The Wrist and Its Disorders. Philadelphia, WB Saunders, 1997.)*

3. The radioscapholunate ligament (ligament of Testut) functions more as a neurovascular bundle than as a ligament.
4. The short radiolunate ligament originates from the lunate fossa palmar rim. The long radiolunate and short radiolunate ligaments are the primary

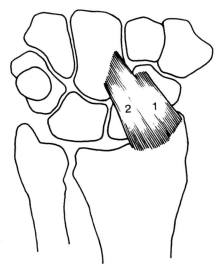

Figure 1-26 ◈ Palmar view: components of the radioscaphocapitate ligament. 1, radioscaphoid component; 2, radiocapitate component. *(From Weber ER: Physiologic bases of wrist function. In Lichtman DM, Alexander AH, eds: The Wrist and Its Disorders. Philadelphia, WB Saunders, 1997.)*

restraint to lunate dislocation in perilunate dislocation.

Ulnocarpal Ligaments (see Fig. 1-25)
1. The ulnocapitate ligament originates from the fovea of the ulnar head and reinforces the lunotriquetral interosseous ligament prior to its insertion before interdigitating with the radioscaphocapitate ligament at its insertion. It is the ulnar component of the arcuate complex.
2. The ulnotriquetral and ulnolunate ligaments facilitate forearm rotation (stabilizing the DRUJ) while maintaining ulnocarpal stability.

Distal Radioulnar Ligaments (Fig. 1-27)
1. The dorsal and volar radioulnar ligaments originate from the dorsal and palmar aspect of the sigmoid notch and insert in the base of the ulnar styloid. The superficial and deep components of these ligaments may act in opposite fashion to confer stability of the DRUJ during pronation and supination by increasing the area of joint contact.
2. The triangular fibrocartilage complex (TFCC) is the most important stabilizer of the DRUJ.
3. In a normal static load situation with neutral ulnar variance, 18% is transmitted to the ulnocarpal joint (82% radiocarpal).
4. The central 80% of the TFCC is avascular and will not heal if torn (Fig. 1-28).
5. The components of the TFCC include the articular disk, the distal radioulnar ligaments, the ulnocarpal ligaments, and the ECU tendinous subsheath. The meniscal homologue is not an important mechanical component of the TFCC.

INTRINSIC LIGAMENTS

1. The scapholunate interosseous ligament is C shaped and covers the dorsal, proximal, and palmar aspect of the articulation (Fig. 1-29).
   a. The dorsal scapholunate ligament is the thickest, strongest, and most important direct stabilizer of the joint.

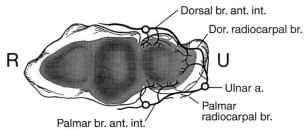

Figure 1-28 ❖ Diagrammatic drawing depicting the vascular supply to the triangular fibrocartilage through the following branches (labeled with abbreviated names): the dorsal and palmar radiocarpal branches of the ulnar artery, the palmar branch of the anterior interosseous artery, and the dorsal branch of the anterior interosseous artery. Note the avascularity of the central and radial aspects of the triangular fibrocartilage. R, radius; U, ulna. *(From Loftus JB, Palmer AK: Disorders of the DRUJ and TFCC. In Lichtman DM, Alexander AH, eds: The Wrist and Its Disorders. Philadelphia, WB Saunders, 1997.)*

b. The proximal membranous portion is composed of fibrocartilage without longitudinal collagen organization.
2. The lunotriquetral interosseous ligament has a similar shape, but the palmar lunotriquetral interosseous ligament is the strongest component. The distal carpal interosseous ligament system consists of dorsal, palmar, and deep ligaments.

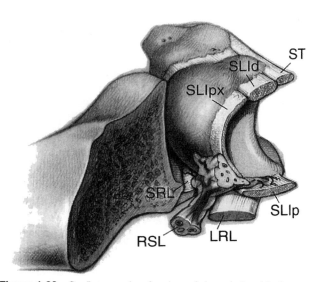

Figure 1-29 ❖ Interpretive drawing of the relationship between the radius and the scapholunate interosseous ligament from a radial and slightly proximal perspective. The drawing is depicted with the radial styloid region and the scaphoid excised. The lunate remains, serving as an attachment for the palmar capsular ligaments, including the long radiolunate (LRL) and short radiolunate (SRL) ligaments. The scapholunate interosseous ligament consists of three regions: dorsal (SLId), proximal (SLIpx), and palmar (SLIp). The radioscapholunate ligament (RSL) is a neurovascular pedicle that separates the palmar and proximal regions of the scapholunate interosseous ligament. Palmar and dorsal scaphotriquetral (ST) ligament fibers form distal extensions of the scapholunate ligament. *(From Berger RA: The gross and histologic anatomy of the scapholunate interosseous ligament. J Hand Surg Am 21:170–178, 1996.)*

❖ **Table 1-5**	
CARPAL KINEMATICS	
Wrist flexion	Distal and proximal carpal rows flex and ulnar deviate
Wrist extension	Distal and proximal carpal rows extend and radially deviate
	Scaphoid rotates 80 degrees
	Lunate rotates 54 degrees
Radial deviation	Distal carpal row extends
	Proximal carpal row flexes
	Scaphoid flexion allows space for trapezium and radial styloid
Ulnar deviation	Distal carpal row flexes
	Proximal carpal row extends
	Palmar position of triquetral facet of hamate (hamate low position)

Kinematics (Table 1-5)

1. There are several theories of carpal kinematics.
2. The capitate is the center of rotation of the wrist joint.
3. The motors of the wrist attach to the metacarpals.
4. Motion starts at the distal carpal row, which acts functionally as a single unit, and is transmitted to the proximal carpal row through ligamentous attachments and compressive forces.
5. There are no direct tendinous attachments to the proximal carpal row.
6. Wrist flexion-extension occurs equally through the radiocarpal and midcarpal joints.
7. Radial-ulnar deviation occurs 60% through the midcarpal and 40% through the radiocarpal joint.

Forearm

Osteology (Fig. 1-30)

The forearm contains two long bones that articulate with each other at the proximal and distal radioulnar joints.
1. Distally, they articulate with the carpus at the wrist joint.
2. Proximally, they articulate with the distal humerus (radial head–capitellum; ulna–trochlea).
3. The radius has two articular surfaces with an intervening shaft.
   a. Proximally, the radial head articulates with the capitellum. The radial tuberosity is the insertion of the distal biceps tendon.
   b. The tuberosity always points opposite to the thumb ray (medial in supination and lateral in pronation).
   c. The proximal radius growth plate appears at age 5 years and fuses between 15 and 18 years.
   d. The shaft of the radius has a gentle curve laterally.
4. The ulna is a long, largely triangular bone with a subcutaneous border.
   a. Proximally, it flares into two processes, the olecranon and the coronoid.

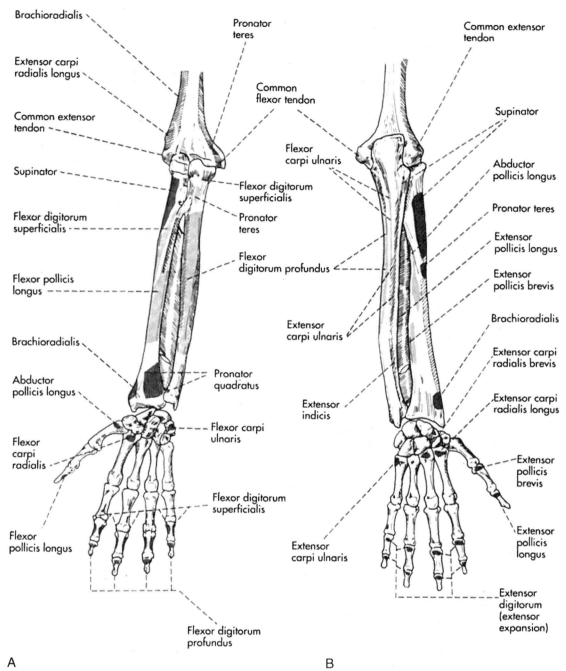

Figure 1-30 ◈ Origins and insertions of muscles of the forearm. *(From Jenkins DB: Hollinshead's Functional Anatomy of the Limbs and Back, 6th ed. Philadelphia, WB Saunders, 1991.)*

b. The olecranon apophysis appears at age 10 years and fuses at 16 years.

c. Distally, the ulnar head articulates with the sigmoid notch of the radius at the DRUJ.

Arthrology

1. The proximal and distal radioulnar joints are involved in forearm rotation.

2. The longitudinal axis of the forearm extends from the center of the radial head proximally to the head of the ulna distally.

3. In pronation and supination, the radius rotates and translates around a fixed ulna.

4. The proximal radioulnar joint is composed of the radial head and the lesser (semilunar) notch of the ulna.

5. The annular ligament confers significant stability to this joint.

Nerve (Fig. 1-31)

CUTANEOUS NERVES

1. The lateral antebrachial cutaneous nerve is the continuation of the musculocutaneous nerve. In the proximal forearm, it is lateral to the cephalic vein. At the radial wrist, its terminal branches are superficial to the cephalic vein.
2. The medial antebrachial cutaneous nerve is a branch of the medial cord of the brachial plexus. Its branches are variable but are at particular risk in medial approaches to the elbow and ulnar nerve (transposition).
3. The posterior antebrachial cutaneous is a branch of the radial nerve and provides sensory innervation to the posterior aspect of the forearm.

RADIAL NERVE

1. The radial nerve enters the arm anterior to the lateral epicondyle after piercing the lateral intermuscular septum approximately 10 cm above the epicondyle. There it lies between the brachialis and brachioradialis.
2. The radial nerve branches into the superficial radial nerve or radial sensory nerve and the posterior interosseous nerve 1 to 3 cm distal to the lateral epicondyle.
3. The ECRB has variable innervation. It is innervated by the radial nerve proper, the posterior interosseous nerve (45%), the superficial radial nerve (25%), and at the bifurcation point (30%).
4. The posterior interosseous nerve then travels under the leading edge of the ECRB tendon, the *arcade of Frohse* (the proximal edge of the supinator), and between the superficial and deep heads of the supinator.
   a. It has been found to be at risk for injury in dorsal approaches to the proximal radius or radial head-neck region.
   b. Its most common order of muscle innervation is (proximal to distal) brachioradialis, supinator, EDC, ECU, EDM, APL, EPL, EPB, and EIP.
   c. When approaching the proximal radius from a lateral approach, the nerve is placed furthest from the radial neck by placing the forearm in full supination.
5. The radial sensory nerve passes through the distal forearm between the brachioradialis and the ECRL. Its terminal branches at the radial wrist lie deep to the cephalic vein.

MEDIAN NERVE

1. The median nerve is made from branches of the medial and lateral cords of the brachial plexus and has contributions from the entire brachial plexus (C5-T1).
2. It lies medial to the brachial artery at the elbow before passing between the deep and superficial heads of the pronator teres muscle. It then runs in the forearm between the flexor digitorum profundus and superficialis muscle bellies.
3. It emerges distally to lie lateral to the palmaris longus tendon and medial to the flexor carpi radialis tendon.
4. The anterior interosseous nerve branches from the lateral aspect of the nerve at the junction of the two heads of the pronator teres.
5. The anterior interosseous nerve runs between the FPL and the FDP and innervates the FPL, FDP to the index and long fingers, and pronator quadratus.
6. The palmar cutaneous branch of the median nerve supplies sensation to the thenar skin and arises from the lateral aspect of the median nerve 0 to 5 cm proximal to the wrist flexor crease.

ULNAR NERVE

1. The ulnar nerve is the continuation of the medial cord of the brachial plexus after giving off its contribution to the median nerve. It receives contributions from the C7 (sometimes), C8, and T1 cervical roots.
2. The ulnar nerve can be compressed in the arm by a thick fascial band between the medial head of the triceps muscle and the medial intermuscular septum (arcade of Struthers). This should not be confused with the ligament of Struthers, which is another structure that causes median nerve entrapment in the distal arm.
3. The ulnar nerve enters the elbow behind the medial epicondyle bound by Osborne's fascia or ligament.
4. The ulnar nerve then passes between the two heads of the FCU to lie between the FDP and the FCU. The nerve then becomes more superficial about 12 cm distal to the medial epicondyle and then travels with the ulnar artery.
5. The ulnar nerve then gives off the dorsal ulnar sensory nerve, which emerges from beneath the FCU about 7 cm proximal to the pisiform.
6. In the distal forearm, the ulnar nerve gives off a branch to the ulnar artery containing sympathetic fibers. This branch is termed the nerve of Henley, and it is believed to be important in the sympathetic control of ulnar artery flow.

ANASTOMOSES

1. The Martin-Gruber anastomosis is present in 10% to 25% of the population.
   a. It is an anastomotic motor fiber connection between the median and ulnar nerves in the forearm.
   b. It is most commonly a median or anterior interosseous nerve connection to the ulnar nerve.
   c. This can lead to an underestimation of an ulnar nerve injury because of its median nerve contribution to traditionally ulnar-innervated musculature.
2. The Riche-Cannieu anastomosis is a motor interconnection between the median and ulnar nerves that occurs distally in the hand.

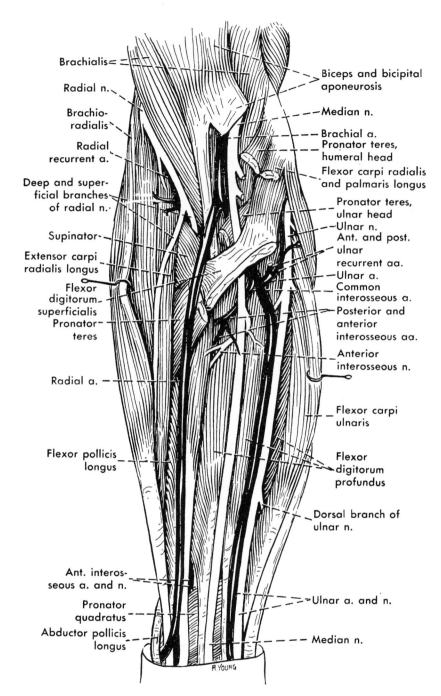

Brachialis

Radial n.

Brachio-
radialis

Radial
recurrent a.

Deep and super-
ficial branches
of radial n.

Supinator

Extensor carpi
radialis longus

Flexor
digitorum
superficialis
Pronator
teres

Radial a.

Flexor pollicis
longus

Ant. interos-
seous a. and n.

Pronator
quadratus

Abductor pollicis
longus

Biceps and bicipital
aponeurosis

Median n.

Brachial a.

Pronator teres,
humeral head

Flexor carpi radialis
and palmaris longus

Pronator teres,
ulnar head

Ulnar n.

Ant. and post.
ulnar
recurrent aa.

Ulnar a.

Common
interosseous a.

Posterior and
anterior
interosseous aa.

Anterior
interosseous n.

Flexor carpi
ulnaris

Flexor
digitorum
profundus

Dorsal branch of
ulnar n.

Ulnar a. and n.

Median n.

Figure 1- 31 ◈ Arteries *(black)* and nerves *(white)* of the forearm. *(From Jenkins DB: Hollinshead's Functional Anatomy of the Limbs and Back, 6th ed. Philadelphia, WB Saunders, 1991.)*

Artery (Fig. 1-31)

1. The brachial artery enters the elbow at the cubital fossa (between the medial and lateral epicondyles, the pronator teres, and the brachioradialis). It divides into the radial and ulnar arteries at the level of the radial neck.
2. The radial artery runs on the pronator teres beneath the brachioradialis and continues to the wrist to lie lateral to the flexor carpi radialis.

3. The ulnar artery lies between the FDS and FDP musculature in the proximal forearm. Distally, it still lies on the volar surface of the FDP but courses between the FDS and FCU tendons.

Interosseous Membrane (Fig. 1-30)

1. The antebrachial interosseous membrane has been described as a quadrangular sheath that extends from the radius to the ulna.

2. With the exception of the proximal band, most of the fibers of the interosseous membrane are directed from the proximal radius to the distal ulna.
3. The central band of the interosseous membrane (interosseous ligament) is responsible for 71% of longitudinal stiffness after radial head excision.
   a. Its anatomic course (proximal radius to distal ulna) may explain the typical pattern of a forearm fracture of both bones.
   b. Other functions of the interosseous ligament have been hypothesized to be load transfer from radius to ulna, origin of flexor and extensor musculature, maintenance of longitudinal forearm stability (Essex-Lopresti injury), and support during forearm rotation.

Muscle and Tendon (Table 1-6)

1. The musculotendinous units of the forearm are arranged in superficial and deep layers.
2. The dorsal surface has the extensor musculature and the volar surface has the flexor musculature.
3. The mobile wad of three as described by Henry consists of the brachioradialis, the extensor carpi radialis longus, and the extensor carpi radialis brevis.
4. An understanding of the cross-sectional anatomy of the forearm is crucial for surgical approaches.

Brachial Plexus (Fig. 1-32 and Table 1-7)

1. Peripheral nerves that innervate the upper extremity largely originate from the cervical roots from

---

❖ Table 1-6

MUSCLES OF THE FOREARM

Muscle	Origin	Insertion	Action	Innervation
Superficial flexors				
Pronator teres (PT)	Med. epicondyle and coronoid	Mid. lat. radius	Pronate, flex forearm	Median
Flexor carpi radialis (FCR)	Med. epicondyle	2nd and 3rd metacarpal bases and trapezium	Flex wrist	Median
Palmaris longus (PL)	Med. epicondyle	Palmar aponeurosis	Flex wrist	Median
Flexor carpi ulnaris (FCU)	Med. epicondyle and post. ulna	Pisiform	Flex wrist	Ulnar
Flexor digitorum superficialis (FDS)	Med. epicondyle and ant. radius	Base of middle phalanges	Flex PIP	Median
Deep flexors				
Flexor digitorum profundus (FDP)	Ant. and med. ulna	Base of distal phalanges	Flex DIP	Median-ant. interosseous/ ulnar
Flexor pollicis longus (FPL)	Ant. and lat. radius	Base of distal phalanges	Flex IP, thumb	Median-ant. interosseous
Pronator quadratus (PQ)	Distal ulna	Volar radius	Pronate hand	Median-ant. interosseous
Superficial extensors				
Brachioradialis (BR)	Lat. supracondylar humerus	Lat. distal radius	Flex forearm	Radial
Ext. carpi radialis longus (ECRL)	Lat. supracondylar humerus	2nd metacarpal base	Extend wrist	Radial
Ext. carpi radialis brevis (ECRB)	Lat. epicondyle of humerus	3rd metacarpal base	Extend wrist	Radial
Anconeus	Lat. epicondyle of humerus	Proximal dorsal ulna	Extend forearm	Radial
Extensor digitorum (ED)	Lat. epicondyle of humerus	Extensor aponeurosis	Extend digits	Radial–post. interosseous
Extensor digiti minimi	Common extensor tendon	Small finger extensor carpi ulnaris	Extend small finger	Radial–post. interosseous
Ext. carpi ulnaris (ECU)	Lat. epicondyle of humerus	5th metacarpal base	Extend/adduct hand	Radial–post. interosseous
Deep extensors				
Supinator	Lat. epicondyle of humerus, ulna	Dorsolateral radius	Supinate forearm	Radial–post. interosseous
Abductor pollicis longus (APL)	Dorsal ulna/radius	1st metacarpal base	Abduct thumb, extend	Radial–post. interosseous
Extensor pollicis brevis (EPB)	Dorsal radius	Thumb proximal phalanx base	Extend thumb MCP	Radial–post. interosseous
Extensor pollicis longus (EPL)	Dorsolateral ulna	Thumb dorsal phalanx base	Extend thumb IP	Radial–post. interosseous
Extensor indicis proprius (EIP)	Dorsolateral ulna	Index finger extensor apparatus (ulnarly)	Extend index finger	Radial–post. interosseous

From Miller MD, Gomez BA: Anatomy. In Miller MD, ed: Miller's Review of Orthopaedics, 3rd ed. Philadelphia, WB Saunders, 2000, p 536.

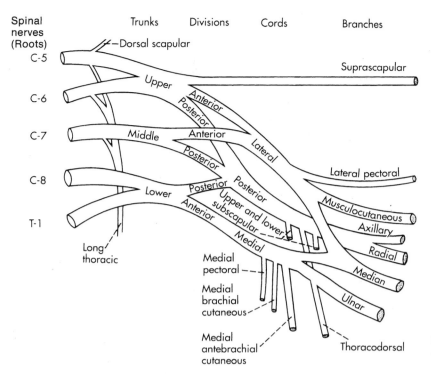

Figure 1-32 ◆ Brachial plexus. *(From Jenkins DB: Hollinshead's Functional Anatomy of the Limbs and Back, 6th ed. Philadelphia, WB Saunders, 1991.)*

C5 to T1. They converge and communicate in the brachial plexus.

2. The brachial plexus lies beneath the clavicle (between scalenus medius and scalenus anterior).

3. There are five subdivisions of the brachial plexus that can be remembered by the mnemonic **R**ob **T**aylor **D**rinks **C**old **B**eer (roots, trunks, divisions, cords, and terminal branches).

4. There are five roots (the ventral rami of C5, C6, C7, C8, T1 [although there are minor contributions from the C4 and T2 roots]), three trunks (upper, middle, lower), six divisions (anterior and posterior divisions of each trunk), three cords (posterior, lateral, and medial, named for their position relative to the axillary artery), and multiple branches but five terminal branches (musculocutaneous, axillary, radial, median, and ulnar nerves) (Table 1-8).

5. There are no nerve branches of the plexus at the level of the division.

6. A prefixed brachial plexus has a large C4 contribution but no contribution from T1.

7. A postfixed brachial plexus lacks C5 contribution but has T2 contribution.

✧ Table 1-7

BRANCHES FROM THE BRACHIAL PLEXUS

	Branches	Nerve Root Contribution	Muscle Innervation
Root	Dorsal scapular nerve	C5	Rhomboid major, minor
	Branch to phrenic nerve	C4, C5	Diaphragm
	Long thoracic nerve	C5, C6, C7	Serratus anterior
	First intercostal nerve	***	
Trunk	Suprascapular nerve	C5, C6	Supraspinatus
	Nerve to the subclavius	C5, C6	Subclavius
Cord	Lateral pectoral nerve	C5, C6, C7	Pectoralis major
	Upper subscapular nerve	C5, C6	Subscapularis
	Thoracodorsal nerve	C7, C8 ± C6	Latissimus dorsi
	Lower subscapular nerve	C5, C6	Subscapularis
	Medial pectoral nerve	C8, T1	Pectoralis minor
	Medial brachial cutaneous nerve	T1	Sensory
	Medial antebrachial cutaneous nerve	C8, T1	Sensory

◆ **Table 1-8**

TERMINAL BRANCHES OF THE BRACHIAL PLEXUS
Nerve Root Contribution

Musculocutaneous n.	C5, C6, C7
Axillary n.	C5, C6
Radial n.	C5, C6, C7, C8, T1
Median n.	C5, C6, C7, C8, T1
Ulnar n.	C7, C8, T1

Bibliography

Berger RA: The ligaments of the wrist: a current overview of anatomy with considerations of their potential functions. Hand Clin 13:63–82, 1997.

Berger RA: The anatomy of the ligaments of the wrist and distal radioulnar joints. Clin Orthop 383:32–40, 2001.

Bianchi H: Anatomy of the radial branches of the palmar arch: variations and surgical importance. Hand Clin 17:139–146, 2001.

Bowers WH: The distal radioulnar joint. In Green DP, Hotchkiss RN, Pederson WC, eds: Green's Operative Hand Surgery, 4th ed. New York, Churchill Livingstone, 1999, pp 986–1032.

Branovacki G, Hanson M, Cash R, et al: The innervation pattern of the radial nerve at the elbow and in the forearm. J Hand Surg Br 23:167–169, 1998.

Brunelli F, Gilbert A: Vascularization of the thumb: anatomy and surgical applications. Hand Clin 17:123–138, 2001.

Coleman SS, Anson BJ: Arterial patterns in the hand based upon a study of 650 specimens. Surg Gynecol Obstet 113:409–424, 1961.

Doyle JR: Extensor tendons—acute injuries. In Green DP, Hotchkiss RN, Pederson WC, eds: Green's Operative Hand Surgery, 4th ed. New York, Churchill Livingstone, 1999, pp 1950–1987.

Freedman DM, Botte MJ, Gelberman RH: Vascularity of the carpus. Clin Orthop 383:47–59, 2001.

Gardner E, Gray DJ, O'Rahilly R: Anatomy: A Regional Study of Human Structure, 2nd ed. Philadelphia, WB Saunders, 1963.

Glickel SZ, Barron OA, Eaton RG: Dislocations and ligament injuries of the digits. In Green DP, Hotchkiss RN, Pederson WC, eds: Green's Operative Hand Surgery, 4th ed. New York, Churchill Livingstone, 1999, pp 772–808.

Hettinger PC, Berger RA: Functional ligamentous anatomy of the trapezium and trapeziometacarpal joint (gross and arthroscopic). Hand Clin 17:151–168, 2001.

Jebson PJL: Deep subfascial space infections. Hand Clin 14:557–566, 1998.

Mazurek MT, Shin AY: Upper extremity peripheral anatomy. Clin Orthop 383:7–20, 2001.

McGinley JC, Kozin SH: Interosseous membrane anatomy and functional mechanics. Clin Orthop 383:108–122, 2001.

McGrouther DA: Dupuytren's contracture. In Green DP, Hotchkiss RN, Pederson WC, eds: Green's Operative Hand Surgery, 4th ed. New York, Churchill Livingstone, 1999, pp 563–569.

Miller MD, ed: Review of Orthopaedics, 3rd ed. Philadelphia, WB Saunders, 2000.

Netter FH: Atlas of Human Anatomy. Summit, NJ, Ciba-Geigy Corporation, 1989.

Strickland JW: Flexor tendons—acute injuries. In Green DP, Hotchkiss RN, Pederson WC, eds: Green's Operative Hand Surgery, 4th ed. New York, Churchill Livingstone, 1999, pp 1851–1897.

Tan ST, Smith PJ: Anomalous extensor muscle of the hand: a review. J Hand Surg Am 24:449–455, 1999.

Viegas SF: Advances in skeletal anatomy of the wrist. Hand Clin 17:1–11, 2001.

Viegas SF: The dorsal ligaments of the wrist. Hand Clin 17:65–75, 2001.

Woo SL, An KN, Arnoczky SP, et al: Anatomy, biology, and biomechanics of tendon, ligament and meniscus. In Simon SR, ed: Orthopaedic Basic Science. Rosemont, Ill, American Academy of Orthopaedic Surgeons, 1994.

Zancolli E: The trapeziometacarpal joint: tenotomy of the accessory tendons in early osteoarthritis. Hand Clin 17:13–43, 2001.

Zook EG, Brown RE: The perionychium. In Green DP, Hotchkiss RN, Pederson WC, eds: Green's Operative Hand Surgery, 4th ed. New York, Churchill Livingstone, 1999.

2

✧ Virak Tan, MD ✧ Aaron Daluiski, MD

TENDON

Basic Science

Structure

Tendons are dense, uniform connective structures that attach muscle to bone. They are made up of complex composite materials consisting of long collagen fibrils embedded in a matrix of proteoglycans (1% to 5% of the tendon's dry weight). There are relatively few cells (fibroblasts) within the tendon, which produce its major constituent—type I collagen (86% of tendon dry weight). Type I collagen contains a high concentration of glycine (~33%), proline (~15%), and hydroxyproline (~15%, almost unique to collagen and often used for identification).

The collagen fibrils are arranged in parallel rows into fascicles. The fascicles are surrounded by loose areolar tissue, the endotenon, which binds them together but allows longitudinal sliding of the fascicles relative to one another. The endotenon also surrounds and supports blood vessels, lymphatics, and nerves. The outer layer of the tendon is the epitenon, a fine fibrous structure that is highly cellular and vascular and that is continuous with the endotendon (Fig. 2-1). The insertion of tendon into bone is through four transitional tissues: tendon, fibrocartilage, mineralized fibrocartilage (Sharpey's fibers), and bone.

Types by Vascular Supply

UNSHEATHED

The unsheathed tendons are covered with paratenon and are also known as vascular tendons. These tendons have a rich capillary network for nutritional supply. Vessels enter from many points in the periphery, travel through intratendinous channels, and anastomose through a longitudinal system of capillaries.

SHEATHED

The sheathed type, also known as avascular tendons, have a mesotenon containing blood vessels (vincula) that supply segments of tendon. As a result, these tendons have avascular regions (watershed areas) that must receive nutrition by diffusion of synovial fluid or by imbibition (pumping process that drives nutrients from the synovial fluid into the tendon proper).

The flexor tendons of the digits are sheathed tendons. The periosteal insertion is a source of blood supply for both sheathed and unsheathed tendons.

Tendon Healing

Initially, all healing was thought to be extrinsic. Currently, tendons are believed to have both an intrinsic and extrinsic capacity to heal, and the relative contribution of each depends on the type of injury and the method of repair. Similar to healing of other biologic tissues, tendon healing involves three phases: inflammatory, fibroblastic (or collagen producing), and remodeling. The events that occur in each of these phases are summarized in Table 2-1. The same cellular and molecular regulations of tendon healing also govern adhesion formation. Cells from the tendon sheath appear to be responsible for formation of adhesions between the tendon and sheath.

Anatomy (see Chapter 1)

Extensor System

The tendons of the extensor system are extrasynovial except at the wrist, where they are surrounded by the retinaculum. The two components are the extrinsic (innervated by the radial nerve) and intrinsic (innervated by the ulnar and median nerves) muscle groups.

EXTRINSIC MUSCLES

The extrinsic muscles include the extensor carpi radialis brevis (ECRB), the extensor carpi radialis longus (ECRL), and the extensor carpi ulnaris (ECU), which extend the wrist. Extrinsic extensors of the hand are the extensor digitorum communis (EDC; variable to the small finger, present in about 50% of cadaver specimens), the extensor indicis proprius (EIP), the extensor digiti quinti (EDQ; the EIP and EDQ are ulnar to the communis tendons on the dorsum of the hand), and the thumb abductor pollicis longus (APL) and extensor pollicis longus and brevis (EPL and EPB). All extrinsic tendons cross the wrist under the extensor retinaculum within six discrete compartments (all fibro-osseous except the fifth, which is fibrous) (Table 2-2 and Fig. 2-2).

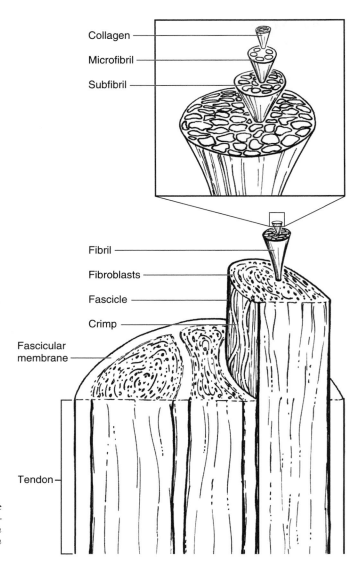

Figure 2-1 ❖ Schematic representation of the structure of the tendon. *(From Woo SL, An K, Frank CB, et al: Anatomy, biology, and biomechanics of tendons and ligaments. In Buckwalter JA, Einhorn TA, Simon SR, eds: Orthopaedic Basic Science, 2nd ed. Rosemont, Ill, American Academy of Orthopaedic Surgeons, 1999.)*

❖ **Table 2-1**

PHASES OF TENDON HEALING

	Inflammatory	Fibroblastic/Collagen-Producing	Remodeling
Time period	3–5 days	1-6 weeks	6 weeks-9 months
Origin of predominant cells	Paratenon	Paratenon Epitenon Endotenon	Endotenon
Molecular activity	Transforming growth factor (TGF)-β (from hematoma) Platelet-derived growth factor synthesis	↑TGF-β Basic fibroblast growth factor accumulation	TGF-β3 (TGF-β agonist) ↑Integrin
Cellular activity	Fibroblast proliferation and migration into injury site Phagocytosis of clot Synthesis of new collagen	Fibrovascular proliferation to form a tendon "callus" (random and disorganized pattern) Collagen and extracellular matrix production Neovascularization	Collagen synthesis continues Collagen fibers reorganize into longitudinal pattern with cross-linking
Strength	Fibrin clot (± sutures)	Granulation tissue	Collagen cross-linking

◆ Table 2-2

EXTENSOR COMPARTMENTS AND INFLAMMATORY CONDITIONS

Compartment	Tendons	Inflammatory Condition
1	APL/EPB (may be multiple compartments)	de Quervain's tenosynovitis
2	ECRL/ECRB	Intersection syndrome
3	EPL (Lister's tubercle)	EPL tendinitis
4	EIP/EDC (EIP ulnar side)	EIP syndrome
5	EDQ	EDQ tendinitis
6	ECU	ECU tendinitis and subluxation

From Miller MD: Review of Orthopaedics, 3rd ed. Philadelphia, WB Saunders, 2000.

INTRINSIC MUSCLES

The intrinsic muscle system (lumbricals and interossei) lies volar to the flexion axis of the metacarpophalangeal (MP) joint but travels dorsally to lie dorsal to the axis of the proximal interphalangeal (PIP) and distal interphalangeal (DIP) joints. Lateral band strain is 10 times more in the hook position than in the full flexion position of the fingers. Just distal to the MP joints, the intrinsic system joins the extrinsic at the level of the PIP joint. At this point, the extensor tendon trifurcates and meets the two lateral bands.

Interossei

There are four dorsal and three volar interossei. The dorsal interossei abduct (Dorsal ABduct—DAB) and the volar interossei adduct (Palmar ADduct—PAD) the digits.

Dorsal Interossei

The first, second, and fourth dorsal interossei have two distinct muscle bellies. The superficial belly of each originates from the adjacent metacarpal shaft and inserts onto the respective proximal phalanx. It is this component that provides primary abduction and weak flexion of the MP joint. Because there are no insertions into the dorsal aponeurosis, they have no effect on the middle or distal phalanx. The deep bellies of the first, second, and fourth originate from the radial side of the index and middle and the ulnar side of the ring metacarpal. They insert onto the dorsal extensor hood through the lateral tendon or lateral band. The third dorsal interosseous has a single muscle belly that inserts onto the dorsal hood of the middle finger. The deep head flexes and weakly abducts the MP joint while extending the PIP and DIP joints through the lateral bands.

Volar Interossei

The three volar interossei arise from the metacarpal shafts and insert onto the dorsal hood on the ulnar side of the index and the radial sides of the ring and small fingers. They cause adduction through their insertion onto the dorsal aponeurosis.

Lumbricals

The first and second lumbricals arise from the index and long profundus tendons; the third and fourth arise dually from the long and ring and the ring and small, respectively. The lumbricals contribute fibers to the extensor hood at the level of the proximal phalanx. They are flexors of the MP joints and "relax their own antagonist" (contraction of the lumbrical relaxes the profundus tendon, facilitating DIP joint extension).

JUNCTURAE TENDINUM

These are fibrous "cross-connections" between the common extensors. They arise and insert just proximal to the MP joint, originating from the long to index and from the ring to both the long and small finger extensor tendons (see Fig. 2-2). The juncturae limit independent digital extension of the ulnar three digits.

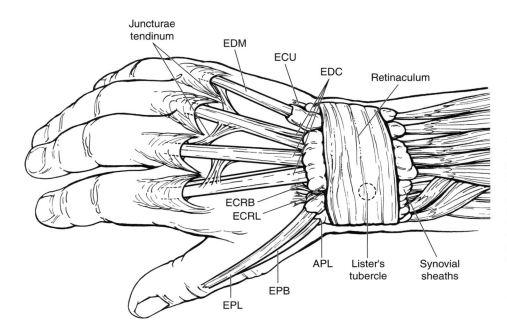

Figure 2-2 ◆ Extensor or dorsal compartments of the extrinsic extensor tendons of the hand. These "compartments" are canals underneath the extensor retinaculum by which the tendons gain entrance to the hand. They are labeled 1 through 6, from radial to ulnar. See also Table 2-2. Also shown on the drawing are juncturae tendinum interconnecting the extensor digitorum communis of the fingers. *(From Doyle JR: Extensor tendons—acute injuries. In Green DP, Hotchkiss RN, Pederson WC, eds: Green's Operative Hand Surgery, 4th ed. New York, Churchill Livingstone, 1999.)*

◆ **Table 2-3**

FINGER JOINT FLEXION AND EXTENSION

Joint	Flexion	Extension
MP	Interossei Lumbricals	EDC (through sagittal bands; can be through central slip if middle phalanx is held in flexed position)
PIP	FDS FDP	Intrinsics (by lateral bands) Central slip of EDC
DIP	FDP	Active—terminal tendon of EDC Passive—oblique retinacular ligament

From Miller MD: Review of Orthopaedics, 3rd ed. Philadelphia, WB Saunders, 2000.

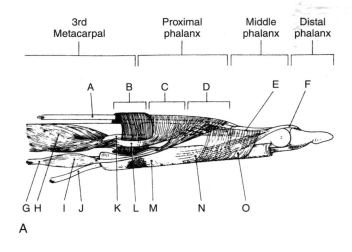

A

This relationship is important clinically; if the long or little finger EDC is lacerated proximal to the juncturae, full extension of these digits may be possible through the action of the ring EDC.

SAGITTAL BANDS

The extrinsic extensor mechanism is centralized over the MP joints by the sagittal bands. At the level of the MP joint, the sagittal bands form a "sling," connecting the extensor tendon to the volar plate. It is through this mechanism primarily (not by direct insertion of the extensor tendon to bone) that MP extension occurs (Tables 2-3 and 2-4).

TRANSVERSE RETINACULAR LIGAMENT

The transverse retinacular ligament (also known as transverse fibers of the interossei, oblique fibers of the dorsal aponeurosis) is a transversely oriented fibrous extension from the interossei over the proximal phalanges arising just distal to the sagittal bands. In contrast to the sagittal fibers, which extend the MP joint, the transverse fibers form a sling that aids in flexing the proximal phalanx (MP flexion) (Fig. 2-3).

DISTAL EXTENSOR MECHANISM

The distal part of the interossei coalesces with the lateral bands and the lumbrical tendon (on the radial side) to form the terminal tendon (inserting onto the distal phalanx) that extends the DIP joint.

LINKED EXTENSION

Extension of the interphalangeal (IP) joints is linked.
1. Actively: pull of the common extensor causes concomitant extension of the PIP (by the central slip) and DIP (by the lateral bands on the terminal tendon) joints.

◆ **Table 2-4**

THUMB JOINT FLEXION AND EXTENSION

Flexion	Extension	Abduction	Adduction
FPB	APL	Opponens pollicis	Adductor pollicis
FPL	EPL	Abductor pollicis brevis (through insertion on base of proximal phalanx)	EPL
Opponens pollicis	EPB		

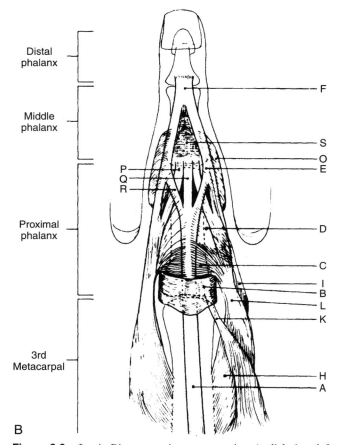

B

Figure 2-3 ◆ **A,** Diagrammatic representation (radial view, left middle finger) of the muscles, tendons, and fascia that directly influence the motion of the finger. **B,** Dorsal aspect of the left middle finger. A, common extensor tendon; B, sagittal band; C, transverse fibers of the interossei; D, oblique fibers of the interossei; E, lateral conjoined tendon; F, terminal tendon; G, flexor digitorum profundus tendon; H, interosseus muscle (second dorsal), deep head; I, lumbrical muscle; J, flexor digitorum superficialis tendon; K, medial tendon, superficial head of second dorsal interosseus; L, lateral tendon of deep head of second dorsal interosseus muscle; M, fibrous flexor pulley; N, oblique retinacular ligament; O, transverse retinacular ligament; P, medial interosseus band; Q central slip of the common extensor; R, lateral slip of the common extensor; S, triangular ligament. *(From Smith RJ: Balance and kinetics of the fingers under normal and pathological conditions. Clin Orthop 104:92-111, 1974.)*

2. Passively: through the oblique retinacular ligament of Landsmeer, which originates on the flexor pulley system at the proximal phalanx (volar to PIP joint) and inserts onto the terminal tendon (dorsal to DIP joint). As the PIP joint extends, the oblique retinacular ligament tightens, causing passive extension of the DIP joint. The oblique retinacular ligament on the ulnar side of the small finger often becomes involved in Dupuytren's contracture, causing small finger PIP flexion and DIP extension. This cord must be addressed at the time of the surgical excision.

INTRINSIC PLUS POSITION

The intrinsic plus position mimics action of the intrinsic system (MP flexion and PIP and DIP extension).

INTRINSIC MINUS POSITION

The intrinsic minus position mimics position of digits if the intrinsic system were to be absent (MP extension and PIP and DIP flexion). It is most commonly seen as a result of nerve palsies.

Flexor System

DISTAL FOREARM

The extrinsic flexor tendons are arranged in three layers in the distal forearm.

1. The superficial layer contains the wrist flexors: flexor carpi radialis (FCR), palmaris longus (PL; absent in up to 25% of the population), and flexor carpi ulnaris (FCU), from radial to ulnar.
2. The intermediate layer contains the flexor digitorum superficialis (FDS).
3. The deep layer contains the flexor digitorum profundus (FDP) and flexor pollicis longus (FPL). The FDS tendons normally arise from independent muscle bundles; therefore, each finger can be flexed independently at the PIP joint. Because there is a common muscle belly for the long, ring, and small profundus tendons, simultaneous flexion of multiple fingers usually occurs. The FDP is the primary digital flexor; the FDS and the interossei combine for forceful flexion (see "Quadriga").

WRIST

The three wrist flexors cross the joint outside the carpal canal. The FCR travels in the groove of the trapezium to insert on the volar aspect of the index metacarpal. The PL fans out at the level of the wrist and continues distally as the palmar fascia. On the ulnar side of the wrist, the FCU inserts onto the pisiform, hook of the hamate, and fifth metacarpal bone. The nine extrinsic digital flexor tendons (FDS × 4, FDP × 4, and FPL) cross the wrist beneath the transverse carpal ligament (i.e., within the carpal tunnel) along with the median nerve.

PALM

At the level of the distal palmar crease, the profundus tendons lie deep to their respective superficialis tendons and as paired tendons enter their flexor sheaths for the remainder of their course to each digit. The FPL is also contained in a synovial sheath. The lumbricals originate from their corresponding FDP in the palm.

DIGIT

The FDP and FDS enter the digital sheath at the level of the metacarpal neck.

1. Within the proximal tendon sheath, the FDS tendon splits into radial and ulnar slips and wraps around the profundus tendon. The two slips then rejoin dorsal to the FDP at Camper's chiasma (Latin for "crossing") and finally insert into the proximal half of the middle phalanx as two slips again (Fig. 2-4). This decussation allows the FDP tendon to pass more distally to insert on the volar aspect of the distal phalanx.
2. Tendon sheath
   a. The flexor tendons are contained within the flexor tendon sheaths. The sheaths are lined by

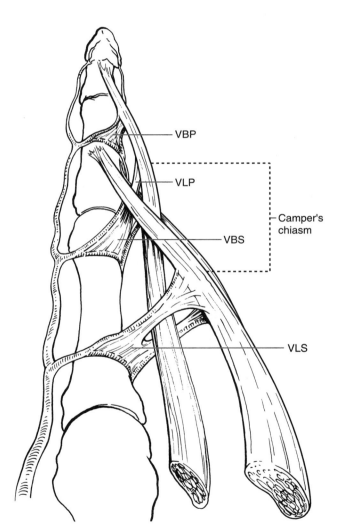

Figure 2-4 ◈ Schematic drawing of the flexor tendons of the hand. At the level of the proximal phalanx, the superficialis tendon bifurcates around the profundus (known as Camper's chiasm) before inserting onto the middle phalanx. Vincula carry blood supply to the flexor tendons within the digital sheath. VBP, vinculum breve profundus; VLP, vinculum longum profundus; VBS, vinculum breve superficialis; VLS, vinculum longum superficialis. *(From Strickland JW: Flexor tendons—acute injuries. In Green DP, Hotchkiss RN, Pederson WC, eds: Green's Operative Hand Surgery, 4th ed. New York, Churchill Livingstone, 1999.)*

visceral and parietal synovial layers, which provide protection, nutrition, and a smooth gliding surface for the flexor tendons. They also function to hold the tendons in close apposition to the phalanges. For the index, middle, and ring fingers, the sheaths begin at the level of the metacarpal neck. The thumb and small finger tendon sheaths are in direct communication with the radial and ulna bursae, respectively.

b. Vincula (see Fig. 2-4), folds of mesotenon on the dorsal surface of the flexor tendons, carry nutrient vessels from the paired digital arteries. There are short and long vincula for each tendon. An intact vinculum can flex the PIP joint when both flexor tendons are completely severed.

c. The pulleys are fascial condensations overlying the flexor tendon and sheath that form the fibro-osseous flexor pulley system (Fig. 2-5).

   i. In the fingers, there are eight pulleys, five annular (A1 to A5) and three cruciate (C1 to C3).

   ii. The odd-numbered annular pulleys arise from the volar plates of the MP, PIP, and DIP joints ("odds over joints").

   iii. The even-numbered annular pulleys arise from the periosteum of the middle and distal phalanges.

   iv. The A2 pulley is located at the proximal part of proximal phalanx ("proximal-proximal"). The A4 pulley is located at the middle of the middle phalanx ("middle-middle").

   v. The cruciate pulleys are thin and collapsible, which allows the annular pulleys

to approximate each other during digital flexion. The C1 pulley lies between the A2 and A3, the C2 between the A3 and A4, and the C3 between the A4 and A5.

vi. The A2 and A4 are the most important pulleys and should be preserved or reconstructed, when possible. Both of these pulleys act to prevent bowstringing and increase the mechanical advantage of flexor tendons. Any alteration that increases the distance of the flexor tendon from the axis of the joint will increase the moment arm (torque). In addition, a greater linear excursion of the tendon will be required for the same amount of finger flexion (Fig. 2-6). Disruption of the A2 or A4 pulley may lead to flexor tendon bowstringing, limited active flexion, or flexion contracture. Loss of the A4 pulley leads to greater efficiency of flexion deficit compared to the A2 pulley.

vii. Proximal to the A1 pulley, condensation of the palmar fascia leads to the formation of the palmar aponeurosis pulley, which is thought to be important when the integrity of the other pulleys is lost (see Fig. 2-5).

viii. In the thumb, there are only two annular pulleys (A1 and A2 overlying the MP and IP joints, respectively) and one oblique pulley. The oblique pulley is centered on the proximal phalanx and is in continuity with fibers from the adductor pollicis insertion.

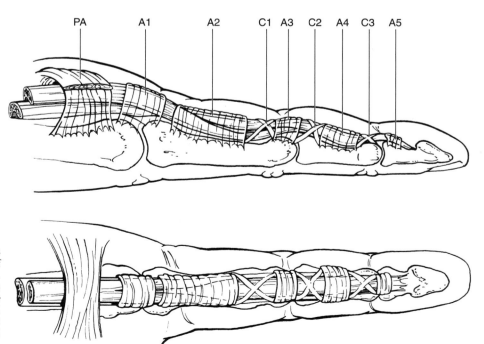

Figure 2-5 ◆ Lateral and volar views of the fibro-osseous pulley system of the flexor tendons. See text for details. PA, palmar aponeurosis pulley. *(From Strickland JW: Flexor tendons—acute injuries. In Green DP, Hotchkiss RN, Pederson WC, eds: Green's Operative Hand Surgery, 4th ed. New York, Churchill Livingstone, 1999.)*

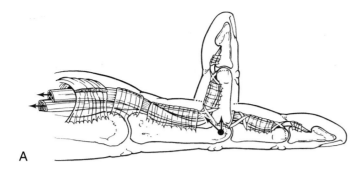

A

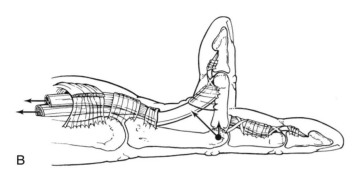

B

Figure 2-6 ◆ Schematic showing the moment arm of the flexor tendon as the finger flexes to 90 degrees. **A,** With an intact pulley system, the moment arm changes minimally because the pulleys hold the tendon close to the center of rotation. **B,** With disruption of the normal pulley system, bowstringing occurs and the moment arm increases significantly, requiring a greater amount of tendon excursion to achieve the same amount of flexion. *(Courtesy of Virak Tan, MD.)*

Tendinopathies

Stenosing Flexor Tenosynovitis (Trigger Finger or Thumb)

There is a discrepancy in size between the tendon and sheath that causes the triggering. It can be classified as nodular or diffuse.

1. Nodular type
   a. Nodular tenosynovitis is due to thickening of the tendon on the distal edge of the A1 pulley.
   b. FPL thickening in a trigger thumb occurs at the sesamoid in the region where the flexor pollicis brevis (FPB) inserts.
2. Diffuse type
   a. Diffuse tenosynovitis is due to diffuse thickening of the flexor tenosynovium, as in rheumatoid arthritis.
   b. In patients with rheumatoid arthritis, the treatment of choice is excision of a slip of the FDS and tenosynovectomy (the A1 pulley should be preserved to avoid increasing the lever arm of the tendon and thus potentiating the flexion deformities at the MP joints).
3. Incidence is higher in patients with diabetes, hypothyroidism, gout, and renal disease. Women are affected more often than are men in a 4:1 ratio.
4. It most commonly affects the thumb, ring finger, or long finger (least often in the index finger).
5. It may present initially as pain and tenderness in the palm without frank locking.
6. Carpal tunnel syndrome is more commonly associated with trigger digits (17% to 23%) than are

disorders such as de Quervain's tenosynovitis and Dupuytren's disease.

7. Treatment includes splinting and nonsteroidal anti-inflammatory drugs (NSAIDs) for mild or early cases, corticosteroid injections, and surgical release of the A1 pulley.
   a. Treatment with corticosteroid injections is successful in 50% to 93% of cases, but there is a high recurrence rate.
   b. Injections are less likely to be successful in patients with diabetes mellitus, those with triggering for longer than 4 to 6 months in duration, and those with diffuse rather than nodular tenosynovitis.
   c. Surgical release of the A1 pulley is indicated in patients whose treatment with multiple injections fails.
      i. The radial digital nerve must be protected during a trigger thumb release because it crosses the area of surgical dissection.
      ii. Percutaneous trigger release often results in scoring of the FDS and is contraindicated for the thumb and index finger because of risk of digital nerve injury.
8. Differential diagnosis must also include locking due to impingement of the collateral ligaments on a prominent metacarpal head condyle. In this setting, the IP joints may be extended while the MP is held in the flexed position (in contrast to triggering due to stenosing tenosynovitis, in which there is limited IP extension with the digit in the locked flexed position). Locking MP joints occur most commonly in the long and index fingers.

de Quervain's (First Dorsal Compartment, APL/EPB) Tenosynovitis

1. de Quervain's tenosynovitis is one of the most common causes of radial-sided wrist pain.
2. The cause may be related to repetitive use, direct trauma, inflammatory arthritis, and os radiostyloideum.
3. The condition is diagnosed by tenderness over the radial styloid with a positive Finkelstein's test (Eichhoff maneuver—pain over the radial styloid when the flexed thumb held in a clenched fist is ulnarly deviated by the evaluator).
4. Treatment includes splinting (forearm-based thumb spica) and NSAIDs for mild or early cases, corticosteroid injections, and surgical release of the first dorsal compartment.
   a. Injection of the tendon sheath with a soluble corticosteroid is successful in 50% to 80% of cases.
   b. Operative treatment entails release of the tendon sheaths of the APL and EPB.
      i. The APL usually has several slips (two to four), and the EPB often has a separate sheath that requires release.
      ii. Complications include subluxation of the compartment (retinaculum released too far radially), persistent symptoms (missed and unreleased EPB sheath), and injury to the lateral antebrachial cutaneous and dorsal sensory radial nerves. Avoid injury to the radial artery (deep to compartment).
      iii. Inadequate decompression of the EPB sheath can be tested by placing the thumb in abduction and passively flexing the MP joint.

Intersection Syndrome

1. Inflammation of the second dorsal extensor tendon compartment presents with pain localized about 4 cm proximal to the wrist.
2. On clinical examination, it feels and sounds like wet leather rubbing on itself (crepitation).
3. There is a history of repetitive use; it is often seen in athletes (weightlifters or rowers).
4. The cause is not friction between the first and second extensor compartments but stenosing tenosynovitis of the second compartment.
5. Treatment includes wrist splinting and NSAIDs for mild or early cases, corticosteroid injections, and surgical release of the second compartment.
6. Operative treatment: longitudinal incision with full release of the second compartment without repair of the retinaculum with postoperative splinting for 2 weeks.

ECU Tendinitis

1. The ECU tendon lies in its own fibro-osseous tunnel. It also moves freely over the ulnar head to allow unrestricted pronation-supination; this mobility places the ECU at risk for tendinitis.
2. Tendon subluxation is evaluated by flexing and extending the wrist while it is held in supination and ulnar deviation.
3. ECU subluxation is often associated with triangular fibrocartilage complex tears.
4. Patients with ECU tendinitis whose conservative treatment fails (splinting and corticosteroid injections) may require tenosynovectomy with sheath release.
   a. Surgical treatment should include arthroscopic assessment of the triangular fibrocartilage complex.
   b. In patients with ECU instability, sheath reconstruction with a slip of extensor retinaculum is necessary to prevent subluxation.

FCR Tendinitis

1. FCR tendinitis is typically caused by overuse; it is more common in women.
2. It can be associated with a spur on the trapezium.
3. Tenderness is usually present over the FCR just proximal to the wrist crease.
4. Linburg's syndrome (tenosynovitis secondary to tendinous connection between the FPL and the index finger FDP found in 25% of cadavers) must be ruled out.
5. Nonoperative treatment includes activity modification, splinting, NSAIDs, and corticosteroid injections.
6. Release of the FCR sheath is considered if nonoperative treatment fails. Avoid injury to palmar cutaneous branch of the median nerve.

FCU Tendinitis

1. FCU tendinitis is secondary to chronic repetitive trauma or calcific tendinitis.
2. Pisotriquetral arthritis must be ruled out.
3. Nonoperative treatment includes splinting, activity modification, NSAIDs, and corticosteroid injections.
4. Operative débridement is rarely required. Aspiration or open excision of calcium deposits is indicated in cases of calcific tendinitis.

Extensor Tendon Injury

General Considerations

1. In acute tendon disruptions, closed injuries are treated closed (splints), and open injuries are treated open (surgical repair).
2. Surgical repair should be performed by use of nonabsorbable material with a core suture (modified Kessler).
3. Open injuries should be treated with irrigation and débridement, tendon and wound repair, and tetanus and antibiotic prophylaxis as needed (see Chapter 11).
4. Partial open tendon injuries should be repaired if more than 50% of the width of the tendon is involved (nonabsorbable grasping core stitch and 4 to 6 weeks of splinting, followed by range of motion). If less than 50% of the width of the

tendon is involved, treat by splinting for 10 to 14 days followed by protected range of motion.

5. Extensor tendon repairs can be immobilized for the duration of the healing.
   a. Extensor tendon repairs proximal to the proximal phalanx are immobilized with the wrist in 45 degrees of extension and the MP joint at 10 degrees of flexion for 4 to 6 weeks before protected range of motion is allowed.
   b. Dynamic extension splinting in the rehabilitation process to allow early motion helps to limit adhesion formation and results in greater return of motion.
6. In general, the more proximal injuries of the hand have a better result than the more distal injuries.
7. Because the extensor system is linked, discontinuity at one joint will lead to increased force of pull at the adjacent joint, leading to a reciprocal deformity in the adjacent finger joint (see "Other Tendon Disorders").
   a. Untreated mallet fingers (DIP flexion) lead to PIP extension (swan-neck deformity).
   b. Untreated central slip injuries (PIP flexion) lead to DIP extension (boutonnière deformity).

Zones

Zones are used to describe the location of tendon injuries of the extensor mechanism. See Tables 2-5 and 2-6 and Figure 2-7. (Remember, "odd joints, even bones.")

ZONE I (MALLET FINGER)

1. Mallet deformities (DIP flexion) are caused by disruption of the terminal tendon. They are typically closed injuries but can be open.
2. Mallet thumbs are rare injuries and easily missed because of multiple extensors of the thumb IP joint. Isolated EPL function can be tested by lifting the thumb off a flat surface while the EPL tendon is palpated proximally.
3. Closed injuries should be treated by continuous DIP extension splint for 6 weeks, followed by 4 weeks of night splinting.
4. Missed injuries should be treated with splinting up to 6 months from the injury.
5. Although splinting is successful most of the time (80%, even with delayed diagnosis), there is a high complication rate (skin problems, noncompliance).

◆ **Table 2-5**

FINGER EXTENSOR INJURIES

Zone	Anatomic Level	Disorder	Treatment
I	DIP	Mallet finger	
		Type I: closed/blunt	Stack splint 6–8 weeks; night splint and wean during 2 weeks
		Type II: laceration	Repair skin and tendon in single layer; splint
		Type III: abrasion with skin loss	See type II
		Type IV	
		A: Transepiphyseal	Splint
		B: Hyperflexion injury (20%–50% articular surface)	Splint ± fix
		C: Hyperextension injury (>50% articular surface; usually with subluxation)	Fix if large enough (over button or tension band); pin DIP if subluxated
II	Middle phalanx	Usually lacerations	<50% involvement: splint 2 weeks and begin protected range of motion
			>50% involvement: repair with nonabsorbable suture; splint DIP in extension × 6 weeks and allow active PIP flexion
III	PIP	Boutonnière lesion (rule out pseudoboutonnière)	Splint PIP in neutral; allow active DIP motion
		Laceration	Repair with modified Kessler, 4-0 suture
IV	Proximal phalanx	Usually partial lacerations	Repair with modified Kessler, 4-0 nonabsorbable suture; repair isolated lateral band lesions
V	MP	Human bite ("fight bite")	Open irrigation and débridement; delayed repair of extensor mechanism in 5–7 days
		Laceration	Modified Kessler, 4-0 nonabsorbable suture; repair sagittal bands
		Closed sagittal band; dislocation of EDC usually ulnar to MP	Within 2 weeks of injury, splint with MP at 20 degrees, IP joints free
VI	MC	Laceration	Repair with core stitch
VII	Extensor retinaculum (carpus)	Laceration; rule out rheumatoid arthritis in closed atraumatic instances	Repair laceration; splint wrist in 45 degrees of extension × 4–5 weeks; fingers free
VIII	Distal forearm	Closed injury rare	Splint incomplete injuries; repair complete lacerations
IX	Mid to proximal forearm	Penetrating injury	Must explore to rule out radial or posterior interosseous nerve lesion vs. tendon laceration; repair muscle belly and nerve

◆ Table 2-6			
THUMB EXTENSOR INJURIES			
Zone	**Anatomic Level**	**Disorder**	**Treatment**
I	IP joint	Mallet thumb	
		Closed	Splint 6–8 weeks; night splint and wean during 2 weeks
		Laceration	Repair skin and tendon in single layer; splint
II	Proximal phalanx	EPL laceration	Repair with nonabsorbable suture; static IP splint in extension × 6 weeks
III	MP joint	EPL and EPB laceration	Repair both with modified Kessler, 4-0 suture; dynamic splinting with wrist in extension, CMC neutral, MP at 0 degrees; allow active flexion
IV	MC	EPL and EPB lacerations	See thumb zone III
V	CMC joint	EPB and APL (multiple slips)	Modified Kessler, 4-0 nonabsorbable suture; repair all slips

6. In association with an avulsion fracture of the distal phalanx (bony mallet), consideration should be given to fracture fixation if there is DIP joint subluxation or if the fracture fragment is more than 50% of the articular surface.

7. In open injuries, repair of skin and tendon in a single layer is recommended for clean lacerations. Degloving injuries should be treated with tendon and skin grafting.

ZONE II (OVER MIDDLE PHALANX)

1. Injuries over the middle phalanx are typically due to lacerations, but tendon injury is often only partial.

2. These should be surgically repaired if more than 50% of the width of tendon is disrupted.

ZONE III (CENTRAL SLIP OVER THE PIP JOINT)

1. Diagnosis can be subtle, requires careful examination, and is often missed in the emergency department. Patients often present with swelling of the PIP joint, mild PIP extension lag (>15 degrees loss), and weak extension against resistance.

2. Radiographs may show PIP subluxation.

3. Treatment for closed injuries includes PIP extension splint with DIP free for 6 weeks. DIP flexion exercises are initiated while the PIP is held extended to allow dorsal translation of the lateral bands.

4. In association with an avulsion fracture of the middle phalanx, consideration should be given to fracture fixation if there is PIP joint subluxation or if the fracture fragment is more than 40% of the articular surface.

5. Open injuries should be treated with open tendon repair, including primary repair or reconstruction by use of a slip of lateral band and temporary K-wire pinning of the PIP joint in full extension. Degloving injuries should be treated with tendon and skin grafting.

6. Missed closed injuries should be treated with a splint for up to 6 months after injury.

ZONE IV (OVER PROXIMAL PHALANX)

1. Injuries over the proximal phalanx are typically due to lacerations, but tendon injury is often only partial.

2. These should be surgically repaired if more than 50% of the width of tendon is disrupted.

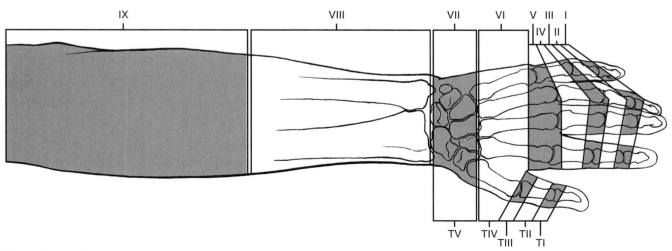

Figure 2-7 ◆ Zone of injury for extensor tendons. *(From Doyle JR: Extensor tendons—acute injuries. In Green DP, Hotchkiss RN, Pederson WC, eds: Green's Operative Hand Surgery, 4th ed. New York, Churchill Livingstone, 1999.)*

ZONE V (OVER MP JOINT)

1. Open injuries should always suggest human bites. (see Chapter 11.)
2. Radiographs to rule out metacarpal head fractures, tooth fragments, or foreign bodies are necessary.
3. Early and aggressive (and sometimes multiple) irrigation and débridement in the operating room with appropriate intravenous antibiotic coverage is indicated. Tendon repair and wound closure are delayed for 5 to 7 days after irrigation and débridement. The tendon laceration is typically proximal to the skin laceration, and thus careful wound exploration is necessary. The joint should be explored for foreign bodies.
4. Injuries that involve the sagittal band may result in extensor mechanism subluxation.
   a. The radial sagittal band of the long finger is most commonly ruptured, causing ulnar subluxation of the extensor mechanism.
   b. The patient presents after a blunt injury with inability to actively extend the MP joint fully and ulnar subluxation of the finger.
   c. Acute injuries are treated with immobilization with the MP joints held in extension.
   d. Chronic injuries are treated surgically with the option of sagittal band repair or reconstruction with a distally based slip of the extensor mechanism or juncturae tendinum. Later than 2 weeks, injuries often require reconstruction.
5. In the thumb, injuries involve the APL and EPB tendons, requiring repair of multiple slips. Exploration and repair of the superficial radial nerve are necessary.

ZONE VI (OVER METACARPAL)

1. Injuries over the metacarpals have a better prognosis than the more distal injuries.
2. The injury is often confused with peritendinous fibrosis (also called factitious lymphedema of the hand) that should be treated conservatively.
3. These should be surgically repaired if more than 50% of the width of tendon is disrupted.

ZONE VII (OVER WRIST JOINT)

1. Injury over the wrist joint typically involves a concomitant laceration of the extensor retinaculum.
2. Distal radius fractures can lead to attritional rupture of the EPL, typically treated with EIP to EPL transfer (no deficit of independent index finger extension after transfer). EIP is harvested proximal to the sagittal band with little donor deficit.

ZONE VIII (OVER FOREARM)

Repair of the tendon at the myotendinous junction is often difficult. It is necessary to find the intramuscular raphe to obtain a good repair.

ZONE IX (OVER PROXIMAL FOREARM)

1. Most require exploration because the laceration can be due to injury to either the posterior interosseous nerve or the proximal muscle belly, both of which require repair.

2. It is necessary to explore all wounds carefully because the size of the laceration may be misleading with regard to the internal injury.
3. Repair muscle belly lacerations with absorbable suture by a figure-of-eight or mattress stitch.

Results

Good to excellent results: zone IV, 43%; zone V, 83%; zone VI, 65%.

Flexor Tendon Injury

The spectrum of flexor tendon injuries includes lacerations, avulsions, and spontaneous ruptures. Depending on the location and mechanism of injury, the severity can range from partial tendon laceration to multiple tendon involvement with concomitant neurovascular injuries.

Physical Examination

1. In the relaxed state, the digits with intact flexor tendons should form a cascade of semiflexion. A digit with a severed flexor tendon will cause the affected finger to be more extended, disrupting the resting cascade.
2. Both the FDS and FDP of each digit must be tested separately for both active and passive range of motion and strength. To test the FDS integrity, the profundus tendons must be immobilized by holding all the uninvolved fingers in full extension. This maneuver isolates the superficialis function. A deficiency of the little finger FDS is displayed in 34% of normal individuals; they cannot fully flex the PIP in isolation.
3. The skin laceration does not always correlate with the level of the flexor tendon disruption. Lacerations that occur with the finger in flexion will result in the tendons being cut more distally than the skin. Tendons cut with the finger in extension tend to be cut at the level of the skin laceration. Lacerations on the palmar aspect of the finger will almost always injure the FDP before the FDS.
4. A careful neurovascular evaluation is critical to assess further injury.
5. Partial tendon lacerations may be difficult to diagnose but are suggested by pain and weakness with resisted range of motion. Magnetic resonance imaging and ultrasonography are helpful diagnostic aids in these cases.

Timing of Repair

1. Delayed primary repair (within a few days after injury) has results similar to or better than those of emergent primary repair.
2. To prevent proximal retraction of the severed tendons, forearm and wrist should be placed in a forearm-based dorsal splint with the wrist in slight flexion (~20 degrees), the MP joints at 50 degrees or more of flexion, and the DIP and PIP joints extended.

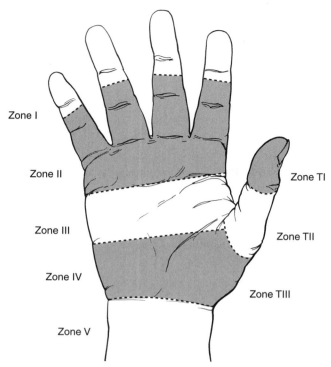

Zone I

Zone II

Zone TI

Zone III

Zone TII

Zone IV

Zone TIII

Zone V

Figure 2-8 ✦ Zone of injury for flexor tendons. *(From Green DH, Hotchkiss RM, Pederson WC: Green's Operative Hand Surgery, 4th ed. New York, Churchill Livingstone, 1998.)*

Zones

Zones are used to describe the location of tendon injuries of the flexor mechanism. The thumb has zones I through III different from those of the fingers, but zones IV and V are the same. The relevance of the zonal distinction was more important in the past when zone II injuries were not repaired primarily (Fig. 2-8).

ZONE I (distal to the FDS insertion for the digits; region of the FPL insertion for the thumb)

1. Only one tendon (FDP or FPL) is present and can be injured ("one tendon in zone I"). Primary end-to-end repair is preferred. If the distal stump is very short or nonexistent, direct reattachment of the proximal stump to the bone (by the pull-out suture over a button technique or suture anchors) may be performed. Advancement of the tendon greater

than 1 cm should be avoided to prevent quadriga effect or flexion contracture.
2. After 3 to 4 weeks, direct repair of the tendon ends may not be possible. In this instance, the choice of treatment includes benign neglect, DIP tenodesis or fusion, and free tendon grafting (rarely indicated; see "Salvage Procedures").
3. FDP avulsion (jersey finger) represents an avulsion injury in zone I.
   a. The diagnosis is often missed initially, the injury usually dismissed as a sprain or jammed finger. The mechanism is forced extension of the digit during maximal contraction of the profundus muscle.
      i. It is most common in male athletes.
      ii. The ring finger is involved in 75% of cases (reported in all fingers, including the thumb).
      iii. Patients present with an inability to flex the DIP joint (MP and PIP joint flexion is intact).
   b. Prognosis depends on the following:
      i. Amount of proximal tendon retraction.
      ii. Remaining blood supply to the tendon.
      iii. Time interval between injury and treatment.
      iv. Radiographic presence and size of a bone avulsion fragment.
   c. These injuries have been classified into three main types (Table 2-7).
      i. Type I: tendon retraction into the palm. Retrieval and reattachment of the tendon must be done within 7 to 10 days before contracture and degeneration. The tendon can be retrieved by inserting a catheter through the pulley system in a retrograde manner. The tendon stump is then sutured to the end of the catheter and delivered distally. Attachment to bone can be accomplished by the pull-out suture/button technique or bone anchor.
      ii. Type II: tendon retraction to PIP joint (most common). The tendon avulses with a fleck of bone, which is caught up at the A3 pulley (occasionally seen on a lateral radiograph). There is less retraction, probably related to the vincula, and therefore repair is possible up to 6 weeks. The technique for reattachment is as described for

✦ Table 2-7			
LEDDY CLASSIFICATION OF PROFUNDUS AVULSION INJURIES			
Type	**Tendon Retraction Level**	**Repair**	**Interval / Treatment**
I	Palm	(Dysvascular)	7–10 days
II	PIP joint (held by vinculum longum)		3 months
III	A4 pulley (held by bone avulsion fragment)	Open reduction and internal fixation of fragment	
IIIa	Type III but profundus also avulses off fracture fragment	Treatment based on level of tendon retraction	

From Miller MD: Review of Orthopaedics, 3rd ed. Philadelphia, WB Saunders, 2000.

type I. Some type II jersey fingers turn into type I when they are not repaired in a timely fashion.

   iii. Type III: minimal tendon retraction. The A4 pulley prevents the large avulsed bone fragment from retracting proximally. On radiography, the fragment can be seen just proximal to the DIP joint. Treatment is open reduction and fixation in the acute and subacute stages. Repair may be possible up to 3 months from injury. For the chronic cases, DIP arthrodesis or tendon grafting (rarely, see "Salvage Procedures") is indicated.

ZONE II (the area between zone I and the metacarpal neck for the fingers; the region from the neck of the proximal phalanx to the neck of the metacarpal in the thumb)

Both the FDS and FDP exist in zone II ("two tendons in zone II"), and both are usually injured.

1. Zone II is historically known as no-man's land because injuries in this region tended to have poor results.
2. After the tendon repair, any lacerations of the digital nerves should be repaired. On occasion, digital artery repair is also necessary.
3. When both tendons are disrupted, the standard is to repair the FDS in addition to the FDP because it
   a. results in better balance of the injured finger.
   b. spares the long vinculum of the superficialis.
   c. prevents a hyperextension deformity at the PIP joint.
   d. adds strength to the finger.
   e. provides a smooth gliding bed for the profundus repair.
4. FDS avulsions are less common than FDP avulsions. These patients often exhibit limited PIP motion and a mass at the A1 pulley. Treatment may require tendon excision and tenolysis.

ZONE III (the region between the distal palmer crease and the distal edge of the transverse carpal ligament [origin of lumbricals] for the fingers; the region of the thenar muscles for the thumb)

There is relatively good prognosis for injuries in this zone. The FPL is rarely injured in this zone because of the overlying thenar muscles.

ZONE IV (carpal tunnel)

In this region, tendon can be injured in various combinations. There is usually injury to the median and possibly ulnar nerve. Primary repair of all severed structures should be done before muscle contracture occurs. Postoperatively, the wrist should be immobilized in neutral (not flexion) to prevent bowstringing. Despite early repair, functional recovery is guarded.

ZONE V (the region of the distal forearm from the proximal edge of the transverse carpal ligament to the musculotendinous junction of the flexors)

Lacerations in this zone can involve the wrist and digital flexors as well as neurovascular structures (i.e., "spaghetti wrist"). Tendon repairs in this zone can be performed with just core sutures (epitenon sutures are unnecessary), but care must be taken to suture the corresponding ends together with the correct orientation. Prognosis is more favorable unless there are concomitant neurovascular injuries.

Suture

Numerous studies with use of various in vivo and in vitro models have examined the effect of different suture techniques. Although direct comparison of the studies is difficult, the following general conclusions can be drawn.

1. Strength is directly related to the number of suture strands crossing the repair site (in clinical practice, most use four strands).
2. Larger suture calibers increase the strength of repair (in clinical practice, most use 3-0 or 4-0 caliber nonabsorbable sutures).
3. Locking loops add little strength and may actually lead to collapse and gapping at moderate tensile loads (many tendon suture techniques have been described, but the most widely used is the modified Kessler-Tajima technique).
4. The weakest link in the repair is the suture knot.
5. Braided synthetic 3-0 or 4-0 sutures are probably the best for repairs because of ease of placement, adequate strength, and minimal stretching (low elasticity).
6. Continuous circumferential running epitendinous suture can add 10% to 50% strength to the core sutures. It also reduces gapping at the tendon ends. The 6-0 synthetic monofilament is commonly used.
7. Dorsal placement of core sutures yields greater tensile strength than volar placement.

Prognostic Factors

1. Clean, sharp lacerations do better than does tendon disruption caused by crush injuries.
2. Zone II injuries have the worst results.
3. Younger patients do better than older ones. Small children can have poor results because of the small size of the injured structures and the patient's inability to cooperate with the postoperative rehabilitation protocol.
4. Adhesion formation portends a worse prognosis. The following factors contribute to adhesions:
   a. Severity of injury (crush component).
   b. Poor surgical technique (pinching, crushing, or excessive touching of the tendon ends or sheath).
   c. Gapping at the repair site, especially of more than 3 mm.
   d. Tendon ischemia (disruption of the vincula and sheath).
   e. Immobilization after repair.

Contraindications to Primary Repair

The following are contraindications to primary repair:
1. Severe multiple soft tissue injuries to the finger and palm.

2. Significant skin defect over the flexor tendon system.
3. Contaminated (or potentially contaminated) wound.

In these cases, it is more prudent to address the soft tissue and wound problems before the tendon repair. Any chance of achieving a good result requires a healthy bed for the tendon repair.

Sheath Repair

At present, sheath repair during the time of primary tendon repair remains a controversial issue. There is a belief that sheath closure leads to less adhesion formation; however, there are conflicting clinical studies to this effect. Therefore, the current recommendation is that repair of the flexor tendon sheath be attempted but no extraordinary measures taken if this cannot be achieved readily. In the latter case, the sheath should be trimmed back to prevent incarceration of the tendon.

Partial Tendon Laceration

Lacerations less than 60% of the tendon width do not need to be sutured. Those greater than 60% should be repaired to prevent possible entrapment, complete rupture, and triggering. Some authors think that tendon lacerations up to 95% have better results with conservative treatment. These authors recommend limited trimming of the tendon edges or pulley release to prevent triggering but no suture in the substance of the tendon itself.

Postoperative Rehabilitation

1. The goal of flexor tendon rehabilitation is to start early controlled mobilization. It is known that repaired tendons subjected to early motion have greater tensile strength, excursion, and function than do those treated with immobilization. In addition, motion after repair leads to increased gliding, decreased adhesions, and increased collagen fibril size.
2. Tendons immobilized after repair have decreased tensile strength in 5 days to 3 weeks. This decrease in strength is not appreciable when early controlled mobilization programs are used.
3. Different mobilization protocols have common features:
   a. During periods of rest, the wrist and MP joints are splinted in a position of flexion; the PIP and DIP joints are extended.
   b. Use of the hand is not permitted for 6 to 8 weeks.
   c. Most protocols are not applicable for patients who are noncompliant or uncooperative.
   d. A well-trained hand therapist should supervise the rehabilitation program.
4. There are three common early controlled-motion programs.
   a. Active extension with rubber band flexion (modified Kleinert). This is a dynamic splinting program in which a rubber band outrigger is attached to a dorsal block splint with the wrist and MP joint in flexion and the IP joint in extension. The rubber band passively flexes the digits, but the patient is allowed to actively extend up to the limit of the splint. Modifications such as bars and "synergistic" wrist extension-flexion splints can be added to improve composite digital motion (Fig. 2-9).
   b. Controlled passive motion (modified Duran). This program allows passive motion of the digits (by either the patient or therapist) in the resting splint. Active motion is started 4 weeks after repair. At 6 weeks, blocking exercises are started and passive stretching of a flexion contracture is performed. Neuromuscular stimulation can also be safely added to the treatment of tendon repair at 5 to 6 weeks postoperatively. At 8 to 10 weeks, strengthening exercises are instituted. The proposed advantage is that there is less likelihood of flexion contractures than with the modified Kleinert protocol (Fig. 2-10).
   c. Controlled active motion. This protocol is based on the fact that wrist extension and MP flexion produce the least tension on the repaired tendon, especially during active digital motion. During therapy, the resting splint is exchanged for a tenodesis splint. The patient is

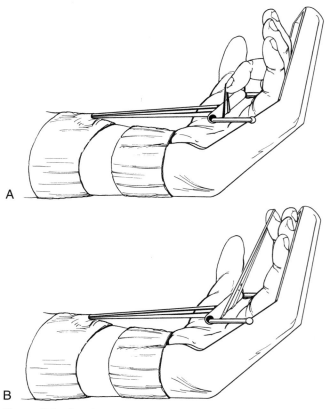

Figure 2-9 ❖ Flexor tendon rehabilitation protocol consisting of active finger extension and passive flexion with rubber bands (modified Kleinert). *(From Strickland JW: Flexor tendons—acute injuries. In Green DP, Hotchkiss RN, Pederson WC, eds: Green's Operative Hand Surgery, 4th ed. New York, Churchill Livingstone, 1999.)*

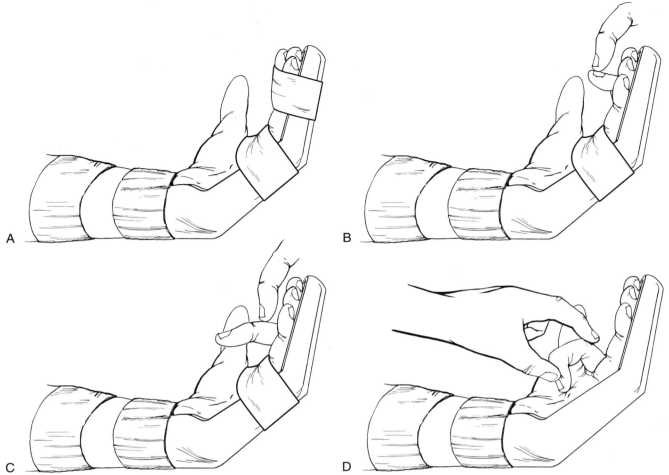

A

B

C

D

Figure 2-10 ◈ Flexor tendon rehabilitation protocol with controlled passive motion (modified Duran). *(From Strickland JW: Flexor tendons—acute injuries. In Green DP, Hotchkiss RN, Pederson WC, eds: Green's Operative Hand Surgery, 4th ed. New York, Churchill Livingstone, 1999.)*

allowed motion at the wrist from full flexion to 30 degrees of extension, provided that MP joints are maintained beyond 60 degrees of flexion. With the wrist extended, the IP joints are then passively flexed, and the patient is instructed to hold that position for 5 seconds, then to release ("place and hold" technique) (Fig. 2-11).

Flexor Tendon Injuries in Children

These injuries are approached with the same principles as in adults. Repair of flexor tendons in the skeletally immature child has the added importance of promoting normal digital growth. The few differences of tendon repair between the adult and child are the smaller structures injured and the inability to institute a structured early motion program in children. Repairs in children usually require smaller core sutures (5-0 caliber), and postoperative care consists only of immobilization for 4 weeks. A longer period of immobilization leads to poorer results.

Complications of Flexor Tendon Repair

The results of flexor tendon repair are unreliable (particularly in zone II), and complications are common. The exact rate of complications is not well documented in the literature.

1. Rupture
    a. Rupture of the tendon repair is usually related to overly aggressive use of the hand.
    b. The rate of rupture for zone I and zone II repairs (postoperative active motion protocol) is approximately 4% to 6% in the fingers and 17% in the thumb.
    c. Rupture of repair commonly occurs when patients are noncompliant with the therapy program or when they are advanced to more forceful active motion.
    d. Differential diagnosis includes flexor tendon adhesions. Magnetic resonance imaging (most accurate) or ultrasonography can be helpful in confirming the diagnosis.

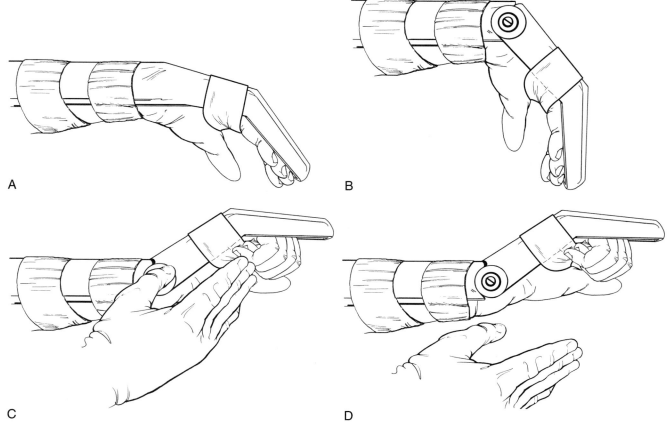

A

B

C

D

Figure 2-11 ◆ Flexor tendon rehabilitation protocol with controlled active motion. *(From Strickland JW: Flexor tendons—acute injuries. In Green DP, Hotchkiss RN, Pederson WC, eds: Green's Operative Hand Surgery, 4th ed. New York, Churchill Livingstone, 1999.)*

   e. The preferred treatment of acute rupture is prompt re-exploration and repeated repair.

2. Joint contracture of the PIP or DIP is the most frequent late complication of flexor tendon repair. This must be distinguished from tendon adhesions. The complication is prevented by modification of the therapy program to permit more extension. A flexion contracture of the PIP joint that develops after flexor tendon repair is treated with extension stretching or serial extension splinting starting at 6 weeks postoperatively.

3. Tendon adhesions may occur despite the best possible repair and postoperative rehabilitation. On examination, there will be greater passive flexion of the digit compared with active flexion. The failure of the tendon to glide usually requires secondary tenolysis. The timing of the tenolysis is based on exhaustion of vigorous therapy, normal or nearly normal passive joint range of motion (i.e., no joint contracture), and wound equilibrium. This usually requires 3 to 6 months or more after the last operative procedure.

Salvage Procedures

When failed repairs result in tendon discontinuity, scarring, or destruction of the sheath or pulley system, a salvage procedure may be indicated.

   Autogenous tendon grafts used in these procedures include PL, plantaris, long extensors of the lesser toes, EIP, extensor digiti minimi, and ring FDS. Use of intrasynovial tendon grafts, such as the toe flexors, has shown less adhesion formation than with extrasynovial grafts.

Primary Tendon Graft of FDP

Primary tendon grafting may be considered when delayed primary repair is not possible because of retraction of tendon ends (usually after 3 to 4 weeks). This option should be discussed with the patient thoroughly (especially if there is normal motion at the PIP joint from an intact FDS) and is rarely performed because the patient can be made worse if the procedure fails.

1. The indications should be limited to young patients, to those with good digital range of motion who require active DIP flexion, and to ulnar digits for power grip.

2. The graft should be passed through the FDS decussation. If the fit is too tight, the graft may be passed around Camper's chiasm, or one slip of FDS can be removed.

3. Under no circumstance should both slips of a functional FDS tendon be sacrificed during the procedure.

4. The distal end of the graft should be attached to the distal phalanx; the proximal anastomosis should be performed proximal to zone II.

STAGED RECONSTRUCTION

In cases in which primary repair or tendon grafting is likely to result in a poor outcome (severe initial trauma, failed previous surgeries, incompetent pulley system), staged flexor tendon reconstruction may be considered. The surgeon and patient must be aware of the complexity of the problem. Many times, arthrodesis or amputation may be the better choice.

Stage 1

The goal of this stage is to create a healthy bed for tendon gliding within a new sheath. The remaining flexor tendon is excised (except for the stump of the FDS, which can be used for pulley reconstruction, and the stump of the FDP to attach the implant and tendon graft). Joint releases and nerve repairs are performed as necessary. The silicone Hunter tendon implant is inserted under the remaining pulleys in a retrograde fashion (a new sheath will form around the implant). The distal end is attached to the FDP stump, and the proximal end is left subcutaneous in the distal forearm. If there is bowstringing of the implant with traction, appropriate pulley reconstruction is performed. Options for pulley reconstruction include a distally based slip of FDS and a free graft. The graft may be woven at the rim of the volar phalanx through the residual pulley. The free graft may be encircled around the phalanx superficial to the extensor mechanism at the middle phalanx and deep to the extensor mechanism at the proximal phalanx. Reconstructed flexor tendon pulleys should be widely spread to decrease tension on the pulley-tendon. Passive motion is started in the early postoperative period to enhance range of motion and to promote excursion of the implant within the new tendon bed. The time interval until the second stage is usually 3 months.

Stage 2

In the second stage, the autogenous tendon graft is sutured to the implant at the proximal end and drawn into the newly formed sheath by pulling the distal end of the implant. The distal end of the graft is then attached to the distal phalanx and the proximal end to a donor motor muscle in the distal forearm (allows better gliding).

Complications of Staged Reconstruction

1. Silicone synovitis (8%) may be associated with buckling or binding of the implant. Treatment is to decrease therapy, but an early stage 2 procedure may be required.
2. Infection requires removal of the implant and appropriate antibiotic treatment.
3. Mechanical failure can rarely occur at the distal end of the implant. Avoid suturing of the proximal end to a motor muscle unit.
4. Rupture of the tendon graft can occur at either juncture but more commonly occurs at the distal attachment. Early recognition with reattachment is recommended. If advancement of the distal end to the distal phalanx is not possible, it can be attached to the middle phalanx to create a "superficialis finger."
5. Late flexion deformity.

Tendon Rupture

Spontaneous nonrheumatoid tendon ruptures in the hand are infrequent in clinical practice. They usually occur after a traumatic event or are due to attrition at bone ridges (fracture, osteophytes, malunion, nonunion) or hardware prominences. Rare causes of rupture include crystalline deposition diseases (gout, calcium pyrophosphate dihydrate crystal deposition disease), tumor or tumor-like conditions of the bones (intraosseous cyst, enchondroma, von Recklinghausen's disease), avascular necrosis of the lunate (Kienböck's disease), tuberculosis, and electrical injury.

Both the digital extensor and flexor tendons can be involved. In the nontraumatic cases, patients can be asymptomatic before the rupture. Diagnosis may be challenging given the minimal premorbid symptoms, and peripheral nerve palsies (e.g., posterior interosseous nerve syndrome) should be ruled out. Treatment depends largely on the nature, location, and quality of the ruptured tendon and the patient's disability. In traumatic cases, primary repair may be possible and is preferable.

Tendon Transfers

Indications

Indications for tendon transfer are to replace lost motor function (when it is impossible to repair nerve, tendon, or muscle), to augment diminished muscle power, and to restore the balance between the flexor and extensor systems.

Timing of Transfer

Timing of transfer is variable and depends on the indication, tissue equilibrium, and restoration of sensibility (if possible). For tendon ruptures, it is advisable to perform transfers earlier rather than later. In cases of nerve injuries or repairs, waiting for nerve regeneration is advocated.

Principles of Tendon Transfer

1. Correction of contracture. Maximum passive range of motion of the joints is necessary before any transfer because no tendon transfer will move a stiff joint. The key is contracture prevention.
2. Adequate donor strength
   a. Strength is measured as force (proportional to the cross-sectional area and volume of the muscle) or work (force × length of the musculotendinous unit).
   b. Muscle strength is graded from M1 (no muscle firing) to M5 (normal strength); M3 represents enough strength to resist gravity.
   c. The donor muscle unit should be M4 or M5 to perform its new function because it will lose one grade after the transfer.
   d. Reinnervated muscles should be avoided.
   e. Donor muscles for tendon transfers with the greatest potential force include FCU and brachioradialis.

3. Amplitude of motion (i.e., excursion)
    a. Excursion is proportional to the muscle fiber length.
    b. It should be comparable between the donor and recipient tendons.
    c. General guidelines for excursion by muscle group: wrist flexors and extensors, 33 mm; finger extensors and EPL, 50 mm; finger flexors, 70 mm.
    d. The amplitude can be improved by transferring a monarticular tendon to a multiarticular tendon, such as the transfer of a wrist flexor (33 mm of excursion) to a digital extensor (50 mm of excursion) in a patient with a radial nerve palsy.
    e. Alternatively, excursion can be improved by dissection of tendon or muscle from its attachments (e.g., FCU).
4. A straight line of pull results in better mechanical advantage and is desirable but not always possible to achieve. A transfer that lies close to the axis of rotation of the joint tends to lead to more motion (angular rotation) but less strength (torque).
5. One tendon/one function. If a donor tendon is transferred to multiple recipient tendons, the force and amplitude of excursion are dissipated and the transfer may fail.
6. Expendable donor. Use of the donor tendon must not result in unacceptable loss of function. For example, one functional wrist flexor (FCU or FCR) should be preserved.
7. Synergism. Synergistic transfer, such as a wrist flexor for finger extension (as opposed to a donor wrist extensor), is desirable because normal hand function coordinates wrist flexion with finger extension. Nonsynergistic tendon transfers can be performed, but it is more difficult for the patient to adapt to the transfer.
8. A tendon transferred close to the axis of rotation of the joint will lead to improved motion (angular rotation) but decreased strength (torque).

Selection of Transfers

The selection of transfers is based on the deficits and the available donors. Adherence to the principles of tendon transfer ensures more favorable outcome (children generally do better than adults). See Table 2-8 for the more common transfers in nerve palsies.

Other Tendon Disorders

Chronic Digital Deformities

Because the extensor system is linked, discontinuity at one joint will lead to increased force of pull at the adjacent joint, causing a reciprocal deformity in the adjacent finger joint.

SWAN-NECK DEFORMITY (DIP FLEXION, PIP HYPEREXTENSION)

1. Nonrheumatoid causes of swan-neck deformity include chronic mallet finger and PIP volar plate injury.

2. These injuries lead to stretch of the transverse retinacular ligament, resulting in migration and eventual contracture of the lateral bands *dorsal* to the axis of rotation of the PIP joint. The dorsally displaced lateral bands potentiate the PIP joint hyperextension.
3. In patients with mild, flexible deformity, splinting to prevent PIP hyperextension or DIP flexion can be used.
4. In more severe cases, treatment should address the site of primary disease. Surgical intervention to prevent PIP hyperextension (FDS tenodesis, Fowler's central slip [proximal] tenotomy, spiral oblique retinacular ligament reconstruction) can correct the deformity. If the primary deformity is at the DIP joint, extensor tendon reconstruction or DIP arthrodesis can be performed.

BOUTONNIÈRE DEFORMITY

1. Nonrheumatoid causes of boutonnière deformity include FDP or central slip disruption and alteration in the triangular ligament that holds the two terminal ends of the lateral bands centralized over the middle phalanx.
2. These injuries lead to stretch of the transverse retinacular ligament, resulting in migration and eventual contracture of the lateral bands *volar* to the axis of rotation of the PIP joint. The volarly displaced lateral bands potentiate the PIP joint flexion.
3. In patients with mild, flexible deformity, splinting the PIP in extension while allowing DIP movement is preferable, even if the deformity is chronic.
4. Reconstructive options for patients whose conservative treatment fails include direct repair of the central slip, free tendon graft of the central slip, Fowler's distal tenotomy, and Matev reconstruction (transfer of the ulnar lateral band to the distal stump of the radial lateral band while the proximal aspect of the radial lateral band is sutured to the base of the middle phalanx).
5. Salvage procedures include fusion and arthroplasty if there are arthritic changes in the PIP joint.
6. Chronic boutonnière deformities are initially treated with stretching of the oblique retinacular ligament and extension splinting of the PIP joint until it has full passive extension before operative management is considered.

Digital Stiffness

Limited range of motion of a digit may be related to a variety of factors. The cause can often be determined on physical examination. It is critical to differentiate stiffness resulting from joint contracture (limited active and passive motion regardless of the position of the adjacent joints) from stiffness secondary to tendon scarring or imbalance (joint motion dependent on the position of adjacent joints).

EXTRINSIC TIGHTNESS

Extrinsic extensor or flexor tightness may be due to trauma or shortening of the extrinsic tendon during repair. Extrinsic extensor tightness is manifested as

✦ **Table 2-8**

COMMON TENDON TRANSFERS FOR NERVE PALSIES

Palsy	Deficit	Transfer	Alternative Transfer	Comments
Radial	Wrist extension	PT to ECRB	FCR to ECRB	Need at least one wrist flexor (excluding PL)
	Finger extension	FCU to EDC II-V	FDS III-IV to EDC II-V FCR to ECD II-V	Limited ability to make fist and flex wrist simultaneously
	Thumb extension	PL to EPL (rerouted)	FDS III to EPL	
Posterior interosseous nerve	Finger extension	FCR to EDC II-V	As above	FCR rather than FCU to limit wrist radial deviation
	Thumb extension	PL to EPL		
Low median	Thumb opposition	FDS IV to AbPB	EIP to AbPB AbDM to AbPB (children) PL to AbPB (weaker)	Opposition also requires thumb adductor and short flexors Opposition may be preserved with ulnar-innervated FPB (superficial head) Pulley should be in the region of the pisiform
High median	Thumb IP flexion	BR to FPL		FDS and PL unavailable for transfer
	Index finger and long finger flexion	FDP IV-V to FDP II-III (side-to-side)	ECRL to FDP II-III (more power, less excursion)	Anterior interosseous nerve palsy: BR to FPL, FDP IV-V to FDP II-III
	Thumb opposition	EIP to AbPB	EDQ to AbPB	
Low ulnar	Hand intrinsics (interossei and ulnar lumbricals)	FDS to lateral bands	ECRL to lateral bands EDQ and EIP to lateral bands (Fowler) FCR + graft to lateral bands	Transfer to lateral bands may cause swan-neck deformities.
	Thumb adduction	ECRL + graft to AdP	BR + graft to AdP	Therefore, transfer grafts to flexor tendon sheath instead in patients with hypermobile joints.
	Index finger abduction	EIP to 1st DIO	AbPL to 1st DIO ECRL to 1st DIO	
High ulnar	Low ulnar nerve deficits (plus)	Same as above		
	Ring finger and small finger FDP	FDP II-III to FDP IV-V (side-to-side)		
Low median and Ulnar	Thumb adduction	BR + graft to abductor tubercle of thumb		
	Thumb abduction	EIP to AbPB		
	Index finger abduction	AbPL to 1st DIO		
	Clawed fingers	ECRL or BR + graft to A2 pulleys		
High median and Ulnar	Low median and ulnar deficits (plus)	Same as above, except for clawed fingers		
	Thumb IP flexion	BR or EIP to FPL		
	Finger flexion	ECRL to FDP		
	Clawed fingers	Tenodesis of MP joints		
	Wrist flexion	ECU to FCU		
Brachial plexus	Elbow flexion	Steindler flexorplasty—flexor pronator mass transferred proximally	Bipolar latissimus transfer Pectoralis major transfer Triceps transfer Sternocleidomastoid transfer	

Modified from Miller MD: Review of Orthopaedics, 3rd ed. Philadelphia, WB Saunders, 2000.

limited flexion of the IP joints while the MP joint is held in flexion. In addition, there is improved flexion of the IP joints while the MP joint is held in extension. In contrast, extrinsic flexor tightness causes limited extension of the IP joints while the MP joint is held in extension and greater extension of the IP joints when the MP joint is held in flexion.

Intrinsic Tightness

Intrinsic tightness is usually the result of trauma or improper immobilization of the hand. Burns and stroke are also common causes. The patient complains of stiffness and pain, and the result of a Bunnell intrinsic tightness test is positive. To perform the test, the examiner passively flexes the MP joint (to relax the intrinsics) to determine the flexibility of the IP joints. This is compared with IP joint flexibility with the MP joint held in extension (to stretch the intrinsics). If there is limited IP joint flexion with the MP joint in extension compared to IP joint flexion with the MP joint in flexion, the test result is positive for intrinsic tightness. The treatment initially consists of aggressive range of motion therapy. However, patients may require intrinsic muscle releases if they do not improve.

Quadriga

1. Quadriga is related to the common origin of the long, ring, and small finger profundus muscles. The index profundus has an independent muscle origin and is less likely to be affected.
2. Quadriga may be post-traumatic or postsurgical related to *functional or anatomic shortening* of one of the profundus tendons. The patient has incomplete active flexion of the unaffected digits because the shortened tendon will achieve full excursion before the unaffected tendons do. Because of the common origin, the unaffected tendons cannot complete the normal excursion, and incomplete composite flexion is observed clinically. The patient may complain of weakness during grip. Conversely, as the fingers are extended, the affected digit will not achieve full extension because it is functionally shorter and more taut than the unaffected digits.
3. The clinical scenarios in which this could happen include the following:
   a. Suturing of the FDP to the extensor tendon after a tip amputation.
   b. Distal advancement of the FDP during repair.
   c. Scarring of the FDP after an amputation.
   d. Improper tensioning of a tendon graft (too short).
4. The treatment options include tenolysis, tendon lengthening, and tenotomy of the affected tendon.

Lumbrical Plus Finger

1. The lumbrical plus finger is related to *functional or anatomic shortening* of one of the lumbricals relative to its corresponding profundus tendon.
2. In an attempt to flex the DIP joint, contraction of the profundus muscle places traction on the shortened lumbrical because the origin of the lumbrical

is on the profundus tendon itself. Tension on the shortened lumbrical leads to paradoxical extension of the IP joints.
3. The clinical scenarios in which this could happen include the following:
   a. Proximal migration of the FDP tendon after an amputation or after an unrecognized avulsion. The proximally migrated FDP will stretch the lumbrical.
   b. Scarred lumbrical.
   c. An excessively long flexor tendon graft to the distal phalanx during tendon reconstruction.
4. Treatment consists of surgical release of the affected lumbrical or lateral band.

Pulley Rupture

1. The flexor pulleys can be injured in isolation or in association with flexor tendon injuries (more common).
2. Closed ruptures are seen in mountain climbers who present with swelling and an inability to flex the affected digit fully.
3. Reconstruction is recommended for the A2 and A4 pulleys to prevent bowstringing, loss of mechanical advantage, and flexion contracture of the finger.
4. The choice of material includes remnant pulley, FDS stump, volar plate, extensor retinaculum, and free tendon graft.
5. The reconstructed pulley should be strong enough to withstand vigorous testing on the operating table and wide enough to decrease tension on the pulley-tendon interface.

"Saddle" Syndrome

1. Adhesions between the interosseous and lumbrical tendons at the level of the MP joint can occur after crush injuries.
2. Patients complain of pain between the metacarpal heads and discomfort with IP joint flexion with the MP in extension.
3. Treatment with corticosteroid injections or tenolysis can be helpful in addressing symptoms.

Distal Biceps Tendon Rupture

1. Distal biceps tendon rupture is most likely to occur in the fourth to sixth decades of life in men.
2. Nonoperative treatment may result in 50% weakness of elbow flexion and supination strength.
3. Operative repair may be performed by a one- or two-incision technique.
4. A hinged dynamic brace with an extension block at 30 degrees is used postoperatively for 6 weeks, followed by progressive range of motion.
5. Repair can be complicated with proximal radioulnar synostosis, more common with the two-incision technique.
6. Chronic biceps tendon ruptures may require tendon reconstruction. Options for tendon graft include semitendinosus or fascia lata autograft and allograft.

Bibliography

al Qattan MM: Conservative management of zone II partial flexor tendon lacerations greater than half the width of the tendon. J Hand Surg Am 25:1118–1121, 2000.

Baker DS, Gaul JS Jr, Williams VK, Graves M: The little finger superficialis—clinical investigation of its anatomic and functional shortcomings. J Hand Surg Am 6:374–378, 1981.

Burton RI, Melchior JA: Extensor tendons—late reconstruction. In Green DP, Hotchkiss RN, Pederson WC, eds: Green's Operative Hand Surgery, 4th ed. New York, Churchill Livingstone, 1999, pp 1988–2021.

Canovas F, Nicolau F, Bonnel F: Avulsion of the flexor digitorum profundus tendon associated with a chondroma of the distal phalanx. J Hand Surg Br 23:130–131, 1998.

Davis TRC, Barton NJ: Median nerve palsy. In Green DP, Hotchkiss RN, Pederson WC, eds: Green's Operative Hand Surgery, 4th ed. New York, Churchill Livingstone, 1999, pp 1497–1525.

De Smet L, Baeten Y: Closed rupture of both flexor tendons of the fifth finger due to a calcium hydroxyapatite deposit in the carpal tunnel. Acta Orthop Belg 64:336–338, 1998.

Doyle JR: Extensor tendons—acute injuries. In Green DP, Hotchkiss RN, Pederson WC, eds: Green's Operative Hand Surgery, 4th ed. New York, Churchill Livingstone, 1999, pp 1950–1987.

Doyle JR: Dynamics of the flexor tendon pulley system. In Hunter JM, Schneider LH, Mackin EJ, eds: Tendon and Nerve Surgery in the Hand: A Third Decade. St. Louis, Mosby, 2001, pp 254–262.

Drape JL, Silbermann-Hoffman O, Houvet P, et al: Complications of flexor tendon repair in the hand: MR imaging assessment. Radiology 198:219–224, 1996.

Elliot D, Moiemen NS, Flemming AF, et al: The rupture rate of acute flexor tendon repairs mobilized by the controlled active motion regimen. J Hand Surg Br 19:607–612, 1994.

Frakking TG, Depuydt KP, Kon M, Werker PM: Retrospective outcome analysis of staged flexor tendon reconstruction. J Hand Surg Br 25:168–174, 2000.

Green DP: Radial nerve palsy. In Green DP, Hotchkiss RN, Pederson WC, eds: Green's Operative Hand Surgery, 4th ed. New York, Churchill Livingstone, 1999, pp 1481–1496.

Hallock GG: The Mitek Mini GII anchor introduced for tendon reinsertion in the hand. Ann Plast Surg 33:211–213, 1994.

Harrison SH: Delayed primary flexor tendon grafts of the fingers. A comparison of results with primary and secondary tendon grafts. Plast Reconstr Surg 43:366–372, 1969.

Joyce ME, Lou J, Manske PR: Tendon healing, molecular and cellular regulation. In Hunter JM, Schneider LH, Mackin EJ, eds: Tendon and Nerve Surgery in the Hand: A Third Decade. St. Louis, Mosby, 2001, pp 286–296.

Omer GE: Combined nerve palsies. In Green DP, Hotchkiss RN, Pederson WC, eds: Green's Operative Hand Surgery, 4th ed. New York, Churchill Livingstone, 1999, pp 1542–1556.

Omer GE: Ulnar nerve palsy. In Green DP, Hotchkiss RN, Pederson WC, eds: Green's Operative Hand Surgery, 4th ed. New York, Churchill Livingstone, 1999, pp 1526–1541.

Saitoh S, Kitagawa E, Hosaka M: Rupture of flexor tendons due to pisotriquetral osteoarthritis. Arch Orthop Trauma Surg 116: 303–306, 1997.

Schneider LH: Flexor tendons—late reconstruction. In Green DP, Hotchkiss RN, Pederson WC, eds: Green's Operative Hand Surgery, 4th ed. New York, Churchill Livingstone, 1999, pp 1859–1945.

Schultz RO, Drake DB, Morgan RF: A new technique for the treatment of flexor digitorum profundus tendon avulsion. Ann Plast Surg 42:46–48, 1999.

Smith RJ: Balance and kinetics of the fingers under normal and pathological conditions. Clin Orthop 104:92–111, 1974.

Stamos BD, Leddy JP: Closed flexor tendon disruption in athletes. Hand Clin 16:359–365, 2000.

Strickland JW: Flexor tendon injuries: I. Foundations of treatment. J Am Acad Orthop Surg 3:44–54, 1995.

Strickland JW: Flexor tendon injuries: II. Operative technique. J Am Acad Orthop Surg 3:55–62, 1995.

Strickland JW: Flexor tendons—acute injuries. In Green DP, Hotchkiss RN, Pederson WC, eds: Green's Operative Hand Surgery, 4th ed. New York, Churchill Livingstone, 1999, pp 1851–1897.

Strickland JW: Development of flexor tendon surgery: twenty-five years of progress. J Hand Surg Am 25:214–235, 2000.

Valenti P, Gilbert A: Two-stage flexor tendon grafting in children. Hand Clin 16:573–578, viii, 2000.

Vaz FM, Belcher HJ: Rupture of the tendon of flexor digitorum profundus in association with an enchondroma of the terminal phalanx. J Hand Surg Br 23:548–549, 1998.

Woo SL, An K, Frank CB, et al: Anatomy, biology, and biomechanics of tendons and ligaments. In Buckwalter JA, Einhorn TA, Simon SR, eds: Orthopaedic Basic Science, 2nd ed. Rosemont, Ill, American Academy of Orthopaedic Surgeons, 1999.

3

✧ Tamara D. Rozental, MD ✧ David R. Steinberg, MD

SKIN AND SOFT TISSUE DEFECTS

Nails

Anatomy (Fig. 3-1)

Definitions

The *perionychium* is composed of the *nail bed* (germinal and sterile matrices) and surrounding soft tissue.

The *hyponychium* is the junction of the nail bed and the skin at the most distal aspect of the finger. It functions as a barrier to infection.

The skin on the dorsum of the nail is termed the *nail wall*, and the *eponychium* (cuticle) is a thin membrane extending from the nail wall to the dorsal aspect of the nail plate.

The *paronychium* extends along the lateral edge of the nail and the eponychium.

The *lunula* is the white arc distal to the eponychium.

The *nail bed* (matrix) is composed of the germinal matrix and the sterile matrix.

The *nail fold* is the area where the proximal nail fits and is composed of a ventral floor and dorsal roof.

The *germinal matrix* extends from the nail fold to the lunula. It is primarily responsible for generating most (90%) of the nail plate. As the germinal matrix produces more nail, the nail plate progresses distally on the sterile matrix.

The *sterile matrix* extends distal to the lunula to the hyponychium. It provides adherence to the nail plate, adds a squamous epithelial layer, and is responsible for thickening the nail plate. The dorsal nail fold also adds a little to the nail plate thickness.

The blood supply to the nail bed comes from two terminal branches of the volar digital artery. The nerve supply is from the dorsal branch of the digital nerve.

Epidemiology of Nail Injuries

Injuries are most common in children and young adults. The long finger is most commonly involved. Most injuries are simple lacerations, and 50% involve a fracture of the distal phalanx. Crush and avulsion injuries have a worse prognosis, as do those associated with phalanx fractures.

Acute Injuries

SUBUNGUAL HEMATOMA

Disruption of the nail bed within an intact nail plate often leads to the formation of a subungual hematoma. Because there is bleeding into a compartment with little compliance, subungual hematomas can cause significant pain. Some authors recommend evacuation of the hematoma if it occupies 25% to 50% of the surface of the nail, whereas others recommend intervention in cases of severe pain regardless of the size of the area involved. Evacuation is achieved by creating a hole in the nail plate with a heated drill or paper clip. This hole should be large enough to allow continued drainage. Alternatively, the nail plate can be removed, the hematoma evacuated, and the nail plate replaced and sutured in position.

SIMPLE NAIL BED LACERATIONS

A hematoma that involves more than 50% of the visible nail and avulsions of the nail from the nail fold are signs of potential nail bed injury. In these cases, consider nail plate removal and nail bed exploration. Irregularities should be trimmed and lacerations repaired with absorbable suture (6-0 chromic gut). If possible, the nail is cleaned and replaced in the nail fold to provide a smooth surface for the nail bed during healing. If the nail is too damaged, a nail substitute (silicone, foil, gauze) can be introduced into the nail fold. In cases of late presentation, nail beds can be explored and repaired up to 7 days after injury. After that, reconstructive procedures are warranted. Good to excellent results are expected in 90% of patients treated acutely. Results are less optimal if the injury is associated with a distal phalanx fracture.

STELLATE LACERATIONS

These are treated in a fashion similar to simple lacerations with accurate approximation of the stellate points.

LACERATIONS WITH FRACTURES OF THE DISTAL PHALANX

A fracture of the distal phalanx has the highest predictive value for a nail bed laceration. If the fracture is

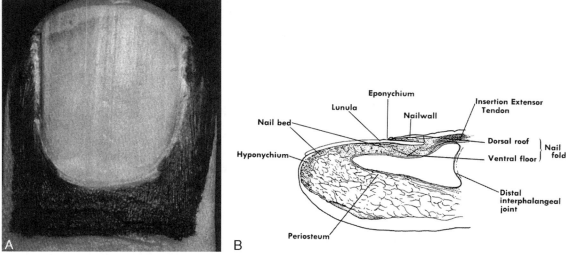

Figure 3-1 ◆ Anatomy of the nail. *(From Zook EG: Anatomy and physiology of the perionychium. Hand Clin 6:1–9, 1990.)*

nondisplaced, the laceration should be repaired and the nail replaced as a splint. Displaced fractures should be reduced and, if unstable, fixed with K-wires. Once the fracture is stable, the nail bed laceration is repaired in the standard fashion.

NAIL BED AVULSION

Avulsions of the sterile matrix are more frequent than those of the germinal matrix. Nail bed avulsions often leave a fragment of nail bed attached to the undersurface of the nail plate. When large fragments of matrix are attached to the nail, the outer edge of the nail bed can be dissected free, facilitating suture placement and repair (Fig. 3-2). For small fragments, the nail with attached nail bed should be replaced without attempting separation. All retrievable fragments of nail bed should be replaced as free grafts. If more material is needed, free full-thickness and particularly split-thickness nail grafts from adjacent digits or toes (usually the second toe) have shown excellent results.

Late Reconstruction

NONADHERENCE

Nonadherence is the most common post-traumatic deformity. Transverse or wide scars of the sterile matrix cause the nail to loosen distal to the scar. Distal nonadherence is not a problem unless dirt buildup underneath causes infection. More proximal nonadherence often results in an unstable, painful nail. Treatment consists of scar resection and nail bed closure. If the nail bed closure results in significant tension, the defect should be closed with split-thickness sterile matrix graft from an adjacent area or toe.

RIDGES

Ridges are caused by scar under the nail bed. Correction requires excision of the scar and smoothing of the irregularity to create a flat nail bed.

SPLIT NAIL

The split nail is caused by a ridge or longitudinal scar in the germinal or sterile matrix. The scar is usually too wide for excision and primary repair of the defect. Sterile matrix scars should be removed and covered with split-thickness nail bed grafts. Germinal matrix scars require full-thickness grafts for nail production.

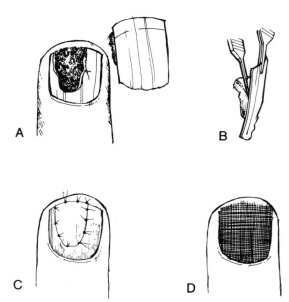

Figure 3-2 ◆ **A,** Nail avulsed from digit with underlying deep nail matrix avulsion. **B,** Inspection in these situations many times reveals the nail matrix still attached to the avulsed nail plate. This should be shaved away for use as a free graft. **C,** The avulsed segment is properly aligned and sutured to the defect. **D,** The avulsed nail should be replaced to cover the defect. If the nail plate is too damaged, the dressing should be fine mesh gauze or other nail substitute. *(From Shepard GH: Management of acute nail bed avulsions. Hand Clin 6: 39–57, 1990.)*

CORNIFIED NAIL BED

Patients in whom the germinal matrix has been removed often have problems with keratinized material growing from the sterile matrix. This is treated by removal of the sterile matrix and coverage with a split-thickness skin graft.

NAIL CYSTS AND SPIKES

Nail cysts and spikes follow incomplete removal of the germinal matrix after amputation of a fingertip. Treatment consists of removal of the cyst or spike and complete excision of the germinal matrix.

HOOK NAIL

Hook nail most commonly occurs after fingertip amputation with loss of bone support for the nail. This is best prevented by not pulling the nail bed over the distal phalanx in closing a distal finger amputation. Primary closure of an amputation without adequate bone support is likely to lead to this deformity. Once the deformity is present, it can be treated by adding support to the nail bed. If the distal nail bed has been pulled over the end of the finger, a V-Y advancement flap, cross-finger flap, or skin graft can be used to replace the soft tissue of the tip while restoring the nail bed onto the dorsum of the bone. Although bone grafts provide good support initially, they tend to be resorbed. Free vascularized toe transfers are the best alternative in trying to preserve nail length, although they are associated with significant donor site morbidity.

Nail Infections (see Chapter 11)

Perionychial infections around the nail are the most common infections of the hand. If detected early, these may be treated with warm soaks and antibiotics. In late cases or after abscess formation, treatment may require incision and drainage with partial or total nail removal. Fungal infections are treated with topical or systemic antifungals (griseofulvin). Bacterial infections with accompanying cellulitis require incision and drainage and subsequent antibiotics. Chronic paronychia, unresponsive to nonoperative management, is treated with removal of nail plate and *marsupialization* (removal of arc-shaped wedge of dorsal nail roof to allow secondary healing). The most likely organisms are mixed gram-negative bacteria and fungus.

Nail Growth Rates

Nail growth takes place at a rate of 0.1 mm/day. It is slower in children younger than 3 years and in adults older than 30 years. The nails of the long fingers grow faster than the nails of the rest of the digits. Fingernails have fourfold faster growth rates than toenails.

Coverage of Soft Tissue Defects about the Hand

Skin Grafts

ANATOMY AND PHYSIOLOGY

Skin is composed of a thick dermis covered by epidermis. The epidermis is composed of five layers: stratum basale, stratum spinosum, stratum granulosum, stratum lucidum, and stratum corneum. The two deepest layers are capable of regeneration of the more superficial cells. Dorsal hand skin is similar to skin found elsewhere in the body, with a continuous layer of epidermis, hair follicles, and sebaceous glands. Palmar skin has deeper ridges and a thicker keratin layer. It does not have pilosebaceous structures but has Meissner and pacinian corpuscles. The vascular supply to the skin comes from a deep and superficial arteriovenous plexus.

Wound healing occurs in four phases: hemostasis, inflammation, proliferation, and remodeling. Partial-thickness wounds, with an intact basement membrane, will heal by re-epithelialization. Loss of a full-thickness segment of skin initiates a process of wound contraction. Fibroblasts migrate into the wound, differentiate into myofibroblasts, and pull the wound edges together, resulting in wound contraction. This decreases the surface area and thus aids the healing process.

TYPES OF SKIN GRAFTS

Full-thickness skin grafts consist of epidermis and the entire thickness of dermis; split-thickness skin grafts consist of epidermis and varying levels of dermis. The advantages of full-thickness skin grafts are better wound bed protection, better sensibility due to greater reinnervation, less wound contracture, and faster maturation. The disadvantages include a higher rate of infection, the need for a better vascularized bed, and a lower survival than split-thickness grafts. The main advantages of split-thickness skin grafts include the ability to survive on beds with limited vascular supply (they require less revascularization) and the ability to cover large defects. Their main disadvantages are suboptimal cosmesis, less durability, and greater propensity for contracture. In general, full-thickness grafts should be used for palmar hand skin grafts, for which better skin quality is needed and contracture is of critical importance. Most dorsal defects can be adequately covered with split-thickness grafts.

CONTRAINDICATIONS TO SKIN GRAFTING

Wound Vascularity

When first applied, skin grafts are nourished by transudate from the wound. Within a few days, the process of vascularization begins. This process requires a relatively well vascularized bed, and grafts placed over denuded bone or tendon have overall lower survival.

Bacterial Content

Surface bacteria are common, but penetration of the bed of the wound with more than 10^5 organisms/g has a high incidence of graft failure.

TECHNIQUE

Wound Preparation

The surface must be débrided of all necrotic tissue. The condition of patients with underlying medical disorders and poor nutritional status should be optimized before the procedure.

Donor Site

The thickness of the desired graft dictates the location of the donor site. Full-thickness skin grafts can be taken from the groin and lower abdomen (for large defects) or from the ipsilateral extremity (small defects). Split-thickness skin graft donor sites include the posterolateral aspect of the trunk and thigh for thicker grafts and the anterior and medial aspects of the thigh for thin grafts.

Graft Harvest

For full-thickness skin grafts, the area of the defect is marked on the donor site. The graft should be 3% to 5% larger than the defect to allow contracture. The graft is then cut out with a small amount of subcutaneous tissue to facilitate wound closure. Grafts should be manually defatted before application. For split-thickness skin grafts, the skin is taken with an adjustable dermatome. Most wounds are covered by grafts 0.015 inch in thickness. Meshing of split-thickness skin grafts extends their surface area and allows drainage of hematoma. This is particularly useful for large defects or contaminated wounds but results in greater wound contracture and less cosmetically pleasing results. Meshed grafts for hand surgery should be limited to large or contaminated wounds.

Donor Site Care

Primary closure is ideal for full-thickness skin grafts. If this cannot be performed, the site should be covered with a split-thickness graft. Split grafts are partial abrasions and heal by re-epithelialization in 7 to 14 days. Hemostasis is achieved with lidocaine- and epinephrine-saturated sponges or with applied thrombin. The wound is then covered with a nonadherent dressing and meshed gauze.

Postoperative Care

Grafts are immobilized to maintain contact between the graft and the bed. A compressive dressing is applied to avoid hematoma. Grafts over concave surfaces tend to lose contact with the bed as fluid accumulates under the graft. This is prevented with a tie-over bolster dressing made with glycerin-soaked cotton, which holds the graft against the wound surface. In general, dressings are left in place for 5 to 7 days. If a hematoma or seroma is noted, the dressing is removed and aspiration performed. The most common causes of graft failure are hematoma and inadequate immobilization. Infection is often a result and not the cause of failure.

Skin Flaps

TYPES OF FLAPS BY VASCULAR SUPPLY

Random-Pattern Flaps

Random-pattern flaps are supported by minute vessels from the subdermal or subcutaneous plexus. The flap is usually raised by incision of three sides and use of the fourth side as a pedicle or base. In general, the length of a random-pattern flap should not exceed the width.

Axial-Pattern Flaps

Axial-pattern flaps receive their blood supply from a single, constant vessel. The area of skin supplied by an axial pedicle is known as the vascular territory, and the area where two territories meet is known as the watershed area. Axial flaps have a larger blood supply than do random flaps and can be made longer. They are also better at resisting infection. The disadvantages are that the vascular pedicle must be preserved and the flap cannot be thinned like random-pattern flaps.

1. Fasciocutaneous flap: axial-pattern flap whose vessels first pass through fascia. Fascia can be transferred without skin, but skin cannot be transferred without fascia.
2. Musculocutaneous flap: axial vessels first supply muscle so muscle can be taken without skin, but skin cannot be taken without muscle.
3. Osteocutaneous flap: axial-pattern flap consisting of skin and bone or a vascularized bone graft without skin.
4. Composite flap: composed of several tissue types, such as a free toe transfer.

TYPES OF FLAPS BY LOCATION

Local Flaps

Local flaps come from skin adjacent to the primary defect. These flaps have qualities similar to the lost skin and are often the most desirable. The highest probability of ischemia is at the tip of the flap.

1. Advancement flap: the pedicle is on the side of the flap opposite the primary defect.
2. Rotational flap: the flap moves laterally and is stretched to cover the primary and secondary defects. All rotation flaps are random-pattern.
3. Transpositional flap: the flap moves laterally, leaving a secondary defect that requires closure (primary or with a new skin cover).

Regional Flaps

Regional flaps come from elsewhere on the limb and may require two operative procedures, one to raise the flap and apply it to the defect and a second to divide the pedicle. The flaps are usually divided at 2 to 3 weeks under local infiltration anesthesia. Early division predisposes to necrosis, and late division can lead to joint stiffness.

Distant Flaps

Distant flaps, from elsewhere in the body, usually require at least two operative procedures unless designed as a free flap (see Chapter 8).

SPECIFIC FLAPS BY LOCATION

Local Flaps

1. Z-plasty (transpositional, random). The sides of the Z-plasty must be of equal length, but the angles may vary. As the angle increases, so does the length along the central limb. The most common is a 60-degree Z-plasty, which gives about 75% of central length. If sufficient skin is not present laterally, multiple Z-plasties can be used sequentially. The longitudinal gain is aggregate, but the transverse loss is not.
2. Axial flag flap (transpositional, axial). The axial flag flap is based on either the dorsal digital (metacarpal) artery or the proper digital artery at the web space of the donor finger, usually either the index or long finger. These flaps are mobile and will reliably cover the volar and dorsal aspect of the proximal phalanx of the index finger or the metacarpophalangeal (MP) joint of the index or long finger (Fig. 3-3).

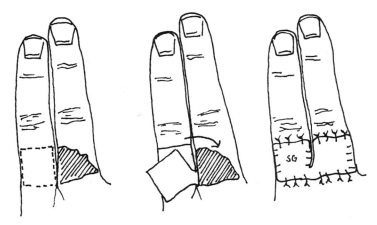

Figure 3-3 ❖ An axial flag flap can be raised from the dorsum of one finger and rotated to cover defects on the dorsal aspect of an adjacent digit. The secondary defect requires skin grafting (SG).

3. Dorsal metacarpal artery flap (transpositional, axial). Dissected from distal to proximal, the pedicle contains the metacarpal artery (first or second), veins, and branches of the radial nerve. This flap is an extension of the axial flag flap: the skin included can extend from the base of the first interosseous space to the proximal interphalangeal (PIP) joint. The flap is most commonly used to cover defects of the thumb and first web space but can also be used for proximal defects of the long and ring fingers. A reversed-flow dorsal metacarpal artery flap can be used for digital defects proximal to the PIP joints and can extend as far ulnar as the fifth metacarpal head.

4. Digital artery island flap (transpositional, axial). This flap is based on the radial or ulnar digital artery. The most useful donors are the long and ring fingers in which digital vessels are codominant and loss of one is less likely to cause problems. Main advantages: restricts the reconstruction to the injured digit, allows early mobilization of the digit, and has minimal cosmetic defect. This is the best axial flap for fingertip amputations.

5. V-Y advancement flap (advancement, random). The V-Y advancement flap is often used for fingertip amputations with dorsal tissue loss (including the thumb). The apex of the V should be at the distal digital crease; the base of the triangle should be as wide as the nail bed. The skin is incised in addition to the periosteal attachments. This flap requires extensive dissection for mobilization while maintaining the vessels and nerve branches supplying the flap. Palmar tissue loss greater than dorsal is a relative contraindication to a V-Y advancement flap (Fig. 3-4).

6. Lateral V-Y advancement flap (advancement, random). Indications for the lateral V-Y advancement flap are similar to those for the V-Y advancement flap. In this case, two flaps are raised, one on the radial side and one on the ulnar side of the digit. They are then advanced toward the midline.

7. Moberg (advancement, axial). This flap is preferably used for thumb tip amputations through the distal phalanx. This flap is preferred for the thumb because the dorsal arterial supply is independent of the volar supply, lessening the chance of dorsal skin necrosis in the thumb compared to the fingers. Defects up to 2.5 cm may be covered. Two parallel flaps are raised just dorsal to the neurovascular bundles and advanced to cover the defect. The secondary defect can be closed either primarily or with a skin graft (Fig. 3-5). If the base of the flap is too proximal, necrosis of the dorsal skin can occur. Flexion of the interphalangeal joint for flap advancement may lead to a flexion contracture.

Regional Flaps (see Chapter 8)

1. Cross-finger flap (random). The cross-finger flap is based on the dorsal aspect of the middle phalanx of the adjacent finger (usually the finger radial to the injured digit except for the index, for which the long finger is used). The flap is tailored to fit a volar primary defect. Indications include fingertip amputations and soft tissue defects that cannot be covered by an advancement flap. The secondary (donor) defect requires full-thickness skin grafting (Fig. 3-6).

2. Reversed cross-finger flap (random). The same principle is employed as in the cross-finger flap, but

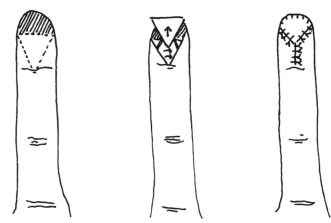

Figure 3-4 ❖ A V-Y advancement flap with its apex at the distal digital crease may be used to cover fingertip defects with dorsal tissue loss.

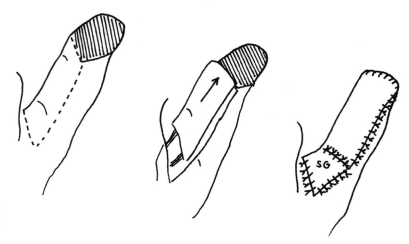

Figure 3-5 ◈ The Moberg advancement flap, composed of the thumb's palmar skin and neurovascular bundles, is useful to cover thumb tip amputations.

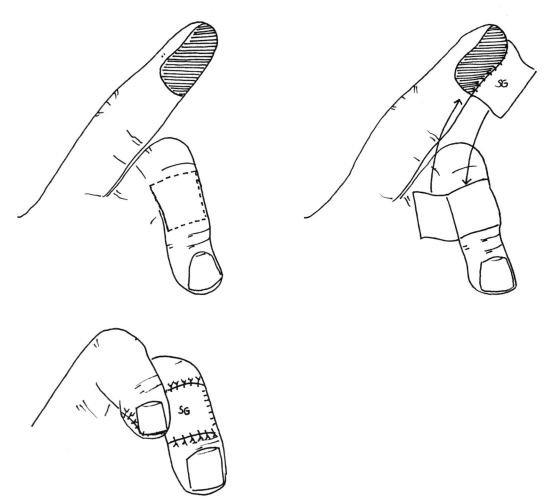

Figure 3-6 ◈ Cross-finger flap. The flap is raised from the dorsum of the middle phalanx and is used to cover fingertip amputations with palmar tissue loss.

this flap is used for dorsal defects. The skin is elevated from the subcutaneous tissues. The flap incorporates the subcutaneous tissues that are swung around its hinge. The superficial surface covers the defect, and the deep layer becomes superficial. The primary defect then requires skin grafting; skin elevated from the donor site initially is used to cover the donor defect.

3. Innervated cross-finger flap (random). In this case, the dorsal branch of the digital nerve of the donor finger on the side away from the injured finger (which innervates the dorsum of the middle phalanx) is divided and joined to the digital nerve of the injured finger on the side opposite the donor digit. Because standard cross-finger flaps usually have excellent sensory results, this is usually not performed.

4. Cross-thumb flap (random). This flap is designed for defects on the radial side of the index finger. The flap is taken from the dorsum of the proximal phalanx. The secondary defect requires skin grafting. To facilitate suturing, skin grafting should be done before the flap is placed over the primary defect (Fig. 3-7).

5. Thenar flap (random). The thenar flap is taken from the proximal radial aspect of the thumb. It is raised at the level of the thenar muscles, with care taken to protect the radial digital nerve. The flap is then sutured to the primary defect, and the secondary site is covered with a full-thickness graft. Advantages over cross-finger flaps include thicker, more durable skin and a less conspicuous donor site. Indications include coverage of transverse and volar oblique wounds at the fingertip (Fig. 3-8). Ulnar thenar flaps can be used for more ulnar defects. Although reports of PIP contractures in the affected digit and tenderness at the donor site exist, these complications are similar in number to those seen with all cross-finger flaps. Most surgeons still prefer this flap for young patients, for whom there is less risk of a PIP contracture.

6. Neurovascular island flap (axial). The main indication for this flap is damage to the pulp of the thumb. It is commonly used for fingertip coverage when restoration of sensibility is crucial (thumb and index finger). It is based on the digital neurovascular bundle and provides good padding, sensation, and blood flow. Any digit with adequate flow in both digital vessels can be a donor, although the ulnar aspect of the long finger is commonly used. The dissection should begin in the palm to check for abnormalities of the vasculature. Because the venous drainage of the flap consists of small, irregular vessels, the pedicle must be raised as one block. The flap is then passed through a tunnel to the primary defect in the thumb. The thumb should be fully abducted and extended to check for kinking of the pedicle. After adequate flow is confirmed,

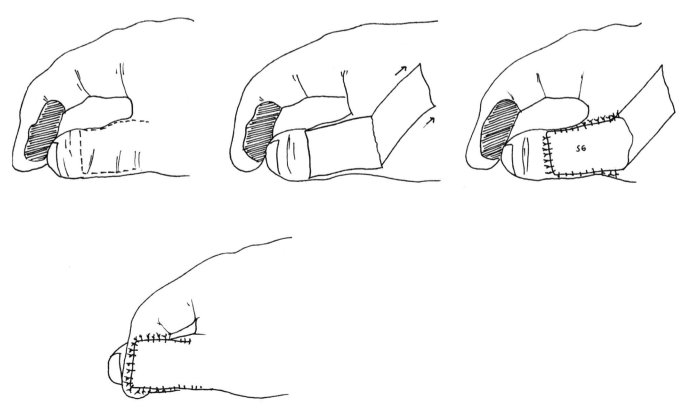

Figure 3-7 ◈ Cross-thumb flap. The flap is raised from the dorsum of the thumb proximal phalanx and is used to cover defects on the radial aspect or pulp of the index finger.

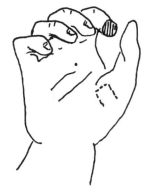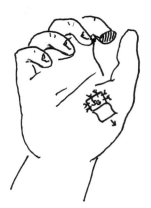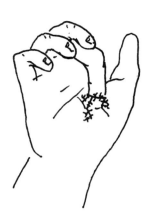

Figure 3-8 ◆ Thenar flap, used mostly in young patients for volar wounds at the fingertip.

the flap is sutured into place; the secondary defect is covered with a full-thickness graft (Fig. 3-9). The main disadvantage is the loss of innervation of the donor digit and decreased circulation and sensation in the ulnar adjacent digit.

7. Fillet flap (axial). This flap is developed from well-vascularized digits that are otherwise going to be sacrificed (secondary to skeletal or neurologic injuries). A longitudinal incision is made along the radial or ulnar side of the digit, and the neurovascular bundle is isolated. The digital skeleton and extensor and flexor tendons are then removed, and the skin flap is placed over the primary defect. The main advantage is the immediate closure of the defect with innervated tissue that may provide normal sensation. This flap is primarily indicated in cases in which severe soft tissue and bone digital injury precludes reconstruction.

8. Scapular flap (axial). The scapular flap is most commonly used as a distant free flap, but it can be raised as an island to cover defects in the axilla (usually after release for burns) as an axial-pattern regional flap.

9. Radial artery forearm flap (axial, fasciocutaneous). This flap is used for defects around the elbow, forearm, or hand. It can be used only if the hand is adequately perfused by the ulnar artery (Allen test). Advantages include good skin quality, mobility, and similarity to the skin of the dorsum of the hand. Disadvantages are a visible defect at the donor site with many wound healing complications and cold intolerance. The radial artery is isolated between the flexor carpi radialis and brachioradialis, and the flap is transposed. If the radial artery requires reconstruction, a cephalic vein graft can be used. The secondary skin defect is usually covered with a split-thickness graft. Another option is to elevate the flap as fascia alone, leaving the overlying skin in place. Distally based radial forearm flaps are possible because of perforators of the radial artery in the distal forearm thus sparing the radial artery. The flap can be obtained as an osteocutaneous flap by harvesting bone from the radius. If bone is harvested, the graft should be less than 10 cm in length and 30% of the cross-sectional area of the radius to prevent fracture. An oval bone graft is harvested because square edges may cause stress risers.

10. Ulnar artery forearm flap (axial, fasciocutaneous). This flap can be used for defects around the elbow or hand. It is not widely used because the ulnar artery provides the major blood supply to the hand in most people. The ulnar artery is isolated between the flexor carpi ulnaris and the flexor digitorum muscles. Advantages: less hairy skin, and secondary defect can often be closed primarily, especially in elderly patients. Disadvantages: ulnar nerve dysesthesias are common secondary to transient nerve ischemia (usually resolve after a few months); the bulk of the flap is greater than the radial artery flap.

11. Reversed posterior interosseous artery flap (axial, fasciocutaneous). The posterior interosseous artery originates from the common interosseous artery in 90% of people and from the ulnar artery in 10% of people. It emerges between the supinator and the abductor pollicis longus and travels distally to anastomose with the anterior interosseous artery. The axis of the flap is along the lateral epicondyle to the distal radioulnar joint with the forearm in pronation. The posterior interosseous artery is first isolated distally, between the extensor carpi ulnaris and the extensor digiti minimi, about 2 cm proximal to the ulnar styloid where it anastomoses with the anterior interosseous artery. Because of its short vascular pedicle and proximal axis of rotation, this flap is limited to dorsal hand coverage, including the first web space and MP joints. Main advantage: it does not sacrifice a major artery. The limiting factor to flap elevation is the nerve branch to the extensor carpi ulnaris muscle.

12. Lateral arm flap (axial, fasciocutaneous). Based on the posterior radial collateral artery. Harvest leads to numbness in the posterolateral elbow due to transection of the lateral cutaneous nerve. Can be elevated 6 cm distal to the lateral epicondyle.

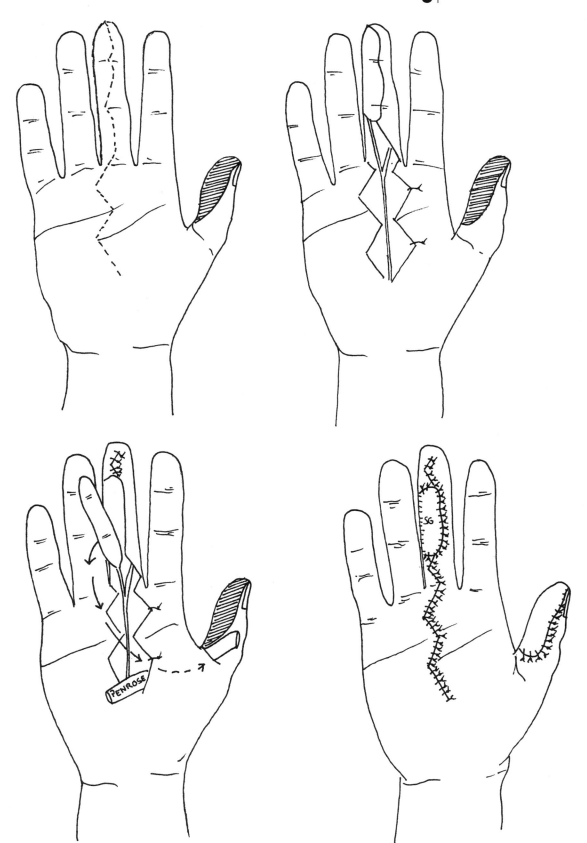

Figure 3-9 ◈ The neurovascular island flap is commonly used to cover thumb pulp defects. The flap is based on the digital neurovascular bundle and is tunneled to the primary defect in the thumb.

Distant Flaps

1. Groin flap (axial, fasciocutaneous). Indications include a large soft tissue defect, the lack of adequate vessels for a free flap, and an incomplete carpal arch precluding the use of forearm flaps. Based on the superficial circumflex iliac arteries (branches of the femoral artery), the flap is centered 2 cm distal to the inguinal ligament. Once the flap is elevated and sewn into a tube, the secondary defect is closed primarily and the hand is placed into the groin. The flap is then sewn over the primary deficit. This flap is usually sectioned 3 to 4 weeks after placement. Disadvantage: immobilization of the entire upper extremity.

2. Latissimus dorsi flap (axial, musculocutaneous). This flap has a wide arc of rotation around its pedicle and is used for reconstruction of the breast, head and neck, abdominal wall, and shoulder. The flap may therefore be used as a regional axial-pattern flap or as a distant free flap. The main blood supply is from the thoracodorsal artery (continuation of the subscapular artery), which gives branches to the chest wall and serratus anterior before dividing into two main branches to the latissimus muscle. The secondary defect should be closed primarily. Disadvantages: brachial plexus neurapraxia from positioning in the operating room, seroma formation postoperatively (use suction drains). No significant loss of function after latissimus flap has been reported. If a small flap is needed, only one of the branches can be divided. Alternatively, a serratus flap, based on a branch from the same vascular pedicle, can be used.

The preferred indications for various skin flaps are summarized in Table 3-1.

POSTOPERATIVE MONITORING AND CARE

Assessment of the color and capillary refill of the flap is essential. Healthy random-pattern flaps are pink; axial flaps are very pale. If arterial flow is insufficient, flaps become pale with a gray tinge. If venous flow is inadequate, flaps become engorged and progressively purple. Patients and nursing staff should be instructed on avoidance of positions that cause kinking of the vascular pedicle. Joints should be mobilized early to avoid stiffness.

Burns

Epidemiology

Approximately 36% of thermal or chemical injuries involve the hand or upper extremity, and 90% of patients with major burns will have involvement of the hands. With early and aggressive treatment, these patients usually have a good prognosis with regard to hand function.

Evaluation

1. First-degree burns involve the epidermis only. Skin is erythematous. These burns require symptomatic treatment only.

2. Second-degree burns involve part of the dermis, and epithelial remnants are spared. Clinical findings include vesicles, swelling, and moist surface. Wounds are hypersensitive to light touch. Both superficial and deep second-degree burns heal spontaneously but may take as long as 6 weeks and may result in hypertrophic scarring and joint immobility. To avoid this, severe burns should be treated by early excision and grafting.

3. Third-degree burns involve the entire dermis. Burns have a leathery appearance and are anesthetic to pinprick or touch. Larger areas of third-degree burns require excision of burned skin, treatment with dressing changes, and delayed skin grafting.

Treatment

FLUID RESUSCITATION

Patients should be adequately resuscitated according to the Parkland formula. Half of the calculated amount of fluid is given in the first 8 hours and the remaining half during the next 16 hours. In general, the palm of the hand is equivalent to 1% of body surface area.

Adults: % body surface area × kg × 2–4 mL of solution

Children: % body surface area × kg × 3 mL of solution

ESCHAROTOMIES

Escharotomies are considered when edema from circumferential burns restricts perfusion. If the burn wounds are supple, there is no need for escharotomy. Edema occurs during the first 36 hours after injury, and the need for escharotomy should be constantly re-evaluated in that time. Capillary pressure in the subcutaneous tissues can be measured with a wick catheter; a pressure of 30 mm Hg or greater requires escharotomy. Other criteria include pain with passive stretch, paresthesias, and loss of Doppler signal over the radial, ulnar, or digital arteries.

Escharotomies are performed at the bedside with intravenous sedation or local anesthesia. An incision on the radial side of the arm and hand is performed first. If adequate flow is not restored, an ulnar incision is then made. Digital escharotomies should be performed for circumferential burns of the fingers. The incisions are made on the ulnar side of each digit except for the thumb and small finger, for which radial incisions are performed to preserve the most important sensory half of the digit. If there is significant edema of the hand, release of the dorsal interossei is performed with incisions between the metacarpals. Escharotomy sites often close by secondary intention; in some cases, skin grafting may be necessary. Care should be taken to closely follow compartment pressures in the hand and forearm and to perform fasciotomies if clinically indicated.

SPLINTING

Splinting burns of the hand is essential to prevent contractures. The burn claw deformity presents with MP extension, PIP flexion, thumb adduction, and wrist flexion. As the hand swells, the MP collateral ligaments tighten and pull the MP joint into extension.

◆ **Table 3-1**

PREFERRED METHODS FOR SPECIFIC SITUATIONS

	Palmar	Dorsal–Larger Defects
Distal to PIP joint	Loss more dorsal—*V-Y advancement* Loss more palmar—Middle/ring—*Digital artery island flap* —<40—female—*Thenar* —male—*Cross-finger* —>40—important—*Neurovascular island* —not important—Revise amputation	*Reversed cross-finger*
PIP joint	*Cross-finger*	*Reversed cross-finger*
Proximal phalanx	Small defect—*Transposition from lateral aspect* Large defect —Palmar alone—*Cross-finger* — +Lateral—Index/middle—*Axial flag* —Ring/small—*Vascular island*	*Reversed cross-finger*
MP joint	Index/middle—*Axial flag* Ring/small—*Vascular island*	Index/middle—*Axial flag* Ring/small—*Vascular island*
Metacarpus or several fingers syndactylized	Useless digit—*Fillet* Small defect—*Vascular island* —*SDMA* Large defect—(*Free lateral arm*) —*Forearm fascia* + skin graft	Useless digit—*Fillet* (*Free lateral arm*)
Thumb	Loss more dorsal—*V-Y advancement* More palmar—<²/₃ pulp—*Moberg* —>²/₃ pulp—(*Neurovascular island* from toe) —*Neurovascular island* —No donor digit, no micro skills —*FDMA or SDMA*	*FDMA* from index *Forearm* (preferably PIA) No donor digit, no vessel —Male—*Infraclavicular* —Female—*Iliac*

FDMA, first dorsal metacarpal artery; PIA, posterior interosseous artery; SDMA, second dorsal metacarpal artery.

From Lister GD, Pederson WC: Skin flaps. In Green DP, Hotchkiss RN, Pederson WC, eds: Green's Operative Hand Surgery, 4th ed. New York, Churchill Livingstone, 1999, p 1839.

Burns over the dorsum of the PIP joints often destroy the extensor mechanism, leaving the flexors unopposed and producing a PIP flexion deformity. The hand should be splinted in the "anticlaw" position with the wrist in neutral, thumb in abduction, MP joints in flexion, and interphalangeal joints in extension. The splint should be removed daily for active and passive range-of-motion exercises. In severe cases, the PIP joints may be pinned in extension with K-wires. These pins are removed as soon as possible to decrease the likelihood of infection. The MP joints should remain mobile.

WOUND CARE

Wounds should be débrided daily and cleaned in water. They should be covered with an antibacterial ointment (silver sulfadiazine or mafenide acetate) and dressed with gauze and elastic netting. Alternatively, nonadherent gloves can be used as dressings and left in place until wounds are healed. If wounds have not healed by 2 to 3 weeks, skin grafting is warranted. Burned skin should be excised until brisk capillary refill is encountered. Once all devitalized tissue has been removed, hemostasis is obtained with epinephrine-soaked sponges or fibrin glue. Split-thickness grafts are commonly used and should, if possible, be unmeshed (less scarring, better cosmetic result). If donor skin is limited, allograft or synthetic products produce satisfactory results. Full-thickness skin grafts are preferred in the palm of the hand due to lower contraction potential.

REHABILITATION

In the first few months after a burn, scar tissue hypertrophies and may limit range of motion. Early involvement of a hand therapist is essential, and patients should perform daily exercises with all joints. Pressure garments are useful in scar management, and Coban wrapping can help control edema.

Chemical Burns

All clothing contaminated with the chemical should be immediately removed and the burns irrigated as soon as possible. Irrigation should be continued for at least 20 to 30 minutes. This dilutes the chemical agent, decreases the rate of the reaction, and restores normal skin pH (alkali burns may require up to 12 hours of irrigation). Persistent chemical contact under the nail may be difficult to treat and may require partial or total removal of the nail. Blisters on finger pads should be débrided to remove adherent chemicals and to allow better irrigation of deeper tissues.

1. Hydrogen fluoride is a common cleaning agent, and burns usually involve contact with the fingertips. Without treatment, the chemical extends into the subcutaneous tissues, binds calcium, and produces osteitis and a chronic wound. Hydrogen fluoride should be neutralized with 10% calcium gluconate applied topically or injected until pain relief is obtained. The mechanism of neutralization

involves the formation of insoluble complexes of calcium and fluoride ions. Because injection of calcium gluconate into the finger pulp can be painful, it can instead be delivered intravenously by a Bier block or intra-arterially with a low-flow pressurized infusion.

2. White phosphorus is used in fireworks and methamphetamine production. Phosphorus particles shower the skin and are oxidized by air. All particles should be removed (copper sulfate will stain particles for easy identification) by irrigation or submersion of the burned extremity under water.

3. Petroleum solvents produce skin irritation and deep dermal slough. Burns are usually poorly recognized but should be treated with dilute soap and water irrigation. These solvents have systemic lung toxicity.

4. Household cleaners are usually composed of multiple alkali chemicals. Burns are treated with water irrigation.

5. Pool cleaners (hydrochloric acid). Water irrigation of reducing agents produces excess heat. Burns should be neutralized with soda lime, skin soap, or magnesium solutions before water irrigation.

6. Industrial cleaners usually contain oxidizing agents. They should be neutralized with milk, egg white, or starch paste before water irrigation.

7. Air bags may contain nitrogen gas to facilitate inflation. Symptoms are usually delayed and include burning sensation, erythema, and blistering. Burns are generally superficial and are treated with analgesics, antihistamines, and topical creams.

8. Burns with elemental sodium should be treated with mineral oil. Water should be avoided because sodium reacts violently with water.

Electrical Burns

Burns from an electric short are usually superficial and are treated like thermal burns. Conduction burns have entrance and exit wounds with massive soft tissue damage in between. The higher the voltage, the greater amount of tissue damage. High voltage is defined as 1000 volts or greater. Resuscitation should focus on the cardiac and respiratory systems; respiratory arrest and ventricular fibrillation are the main causes of death. Because of the potential for myoglobinuria, patients should be adequately hydrated.

For extremity injuries, early fasciotomies and serial débridements are almost always the rule. In children, extensive reconstructions are usually indicated. In adults, severe injuries may be best treated with amputation. Absolute indications for amputation include an insensate limb, life-threatening sepsis, and unsalvageable limb destruction. In cases of bilateral injuries, attempts are made to salvage the least injured hand. Adequate débridement is difficult to achieve because the gross appearance of muscle is not a reliable indicator of its viability. Muscle biopsy and technetium scans have both been used to identify viable muscle. After multiple débridements, flap coverage is often necessary, and although local flaps are preferred, muscle free flaps are commonly used to cover large soft tissue defects.

Radiation Burns

Radiation burns often affect surrounding tissue, so skin grafts and local flaps are not recommended. These are best treated with free flaps. For radiation burns to the thumb, consider a free neurocutaneous toe pulp transfer.

Microwave Burns

Microwave burns are increasingly common in the industrial setting. Adverse effects are primarily thermal because of excess heat production. Systemic effects have also been reported. Hospitalization is recommended to fully evaluate the extent of soft tissue necrosis.

Reconstruction after Burns

CLAW DEFORMITY

Priorities are MP joint motion and good PIP position.

The first stage in MP joint reconstruction often requires resurfacing of dorsal soft tissue with a flap. An alternative involves soft tissue expanders about the dorsal hand to provide skin coverage after excision of the involved skin in the burn scar. Collateral ligament, capsule, and volar plate releases are then performed, depending on the amount of stiffness. PIP flexion contractures in burned hands may require an arthrodesis in 20 to 45 degrees of flexion. Flexion contractures of the wrist are treated with excision of volar scar tissue and skin grafting.

PALMAR CONTRACTURE

This uncommon deformity occurs after grasping of a hot object. The scar tissue should be released and defects covered with full-thickness grafts (ideally taken from the abdomen). PIP contractures in palmar burns require extensive release and often require cross-finger flaps. Aggressive postoperative splinting is essential.

WEB SPACE CONTRACTURES

Web space contracture results from scar involving the dorsal web space. These contractures are classified by extent of involvement and treated with V-M (in contrast to V-Y) plasty, which does not require separation from underlying tissue. In less severe cases or for contractures of the first web space, Z-plasty is the preferred treatment.

ADDUCTION CONTRACTURE

Adduction contracture involves the first web space and results from fibrosis of the adductor and first interosseous muscle (this differs from a web space contracture, which involves only overlying skin). Release of fascia and muscle is necessary until an adequate web space is created. If this is obtained without exposure of deep structures, the defect can be closed with a skin graft; otherwise, a thin flap can be used.

BURN SYNDACTYLY

This is very rare and is similar to congenital syndactyly. Reconstruction requires release along the lateral side of the digits and skin grafts and local flaps.

CONTRACTURE BANDS

Release of hypertrophic scars should be done as needed. Ideally, one should wait for scars to mature (up to 1 year after injury). If mobility of a joint is compromised, however, early release should be performed. The scar tissue is excised, and defects are repaired with local flaps or skin grafts.

AMPUTATION DEFORMITIES

1. Digits can be effectively lengthened by phalangization. This involves deepening of the web spaces with a V-M procedure and skin grafting.
2. Mitten deformity is seen with extensive burns. Treatment focuses on creation of a web space with the opposable digit. The second ray is removed, and the resulting web space is covered with a skin graft or thin flap.
3. Thumb reconstruction. The first stage involves ensuring adequate soft tissue coverage of the first metacarpal and web space.
   a. Pollicization is performed when the thumb does not have enough length to oppose the remaining digits. The index metacarpal is divided proximally. The neurovascular bundle and flexor tendons are isolated and dissected to allow movement; other structures are severed (extensors are later repaired). Bone fixation is obtained with K-wires.
   b. Toe to thumb transfer is also used to gain length. This is a better choice after electrical injury.
   c. Distraction osteogenesis may be used to gain metacarpal length, but complications are common.

NAIL DEFORMITY

Dorsal burns result in eponychial retraction and proximal nail exposure. These areas require coverage to avoid breakdown with daily activities. This usually requires two flaps, one from each side of the digit, transposed to cover the proximal defect.

Frostbite

Pathophysiology

The extremity first responds to cold exposure by vasoconstriction, leading to a decrease in perfusion. Every 10 minutes, there is a transient vasodilation to rewarm the extremity and to prevent freezing. This response is blunted at very cold temperatures. As core temperature falls, blood is shunted away from the skin, leading to a further temperature drop. At 10°C, sensory nerve dysfunction occurs. Ice crystals form at −6°C to −15°C. Most cellular injury results from intracellular dehydration as extracellular ice crystals form. With rewarming, perfusion may be re-established. Capillary thrombosis may prevent perfusion, however, even with restoration of blood flow.

Evaluation

Frostbite can be either superficial or deep. Superficial injuries are characterized by large clear blisters and result in minimal tissue loss. Deep injuries are anesthetic after thawing and are often associated with hemorrhagic blisters after rewarming.

Management

Initial management involves resuscitation with warm intravenous fluid and insulation with blankets or other clothing. The frozen extremity should be treated with rapid rewarming in a water bath at 40°C to 42°C for 30 minutes. After rewarming, elevation is essential to reduce edema formation. Blisters usually form within 6 to 24 hours of rewarming. White blisters should be débrided; hemorrhagic blisters should be drained but left intact. Antibiotics should be administered to prevent superinfection. Radioisotope scans are often used 48 hours after rewarming to direct therapy. Patients without early or late (bone) uptake are likely to progress to amputation. If salvage is attempted, soft tissue defects should be débrided and covered with well-vascularized flaps in the first 10 days after injury.

Late effects of frostbite in children include shortened digits (due to physeal closure at 6 to 12 months after injury) and degenerative changes in the finger joints. The most common angular deformity seen after frostbite injuries in children is radial deviation of the distal interphalangeal joint of the small finger. Growth abnormalities are due to chondrocyte injury in the growth plate. Late sequelae in adults include cold intolerance, hyperhidrosis, trophic changes, and Raynaud's phenomenon.

Miscellaneous

Hyperhidrosis

Hyperhidrosis, overproduction of exocrine sweat glands, exists in generalized and localized forms. Palmar hyperhidrosis can be treated with tap water iontophoresis. Adding anticholinergic agents produces more rapid and longer lasting effects. Botulinum toxin can also be employed. For severe or recalcitrant cases, upper thoracic sympathectomy has excellent results.

Tissue Expanders

Tissue expanders can be used prior to reconstruction of burns to provide autologous skin tissue for coverage. Local tissue response about the expander includes epidermal thickening, fat and muscle atrophy, and an increase in vascularity.

Bibliography

Achauer BM: The burned hand. In Green DP, Hotchkiss RN, Pederson WC, eds: Green's Operative Hand Surgery, 4th ed. New York, Churchill Livingstone, 1999.

Birbeck DP, Moy OJ: Anatomy of upper extremity skin flaps. Hand Clin 13:175–187, 1997.

Brown RE, Zook EG, Russell RC: Fingertip reconstruction with flaps and nail bed grafts. J Hand Surg 24:345–351, 1999.

Browne EZ Jr: Skin grafts. In Green DP, Hotchkiss RN, Pederson WC, eds: Green's Operative Hand Surgery, 4th ed. New York, Churchill Livingstone, 1999.

Ciano M, Burlin JR, Pardoe R, et al: High-frequency electromagnetic radiation to the upper extremity: local and systemic effects. Ann Plast Surg 7:128–135, 1981.

Eaton CJ, Lister GD: Treatment of skin and soft-tissue loss of the thumb. Hand Clin 8:71–97, 1992.

Guy RJ: The etiologies and mechanisms of nail bed injuries. Hand Clin 6:9–21, 1990.

House JH, Fidler MO: Frostbite of the hand. In Green DP, Hotchkiss RN, Pederson WC, eds: Green's Operative Hand Surgery, 4th ed. New York, Churchill Livingstone, 1999.

Lister GD, Pederson WC: Skin flaps. In Green DP, Hotchkiss RN, Pederson WC, eds: Green's Operative Hand Surgery, 4th ed. New York, Churchill Livingstone, 1999.

Markley JM Jr: Island flaps of the hand. Hand Clin 1:689–699, 1985.

Nicholson CP, Grotting JC, Dimick AR: Acute microwave injury to the hand. J Hand Surg 12:446–449, 1987.

Reilly DA, Garner WL: Management of chemical injuries to the upper extremity. Hand Clin 16:215–224, 2000.

Shepard GH: Management of acute nail bed avulsions. Hand Clin 6:39–57, 1990.

Su CW, Lohman R, Gottlieb LJ: Frostbite of the upper extremity. Hand Clin 16:235–247, 2000.

Togel B, Greve B, Raulin C: Current therapeutic strategies for hyperhidrosis: a review. Eur J Dermatol 12:19–23, 2002.

Tredget EE: Management of the acutely burned upper extremity. Hand Clin 16:187–203, 2000.

Van Beek AL, Kassan MA, Adson MH, Dale V: Management of acute fingernail injuries. Hand Clin 6:23–37, 1990.

Wong L, Spence RJ: Escharotomy and fasciotomy of the burned upper extremity. Hand Clin 16:165–174, 2000.

Zook EG: Anatomy and physiology of the perionychium. Hand Clin 6:1–9, 1990.

Zook EG, Brown RE: The perionychium. In Green DP, Hotchkiss RN, Pederson WC, eds: Green's Operative Hand Surgery, 4th ed. New York, Churchill Livingstone, 1999.

4

✧ Jonathan A. Uroskie, MD ✧ Mark E. Baratz, MD
✧ Christopher C. Schmidt, MD

VASCULAR DISORDERS OF THE HAND AND UPPER EXTREMITY

Anatomy

Arterial Supply to the Hand (Fig. 4-1)

1. The subclavian artery (branch from the brachiocephalic trunk on the right and the aortic arch on the left) exits the chest through the costoclavicular space.
   a. The costoclavicular space (thoracic outlet) is bordered by the first rib inferiorly, the clavicle superiorly, the costoclavicular ligament medially, and the anterior scalene muscle anteriorly (Fig. 4-2).
2. The subclavian artery becomes the axillary artery as it passes below the coracoid process.
3. In the arm, the axillary artery gives rise to the brachial and profunda brachii arteries.
4. In the proximal forearm, the brachial artery divides into the radial and ulnar arteries.
5. The ulnar artery gives rise to the common interosseous artery in the proximal third of the forearm.
   a. The common interosseous artery divides into the anterior and posterior interosseous arteries, which travel directly apposed to either side of the interosseous membrane.
   b. The two interossei anastomose distally at the level of the distal radioulnar joint.
6. In the palm, the radial and ulnar arteries anastomose to form the deep and superficial palmar arches (Figs. 4-2 and 4-3). The ulnar artery is the dominant artery in 88% of patients; the radial artery is the dominant artery in only 12% of patients.
7. The radial artery is the predominant contributor to the deep palmar arch.
   a. The deep palmar arch is found 1 cm proximal to the transverse palmar crease.
   b. In 97% of patients, the deep arch is complete with anastomoses between the deep volar branches of the radial and ulnar arteries.
   c. The deep arch gives rise to the volar metacarpal arteries.

8. The ulnar artery divides into superficial and deep branches as it crosses the wrist.
   a. The superficial branch goes on to become the superficial palmar arch; the deep branch joins the radial artery to form the deep palmar arch.

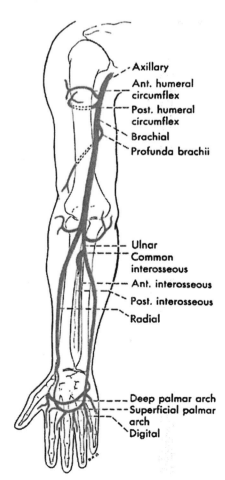

- Axillary
- Ant. humeral circumflex
- Post. humeral circumflex
- Brachial
- Profunda brachii
- Ulnar
- Common interosseous
- Ant. interosseous
- Post. interosseous
- Radial
- Deep palmar arch
- Superficial palmar arch
- Digital

Figure 4-1 ✧ Arterial supply of the upper extremity. *(From Jenkins DV: Hollinshead's Functional Anatomy of the Limbs and Back, 6th ed. Philadelphia, WB Saunders, 1991.)*

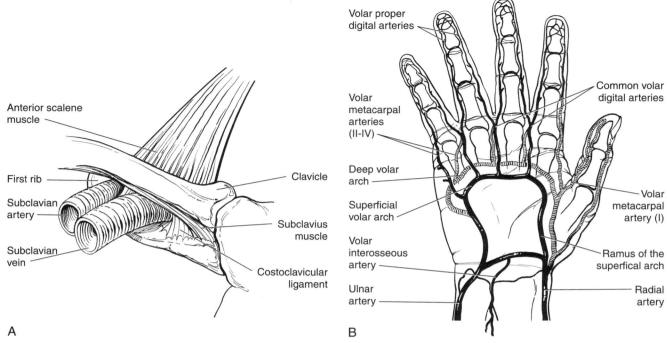

Figure 4-2 ❖ **A,** Vascular anatomy in the costoclavicular space, or thoracic outlet. **B,** Most common vascular anatomy of the hand and digits. *(From Phillips CS, Murphy MS: Vascular problems of the upper extremity: a primer for the orthopaedic surgeon. J Am Acad Orthop Surg 10: 401–408, 2002.)*

   b. The superficial arch is considered complete when the digital arteries from all five digits arise from the arch.
   c. The arch is complete in approximately 79% of patients.
      i. In these cases, diminished flow from the ulnar, the radial, or possibly a persistent median artery potentially could compromise the flow to one or more digits.
   d. The superficial arch gives rise to the common volar digital arteries.
9. In a majority of hands, the blood supply to the digits is derived from both the deep and superficial arches (86% to 98%).
10. A persistent median artery or large interosseous artery may be present. A median artery may be found in approximately 10% of patients.
11. Kaplan's cardinal lines describe surface markings for underlying neurovascular structures. A line drawn from the first web space parallel to the proximal transverse palmar crease is tangent to the deep palmar arch.
12. The volar metacarpal arteries (from the deep arch) and the common volar digital arteries (from the superficial arch) anastomose to form the proper digital arteries.

Arterial Supply to the Wrist (Fig. 4-4)

1. The distal radius is supplied by the radial, ulnar, anterior interosseous, and posterior interosseous arteries.

2. Branches of these arteries are identified by location relative to the extensor compartments and retinaculum.
   a. The supraretinacular vessels lie superficial to the extensor retinaculum.
   b. The intercompartmental vessels lie between extensor compartments.
      i. The 1,2 intercompartmental supraretinacular artery (1,2 ICSRA) arises from the radial artery 5 cm proximal to the radiocarpal joint. It is most commonly used for proximal scaphoid nonunions as a vascularized bone graft.
      ii. The 2,3 intercompartmental supraretinacular artery (2,3 ICSRA) arises from the anterior interosseous artery. It anastomoses with the dorsal intercarpal arch.
   c. The compartmental vessels lie within the extensor compartments.
      i. Fourth extensor compartment artery.
      ii. Fifth extensor compartment artery.
      iii. A vascularized bone graft for Kienböck's disease can be obtained from the distal radius by use of the connection between the fourth and fifth extensor compartment arteries.
   d. Dorsal arterial arches
      i. Dorsal intercarpal arch.
      ii. Dorsal radiocarpal arch.
      iii. Dorsal supraretinacular arch.

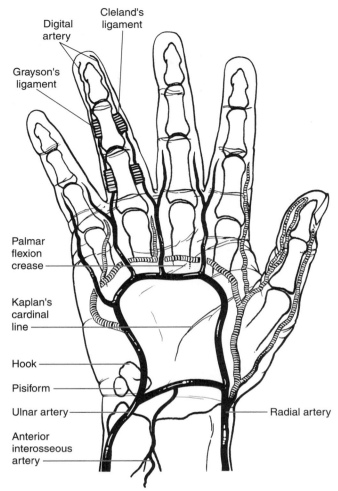

Figure 4-3 ◆ Arterial supply to the hand. *(From Baratz ME, Watson AD, Imbriglia JE: Orthopaedic Surgery: The Essentials. New York, Thieme, 1999.)*

Labels on figure: Digital artery; Cleland's ligament; Grayson's ligament; Palmar flexion crease; Kaplan's cardinal line; Hook; Pisiform; Ulnar artery; Anterior interosseous artery; Radial artery

Evaluation of Vascular Disorders

History

Important aspects of the history to elicit from patients thought to have vascular disorders include the following:
1. Medical history of diabetes mellitus, peripheral vascular disease, or connective tissue disease.
2. The presence of cold intolerance or Raynaud's events.
3. Previous events of fingertip necrosis or ischemia.
4. Family history of blood dyscrasias or other hematogenous abnormalities.
5. History of blunt or penetrating trauma or vascular access for hemodialysis.
6. Occupational exposure to vibratory stimuli or temperature changes.
7. History of drug use, including tobacco, caffeine, and alcohol.

Physical Examination

Physical examination includes a complete evaluation from the neck to the fingertips.

1. Inspection of the hand includes evaluation of color, skin mottling, cyanosis, fingertip ulcerations, and perfusion of the nail beds.
2. Palpation includes the assessment of pulse presence and strength, bruits, and thrills.

ALLEN TEST

1. This is a manual test for assessing competence of the radial and ulnar artery palmar arch anastomoses.
2. The radial and ulnar arteries are simultaneously occluded at the wrist.
3. The patient is asked to open and close the hand while occlusion is maintained to exsanguinate the hand.
4. Once the hand is exsanguinated, the hand is relaxed, compression on one of the arteries is released, and digital perfusion is assessed.
5. The hand should perfuse within 3 seconds.
6. The examination is repeated with release of the other vessel. A delay in reperfusion may indicate an incomplete arch.
7. Digital Allen test. The test can be performed on a single digit by milking the finger from distal to proximal and occluding both digital vessels on the volar aspect of the finger. It is used to assess adequacy of single-vessel circulation.

DOPPLER ULTRASONOGRAPHY

1. Doppler ultrasonography can be used to evaluate vascular perfusion and anatomy.
2. The study can identify areas of occlusion and collateral circulation.

Diagnostic Studies

SEGMENTAL ARTERIAL PRESSURES

1. Combine occlusive cuffs and Doppler units to measure differential arterial pressures along different anatomic segments.

DIGITAL/BRACHIAL INDEX

1. The digital/brachial index is the ratio between the systolic blood pressures measured in the digit and the pressures measured in the arm.
2. A digital/brachial index less than 0.7 indicates decreased blood flow in the digit.

DIGITAL PLETHYSMOGRAPHY (PULSE VOLUME RECORDING)

1. Plethysmography quantitates flow by measuring volume changes in the digit or limb.
2. The tracings demonstrate arterial contractility and vascular perfusion and can help differentiate between occlusion and stenosis.
3. Normal vessels have a triphasic tracing (Fig. 4-5).
   a. Occluded vessels demonstrate tracings with decreased amplitudes because of poor inflow.
   b. Stenotic vessels demonstrate absence of the triphasic waveform because of poor contractility of the vessel as well as mildly decreased amplitudes because of poor inflow.
4. Pulse volume recording is noninvasive and reproducible. It can predict the results of surgical sympathectomy in the hand.

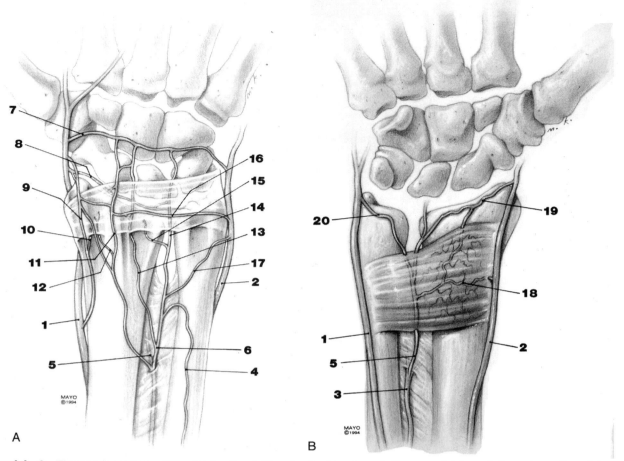

Figure 4-4 ❖ The vascular anatomy of the distal radius. **A,** Dorsal radius blood supply. Two superficial vessels lie on the surface of the extensor retinaculum (the 1,2 intercompartmental supraretinacular artery [ICSRA] [9] and the 2,3 ICSRA [11]). Two deep vessels lie directly on the radius beneath the tendons of the fourth and fifth extensor compartments (the fourth extensor compartment artery [13] and the fifth extensor compartment artery [14]). **B,** The palmar blood supply is provided by two arches connecting the anterior interosseous vessels and the radial artery (palmar carpal arch [19] and palmar metaphyseal arch [18]). 1, radial artery; 2, ulnar artery; 3, anterior interosseous artery; 4, posterior interosseous artery; 5, anterior division of anterior interosseous artery; 6, posterior division of anterior interosseous artery; 7, dorsal intercarpal arch; 8, dorsal radiocarpal arch; 9, 1,2 ICSRA; 10, second compartment branch of 1,2 ICSRA; 11, 2,3 ICSRA; 12, second compartment branch of 2,3 ICSRA; 13, fourth extensor compartment artery; 14, fifth extensor compartment artery; 15, fourth compartment branch of the fifth extensor compartment artery; 16, dorsal supraretinacular arch; 17, oblique dorsal artery of the distal ulna; 18, palmar metaphyseal arch; 19, radial portion of palmar radiocarpal arch; 20, ulnar portion of palmar radiocarpal arch. *(From Mayo Foundation, with permission.)*

Figure 4-5 ❖ **A,** Digital pulse volume recording (PVR) cuff with Doppler probe placed distally above the digital artery. **B,** Normal triphasic PVR waveform. Normal triphasic patterns are seen when the arterial walls are pliable without excessive peripheral resistance, similar to waveforms obtained with a pressure catheter placed in the right atrium. **C,** Occlusive PVR waveform. The amplitude is significantly reduced as a result of diminished inflow. **D,** Stenotic PVR waveform. The triphasic nature of the waveform has disappeared, with a small decrease in amplitude. *(From Phillips CS, Murphy MS: Vascular problems of the upper extremity: a primer for the orthopaedic surgeon. J Am Acad Orthop Surg 10:401–408, 2002.)*

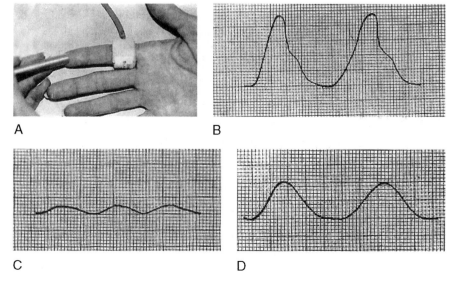

COLOR DUPLEX IMAGING

1. Color duplex imaging is helpful to show thrombosis in large vessels.
2. The study combines ultrasound imaging and color-coded Doppler evaluation.
3. Anomalous vascular anatomy, aneurysms, and other perfusion abnormalities can be identified.
4. Information about direction of flow, periodic versus continuous flow, and response of the vessel wall to the pressure cycle is provided.
5. The study is noninvasive but not as accurate as arteriography.

COLD STRESS TESTING

1. Cold stress testing helps assess the vasomotor and autonomic response of the digit to physiologic stress (cold).
2. The test is used to demonstrate autonomic vascular dysfunction in vasospastic patients.
3. The hand is immersed in cold water or a refrigerator maintained at 8°C for 20 minutes, and the digital skin temperature is measured every 10 seconds.
4. The temperature response with and without local anesthetic can predict the results of surgical sympathectomy in the hand.

Radiographic Studies

ARTERIOGRAPHY

1. Arteriography provides the best anatomic detail of any studies and is considered the "gold standard" for evaluating arterial abnormalities.
2. Radiopaque dye is injected to study the vascular anatomy.
3. Digital subtraction (digital removal of bone and soft tissue shadows) increases the clarity and value of arteriography.
4. It is an invasive procedure with potential problems, including arterial injury at the injection site, vasospasm, and allergy to dye.
5. This invasive procedure has a complication rate of less than 1%.

BONE SCINTIGRAPHY

1. Bone scintigraphy helps assess anatomy and determine and quantify patterns of vascular distribution.
2. The study involves injection of the radionucleotide technetium Tc 99m diphosphonate.
3. Three-phase study
   a. Phase I (2 minutes): radionucleotide arteriogram—helpful in identifying occlusion of major arteries.
   b. Phase II (5 to 10 minutes): soft tissue uptake—helpful in determining the presence of inflammation.
   c. Phase III (2 to 3 hours): bone uptake.
4. Absence of radiotracer distal to a site of occlusion suggests a poor prognosis, whereas presence of radiotracer distal to a site of occlusion indicates collateral flow.

MAGNETIC RESONANCE ANGIOGRAPHY

1. Magnetic resonance angiography is an excellent study for evaluating pathologic changes of soft tissue structures.
2. Anatomic detail is better visualized with angiography.
3. Magnetic resonance angiography can be helpful in assessing the vascular status of carpal bones (scaphoid, lunate, capitate).

Occlusive Vascular Disease

Post-traumatic Occlusive Disease

1. Occlusive vascular disease can be due to trauma, emboli from proximal sources, atherosclerosis, systemic disorders, and hypercoagulable states.
2. Patients complain of pain due to claudication, paresthesias, and cold intolerance.
3. Prognosis is related to etiology.
4. Occlusive vascular disease is usually unilateral in contrast to vasospastic disease, which is often bilateral.

ULNAR ARTERY THROMBOSIS (HYPOTHENAR HAMMER SYNDROME)

1. Hypothenar hammer syndrome is the most common arterial occlusive disorder of the upper extremity.
2. It involves thrombosis of the ulnar artery in the area of Guyon's canal, sometimes with extension into the superficial palmar arch (Fig. 4-6).
3. Hypothenar hammer syndrome usually results from repeated blunt trauma to the base of the hypothenar eminence (typically in laborers).

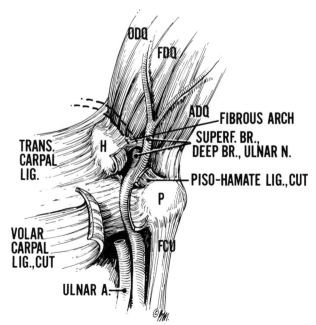

Figure 4-6 ❖ The ulnar nerve courses through Guyon's canal between the volar carpal ligament and the transverse carpal ligament. P, pisiform; H, hamate. *(From Szabo RM: Compression neuropathies. In Green DP, Hotchkiss RN, Pederson WC, eds: Operative Hand Surgery, 4th ed. New York, Churchill Livingstone, 1999.)*

a. Repetitive injury disrupts the elastic lamina in the vessel wall.
b. This leads to aneurysmal dilatation of the vessel and thrombus formation.

Clinical Presentation

1. Patients complain of cold intolerance, pain, and occasionally ischemic changes such as ulceration to the ring and small fingers.
2. The disease is common in men in the fifth decade of life.
3. Pure ulnar sensory involvement is often displayed with decreased sensation and sweating in the ulnar nerve distribution.
   a. There are typically no motor symptoms because of the anatomy of the ulnar nerve in Guyon's canal (see Chapter 1).
   b. The thrombus irritates the periadventitial sympathetic fibers, which can induce vasospasm, further limiting flow.
   c. Embolization of the thrombus can occur, most likely affecting the ring finger because of the takeoff angle of the common digital arteries of the third and fourth web spaces.

Diagnosis

The diagnosis is clinical (history, painless mass on the palm of the hand, positive result of Allen test), but the diagnosis can be supported by pulse volume recordings and color duplex imaging and confirmed by arteriography (Fig. 4-7).

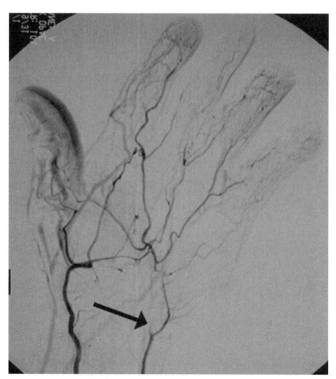

Figure 4-7 ❖ Digital subtraction angiogram of the hand revealing thrombosis of the ulnar artery (arrow) distal to the wrist in a patient with hypothenar hammer syndrome.

Treatment (Table 4-1)

1. Activity modification, smoking cessation.
2. Pharmacologic intervention (calcium channel blockers, α- and β-blockers, intravenous thrombolytics).
3. Cervicothoracic sympathectomy.
4. Surgical reconstruction
   a. Sympathectomy.
   b. Thrombectomy and arterial repair.
   c. Thrombectomy and interpositional vein graft (Fig. 4-8).
   d. Arteriovenous reversal.
5. Re-establishment of circulation may diminish cold intolerance; most patients have residual symptoms.

RADIAL ARTERY THROMBOSIS

1. Radial artery thrombosis is much less commonly seen than ulnar thrombosis.
2. It most commonly occurs on the dorsum of the hand.
3. Deep branches within the snuffbox are often involved.
4. If collateral flow is adequate, ligation of the artery is a treatment option.

Embolic Disease

1. Upper extremity emboli represent 20% of all arterial emboli, and 70% of these are cardiac in origin. Most emboli of arterial origin are derived from the subclavian artery.
2. Patients often present with acute symptoms of pain, pallor, and absence of pulses.
3. Common sources of emboli include the heart, subclavian artery, and superficial palmar arch.
   a. The most common source is the subclavian artery, where damage at the thoracic outlet can lead to thrombus formation and embolic problems (see Chapter 5).
4. The diagnosis is made by history, physical examination, and diagnostic studies like echocardiography and arteriography to determine the source of the emboli.
5. In the acute period, embolectomy and heparinization are recommended if possible. Heparin is continued for 7 to 10 days, followed by 3 months of warfarin treatment.

❖ **Table 4-1**

CLASSIFICATION AND TREATMENT OF VASO-OCCLUSIVE DISEASE

	Level of Injury	Finding	Treatment
I	Internal elastic lamina	Aneurysm	Ligation or reconstruction
		Thrombosis	Ligation or reconstruction
II	Media	Buerger's disease	Reconstruction or sympathectomy
III	Adventitia	Ext. construction	Adventiectomy

Modified from Ruch DS, Koman LA, Smith TL: Chronic vascular disorders of the upper extremity. J Am Soc Surg Hand 1:73–80, 2001.

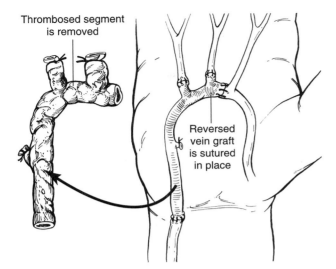

Thrombosed segment is removed

Reversed vein graft is sutured in place

Figure 4-8 ◆ Diagram of reversed vein graft for hypothenar hammer syndrome. *(From Ruch DS, Koman LA, Smith TL: Chronic vascular disorders of the upper extremity. J Am Soc Surg Hand 1:73–80, 2001.)*

a. If embolectomy cannot be performed because of the size of the vessel, thrombolysis with tissue plasminogen activator, streptokinase, or urokinase may be beneficial if it is administered within 36 hours of occlusion.

Aneurysm

1. True aneurysm
   a. A true aneurysm is a dilatation of an arterial vessel wall; the shape is fusiform.
   b. It is composed of all layers of the vessel wall (aneurysm lined by endothelium).
   c. Gradual dilatation of the artery is the most common cause, often related to blunt trauma (e.g., hypothenar hammer syndrome).
   d. The ulnar artery at the level of the hook of the hamate (hypothenar hammer syndrome) is the most common location.
2. False aneurysm
   a. A false aneurysm is a dilatation of the vessel wall as a result of penetrating trauma.
   b. The aneurysm represents a false lumen from delamination; thus, it does not include all layers of the vessel wall (aneurysm not lined by endothelium).
   c. The aneurysm results from traumatic violation of the vessel wall, which leads to hematoma formation. The hematoma fibroses and eventually recanalizes, restoring flow.
3. Mycotic aneurysm
   a. A mycotic aneurysm is a dilatation of the vessel wall as a result of infection.
   b. Subacute bacterial endocarditis leads to septic emboli that lodge in the vessel wall, leading to weakening and aneurysm formation.
   c. Mycotic aneurysms most commonly occur in intravenous drug users.

4. Aneurysms are most often due to embolic phenomena, but an aneurysm can present as an expanding mass.
5. Arteriography is the diagnostic modality of choice and helps determine location of emboli.
6. Surgical treatment is almost always recommended.
   a. Excision and vessel ligation.
   b. Excision and primary vessel repair.
   c. Excision and "patch" grafting.
   d. Excision and interpositional vein graft.

Acquired Arteriovenous Fistula

1. The arteriovenous fistula is created traumatically by penetrating injuries or surgically for dialysis access.
2. An arteriovenous fistula may create ischemic symptoms and "steal" phenomena, which leads to neuropathic symptoms.
   a. Severe cases may lead to high-output cardiac failure.
3. Treatment includes observation, banding of the fistula to reduce flow, ligation, shunt reversal, and neurolysis in cases of severe neuropathy due to steal phenomena.

Atherosclerosis

1. Atherosclerosis typically involves the subclavian artery, more commonly on the left side (3:1).
2. Proximal subclavian stenosis can lead to subclavian steal syndrome, in which blood is shunted away from the brain by reversal of the flow in the vertebral artery to meet the upper extremity demands.
   a. Central nervous system involvement is more common in proximal subclavian stenosis; upper extremity claudication is more common in distal lesions.
3. Plaque formation on the intima of the vessel wall is the common pathologic finding.
4. The diagnosis is made with arteriography.
5. Treatment can include bypass of the stenotic region or endarterectomy.

Arteritis and Systemic Disorders

Thromboangiitis Obliterans (Buerger's Disease)

1. Thromboangiitis obliterans is an inflammatory process of medium to small vessels that leads to occlusion and even segmental obliteration.
2. There is usually more severe disease peripherally.
3. On histologic examination, arterial and venous thrombosis is seen with a significant inflammatory reaction.
4. The cause has been theorized to be a heritable factor, with questionable autoimmune linkage to a hypercoagulable disorder.

PRESENTATION

1. Thromboangiitis obliterans occurs predominantly in adult male smokers in the third decade of life.

2. Presentation is characterized by severe rest pain, cold intolerance, Raynaud's phenomenon, claudication, and digital ischemia with well-demarcated areas of necrosis.
3. The chronic course is painful and protracted, but life expectancy is only slightly shortened.
4. Clinical differentiation from atherosclerosis is made by distal involvement.

DIAGNOSIS

Diagnosis is made with the help of arteriography, but histologic proof of the disease by biopsy is often necessary.

TREATMENT

1. Smoking cessation is the most effective treatment and reduces the incidence of amputations.
2. Pharmacologic treatment with anticoagulants, vasodilators, and prostaglandin inhibitors can be helpful.
3. The role of sympathetic blockade is unknown.
4. Vascular reconstruction can be helpful in some cases.
5. Multiple amputations are often required.

Giant Cell Arteritis

1. Giant cell arteritis mainly involves arteries of the head and the subclavian and axillary arteries.
2. It is most commonly seen in elderly women.
3. The disease is named polymyalgia rheumatica if it is associated with myalgias and arthralgias.
4. Diagnosis is established with a temporal artery biopsy.
5. Treatment includes high-dose steroids and arterial reconstruction if ischemia persists.

Takayasu's Arteritis

1. Takayasu's arteritis commonly involves the subclavian and axillary arteries of young women.
2. Proliferation of the arterial intima leads to stenosis.
3. Treatment includes systemic steroids with a variable response.

Polyarteritis Nodosa

1. Polyarteritis nodosa is a necrotizing arteritis associated with aneurysmal dilatations of small vessels.
2. It has a predilection for arterial bifurcations.

Vasospastic Disease

Raynaud's Disease

1. This vasospastic disease of the small vessels of the digits is of unknown etiology without an association to an underlying disorder.
2. Raynaud's phenomenon is the episodic vasospasm of the digital arteries characterized by progression of symptoms initiated by stress or cold exposure (Table 4-2).
   a. An initial period of blanching from spasm is followed by cyanosis.
   b. Reactive hyperemia results from rewarming, followed by pain and dysesthesias.

❖ Table 4-2
CHARACTERISTICS OF RAYNAUD'S DISEASE
Middle-aged woman without associated medical conditions
Both hands usually involved
Peripheral pulses are usually normal
Stress or cold brings on symptoms
Rarely leads to ischemic changes or gangrene
Intermittent episodes of skin coloration and temperature changes often accompanied by pain

   c. The sequence of finger coloration is white-blue-red.
   d. There is an absence of gangrene and trophic changes.

DIAGNOSIS

This is a diagnosis of exclusion.
1. Allen tests, segmental pressures, and pulse volume recordings are important to rule out associated diagnoses.
2. Laboratory tests to rule out collagen vascular diseases are also important.
3. Arteriography should be considered in patients with unilateral symptoms, progressive gangrene or ulceration, and suspected occlusive or embolic phenomena and when surgical treatment is being considered.
4. Diagnostic criteria include the following:
   a. Characteristic color changes with stress.
   b. Bilateral involvement.
   c. No evidence of occlusive disease.
   d. Absence of an underlying disorder.
   e. At least 2 years' duration.

TREATMENT

1. Smoking cessation (nicotine causes severe vasospasm).
2. Limitation of cold exposure, use of protective garments, and biofeedback.
3. Oral calcium channel blockers offer limited relief.
4. Digital sympathectomy is reserved for patients with recalcitrant symptoms, constant pain, or impending soft tissue loss.
5. Long-term results of sympathectomy are unpredictable.

Raynaud's Syndrome

1. Raynaud's syndrome is defined as Raynaud's disease associated with a specific disorder or known factor.
2. These associated disorders include collagen vascular disorders, hematologic and occlusive diseases, autoimmune disorders, and occupational exposure to cold and vibration (Table 4-3).
   a. Lupus
      i. Lupus can cause segmental arterial occlusion by deposition of antigen-antibody complexes in the vascular endothelium.
      ii. It leads to ischemia at the digital level in patients with superimposed vasospastic disease.

❖ Table 4-3

CAUSES OF SECONDARY VASOSPASTIC DISORDER

Connective tissue disease: scleroderma (incidence of Raynaud's, 80%–90%), systemic lupus erythematosus (18%–26%), dermatomyositis (30%), rheumatoid arthritis (11%)
Occlusive arterial disease
Neurovascular compression: thoracic outlet syndrome
Hematologic abnormalities: cryoproteinemia, polycythemia, paraproteinemia
Occupational trauma: percussion and vibratory tool workers
Drugs and toxins: sympathomimetics, ergot compounds, β-adrenergic blockers
Central nervous system disease: syringomyelia, poliomyelitis, tumors, infarcts
Miscellaneous: reflex sympathetic dystrophy, malignant disease

Modified from Miller MD: Review of Orthopaedics, 3rd ed. Philadelphia, WB Saunders, 2000, p 321.

b. Scleroderma (systemic sclerosis)
    i. Calcinosis is a major part of the disease process.
    ii. Patients with vasospastic disease are part of the CREST syndrome (cutis calcinosis, Raynaud's disease, esophageal strictures, sclerodactyly, telangiectasia).
    iii. Patients can benefit from digital sympathectomy.
c. Rheumatoid vasculitis
    i. Rheumatoid vasculitis is an extra-articular manifestation of rheumatoid arthritis; circulating immune complexes target the vascular endothelium, leading to vasculitis.
    ii. Patients may respond to systemic treatment of rheumatoid arthritis.

TREATMENT (Table 4-4)

1. Smoking cessation and limitation of caffeine intake are recommended. Smoking should cease before elective surgery. Smoking causes decreased serum levels of dopamine.
2. Eliminate environmental factors, avoid cold, dress warmly, and protect the hands.
3. Pharmacologic intervention is aimed at any underlying disorder.
    a. Aspirin and dipyridamole (Persantine) can inhibit platelet aggregation.
    b. Calcium channel blockers and angiotensin-converting enzyme inhibitors are administered to inhibit smooth muscle spasm.
    c. Anticoagulants can prevent thrombosis of small vessels.
    d. Intra-arterial administration of reserpine and sympathetic blockade can also be effective.
4. Surgical treatment
    a. Amputation of necrotic digits.
    b. Sympathectomy (Figs. 4-9 and 4-10)
        i. Sympathectomy is performed in patients who demonstrate improvement after local anesthetic blockade.
        ii. Surgical sympathectomy can be effective, although relief may be short-lived.

❖ Table 4-4

CLASSIFICATION AND TREATMENT OF VASOSPASTIC DISEASE

	Diagnosis	Clinical Finding	Treatment
I	Primary Raynaud's disease	Adequate collateral flow	Nonoperative management
		Inadequate collateral flow	Sympathectomy
II	Secondary Raynaud's disease	Adequate collateral flow	Sympathectomy
		Inadequate collateral flow	Consider bypass graft
III	Thromboangiitis obliterans	Inadequate collateral flow	Bypass graft; consider salvage procedure

Modified from Ruch DS, Koman LA, Smith TL: Chronic vascular disorders of the upper extremity. J Am Soc Surg Hand 1:73–80, 2001.

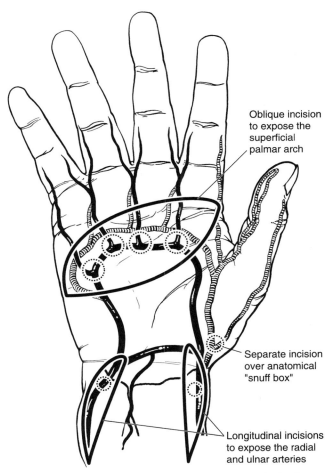

Figure 4-9 ❖ Diagram of sympathectomy for vasospastic disease. *(From Ruch DS, Koman LA, Smith TL: Chronic vascular disorders of the upper extremity. J Am Soc Surg Hand 1:73–80, 2001.)*

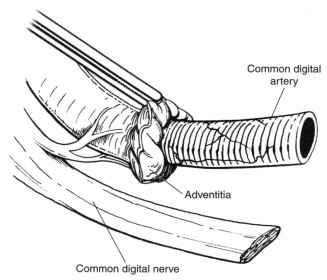

Figure 4-10 ◆ Diagram of adventitial stripping for sympathectomy. *(From Ruch DS, Koman LA, Smith TL: Chronic vascular disorders of the upper extremity. J Am Soc Surg Hand 1:73–80, 2001.)*

    iii. Distal digital sympathectomy is performed by separating the proper digital artery from the common digital nerve and stripping the adventitia of the artery for a distance of 2 cm.

    iv. Digital sympathectomy and vascular reconstruction have good short-term results, but ulcers recur in 20% to 30% in long-term follow-up studies.

    v. The best long-term response from arterial sympathectomy in the hand is in patients with post-frostbite cold intolerance compared with scleroderma and occlusive vascular disease because recurrence of ulcers in these settings is not uncommon.

    vi. Sympathectomy in patients with both occlusive and vasospastic disease will improve nutritional flow to the digits but there will be no change in total flow to the fingertips.

5. Treatment of the underlying disorder.

Vascular Neoplasms (see Chapter 10)

Arteriovenous Malformation

1. Arteriovenous malformations occur when flow is diverted across low-resistance shunts instead of the normal, high-resistance capillary beds.
2. This shunting leads to thickening and dilatation of vessels.
3. Flow can be reversed on the afferent artery, leading to further shunting of the ischemic capillary beds.
4. Collateral circulation is stimulated to compensate for ischemic changes.
5. Signs and symptoms include dilated veins, wounds that fail to heal, pulsatile bleeding, heaviness of the extremity, and pain from ischemia. Other symptoms are hyperhidrosis, hair growth, and increased body temperature.

6. These are most often congenital in nature but may be stimulated by trauma, hormonal changes, infection, or surgical intervention.
7. Arteriovenous malformations can be classified according to the speed of flow.
    a. Slow-flow: usually painless, compressible; can be localized or diffuse.
    b. Fast-flow: usually painful, palpable thrill; do not decompress with limb elevation.
8. Arteriovenous malformations may be associated with other skeletal anomalies.
    a. Klippel-Trenaunay syndrome: capillary, lymphatic, and venous malformations associated with skeletal overgrowth.
    b. Parkes Weber syndrome: capillary, lymphatic, and venous malformations associated with arteriovenous fistulas.
    c. Proteus syndrome: capillary and venous malformations associated with macrodactyly, hemihypertrophy, lipomas, pigmented nevi, and scoliosis.
    d. Maffucci's syndrome: lymphatic and venous malformations associated with multiple enchondromas.
9. Diagnosis is clinical, but Doppler studies, arteriograms, and magnetic resonance angiography can be helpful.

TREATMENT

Treatment depends on symptoms or hemodynamic compromise.

Slow-Flow Arteriovenous Malformation
1. Compression garments.
2. Low-dose aspirin to prevent pain from thrombosis.
3. Embolization.
4. Surgical excision
    a. Indications include functional impairment, pain, nerve compression, and infection.
    b. Failure of excision of the fistula may lead to worsening of symptoms.

Fast-Flow Arteriovenous Malformation
1. Surgical excision
    a. Indications include pain, steal phenomena, ulceration or gangrene, heart failure, and compartment syndrome.
    b. Embolization before surgical excision is helpful.

Hemangioma

1. Hemangioma is a congenital vascular tumor with a characteristic growth cycle; early proliferation is followed by involution.
    a. Endothelial proliferation marks the first phase.
    b. The tumor then grows proportionally to the child.
    c. By the age of 5 years, 50% of lesions will have involuted, and by 7 years, 70% will have involuted.
2. It is the most common vascular tumor of the hand (5% of hand tumors).
3. On examination, hemangiomas are cutaneous or subcutaneous masses with a "spongy" feel to palpation.
    a. They can be compressible or firm.

b. Cutaneous lesions are red; subcutaneous lesions are usually darker blue.

c. These do not change size or turgor with elevation of the limb (in contrast to arteriovenous malformations).

4. Magnetic resonance angiography is the most useful diagnostic adjunct, and Doppler study and arteriography can be helpful.

5. Treatment is based on symptoms. If excision is contemplated, it must be meticulously removed to prevent recurrence.

Glomus Tumors

See Chapter 10.

Acute Vascular Injury

Arterial Injuries

1. Injury to an artery can occur from blunt or penetrating trauma.
   a. Injuries due to blunt trauma may be more difficult to recognize.
   b. Blunt injuries are associated with the development of compartment syndrome.
2. Symptoms depend on the adequacy of collateral circulation.
   a. Collateral circulation can be compromised because of vasospasm of the collateral vessels and abnormal vasomotor responses in cases with concomitant nerve injury.
3. Critical injuries are defined as those in which the arterial injury leads to cell death and the need for amputation.
4. Indications for arterial repair in the upper extremity include the following:
   a. Axillary or brachial artery injury.
   b. Combined radial and ulnar artery injuries.
   c. Radial or ulnar artery injury associated with poor collateral circulation.
5. Relative indications for arterial repair in the upper extremity include the following:
   a. Arterial injury occurring in combination with nerve injury (to diminish the incidence of cold intolerance and to enhance nerve recovery).
   b. Extensive distal soft tissue injury.
   c. Repair of a single forearm artery injury has patency rates between 50% and 90%.
6. In cases of arterial injury associated with long bone fractures, if collateral perfusion is adequate, skeletal stabilization should proceed first. If there is distal ischemia, vascular repair or shunting is given priority.

Osteonecrosis (Avascular Necrosis)

Kienböck's Disease (Lunatomalacia)

CLINICAL PRESENTATION

1. Kienböck's disease is characterized by pain and weakness in the wrist, often without a history of acute trauma.

2. Symptoms may be present for some time before presentation; for this reason, the natural history is not well known.

3. There is loss of wrist joint flexion or extension, with normal pronation-supination.

4. Grip strength is diminished.

5. Kienböck's disease is most common in young adult men (aged 20 to 40 years); it is rare in children.

6. It is rarely bilateral.

ETIOLOGY

1. The etiology is largely unknown.
2. Several possible causes have been proposed.

Vascular

1. Limited local arterial supply to the lunate is compromised by hyperextension or flexion injuries or fracture.
   a. The interosseous supply may be from one or two vessels volarly and dorsally.
   b. In 7% to 26% of lunates, there is only a single blood nutrient vessel (see Chapter 1).
2. Disruption of venous outflow leads to elevated intraosseous pressure, which interferes with vascular flow.

Mechanical

1. Negative ulnar variance.
   a. Ulnar negative variance may increase load and shear stresses on the lunate.
   b. In Hultén's original study, 78% of patients with Kienböck's disease had an ulnar negative variance compared with 23% of the general population.
   c. Other studies have shown that ulnar negative variance occurs with equal incidence in normal individuals and those with Kienböck's disease.
2. Flattened radial inclination.
3. Small lunate.

DIAGNOSIS

1. Plain radiographs are evaluated for sclerosis of the lunate, cystic changes, fragmentation, collapse, and perilunate arthritic changes (Fig. 4-11).
2. Magnetic resonance imaging is helpful in early stages that reveal no changes on plain films.
   a. Loss of marrow fat causes decreased signal on T1-weighted images (Fig. 4-12).
   b. T2-weighted images also reveal low signal intensity.
   c. The signal changes must be diffuse. In cases with focal signal changes (particularly on the proximal ulnar side of the lunate), the diagnosis of ulnocarpal abutment must be strongly considered.
3. Bone scanning was used before the advent of magnetic resonance imaging.

STAGING

See Table 4-5 and Figure 4-13.

TREATMENT

Treatment depends on radiographic stage and ulnar variance (Table 4-6).

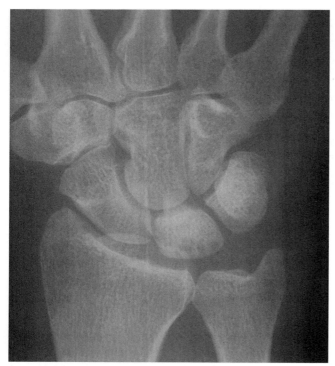

Figure 4-11 ◈ Posteroanterior radiograph of a patient with stage 2 Kienböck's disease. Note increased sclerosis of the lunate without articular collapse.

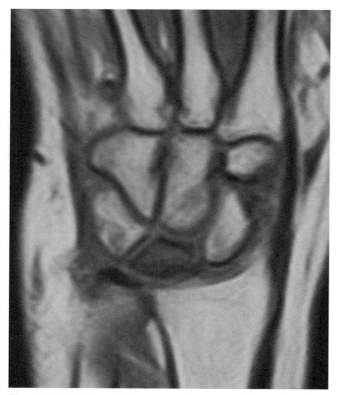

Figure 4-12 ◈ T1-weighted magnetic resonance image of a patient with stage 2 Kienböck's disease. Note diffuse loss of signal intensity of the lunate without articular collapse.

◈ Table 4-5

LICHTMAN CLASSIFICATION OF KIENBÖCK'S DISEASE

Stage 1	Normal radiographic findings, signal intensity changes on magnetic resonance imaging
Stage 2	Lunate sclerosis on plain radiography; fracture lines may be present
Stage 3	Collapse of the lunate articular surface
Stage 3A	Normal carpal alignment and height
Stage 3B	Fixed scaphoid rotation, proximal capitate migration, loss of carpal height
Stage 4	Lunate collapse along with radiocarpal or midcarpal arthrosis

Modified from Allan CH, Joshi A, Lichtman DM: Kienböck's disease: diagnosis and treatment. J Am Acad Orthop Surg 9:128–136, 2001.

Stage 1

1. Cast immobilization is the first option for treatment. Most of these patients are believed to progress to stage 2 in spite of treatment.

Stage 2 to 3A with Ulnar Negative Variance

1. Joint leveling procedures are believed to mechanically unload the lunate, leading to revascularization and prevention of collapse.
2. This can be achieved with radial shortening between 2 and 3 mm (technically simple, low incidence of nonunion) (Fig. 4-14).
3. Ulnar lengthening requires bone grafting, and there is an increased chance of nonunion. It is rarely performed.

Stage 2 to 3A with Ulnar Positive Variance

1. Joint leveling or unloading procedures are also performed.
   a. The radial dome osteotomy decreases lunate contact forces.
   b. Capitate shortening osteotomy (with or without capitohamate fusion) also unloads the lunate (Fig. 4-15).
      i. Load on lunate decreases 66%, but the scaphotrapezial load is increased to 150%.

◈ Table 4-6

TREATMENT OF KIENBÖCK'S DISEASE ACCORDING TO STAGE

Stage 1	Cast immobilization for 3 months
Stage 2 to 3A, ulnar negative variance	Radial shortening; ulnar lengthening; capitate shortening
Stage 2 to 3A, ulnar positive variance	Vascularized bone graft and external fixation; radial wedge or dome osteotomy; capitate shortening
Stage 3B	Intercarpal fusion (scaphotrapeziotrapezoid, scaphocapitate); radial shortening; proximal row carpectomy
Stage 4	Proximal row carpectomy; wrist arthrodesis; wrist denervation

Modified from Allan CH, Joshi A, Lichtman DM: Kienböck's disease: diagnosis and treatment. J Am Acad Orthop Surg 9:128–136, 2001.

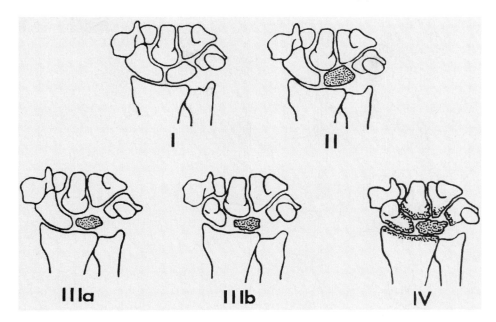

Figure 4-13 ❖ Lichtman stages of Kienböck's disease. Stage I: Normal x-ray, positive MRI or bone scan. A faint fracture may be seen in the lunate body. Stage II: Lunate sclerosis on plain x-ray without evidence of articular surface collapse. Stage IIIa: Lunate fragmentation and articular surface collapse without evidence of carpal collapse. Stage IIIb: Lunate fragmentation and articular surface collapse with loss of carpal height and proximal migration of the capitate. Stage IV: Perilunate degenerative disease. *(From Palmer AK and Benoit MY: Lunate fractures: Kienböck's disease. In Cooney WP, Linscheid RL, Dobyns JH, eds: The Wrist: Diagnosis and Operative Treatment, 1st ed. Philadelphia, Mosby, 1988.)*

    ii. Avascular necrosis of the capitate head and nonunion of the capitate are potential complications.

2. Vascularized grafting (Fig. 4-16)
   a. A vascularized pedicle graft may effectively be taken from multiple areas.
   b. It is commonly taken from the distal radius by use of the connection between the fourth and fifth extensor compartment arteries.
   c. It may also be taken from the second dorsal metacarpal artery.
   d. External fixation after revascularization can help unload the lunate. Temporary unloading may also be achieved by temporary pinning of the scaphotrapeziotrapezoid or scaphocapitate joints.

Stage 3B Radioscaphoid Angle Greater than 60 Degrees
1. Correction of the flexed scaphoid along with intercarpal fusion (scaphotrapeziotrapezoid or scaphocapitate) can decrease load on the lunate and prevent further carpal collapse.

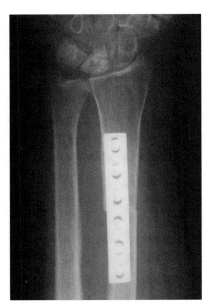

Figure 4-14 ❖ Posteroanterior radiograph of a patient with stage 2 Kienböck's disease treated with a radial shortening osteotomy.

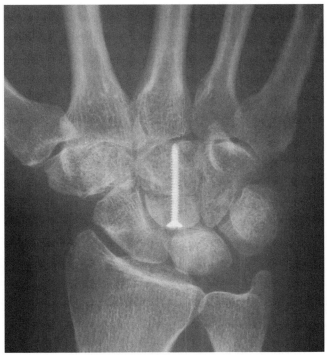

Figure 4-15 ❖ Posteroanterior radiograph of a patient with stage 2 Kienböck's disease treated with a capitate shortening osteotomy internally fixed with a small screw.

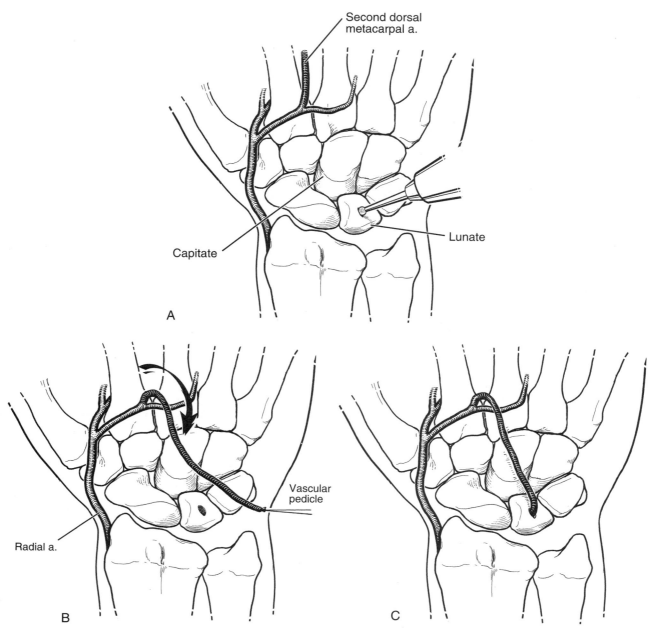

Figure 4-16 ◆ **A,** The lunate is exposed through a limited dorsal midline capsulotomy. **B,** The second dorsal intermetacarpal artery lies between the second and third metacarpals. The vessel is dissected from distal to proximal. The vascular bundle is elevated and held with a suture. **C,** The vascular bundle is passed from dorsal to palmar. *(From Fernandez DL, Gupta R: Vascular bundle implantation for Kienböck's disease. Atlas Hand Clin 4:73–81, 1999.)*

    a. In addition to the fusion, the lunate can be removed and replaced with tendon anchovy to diminish joint irritation.
2. Proximal row carpectomy is a successful salvage procedure; the capitate head must be free of degenerative changes.
3. If mild arthritic changes are present on the capitate head, an interpositional arthroplasty of dorsal wrist capsule in addition to the proximal row carpectomy can be effective.

Stage 4
1. Proximal row carpectomy and wrist arthrodesis are the mainstays of treatment.
2. Wrist denervation alone or in combination with proximal row carpectomy and wrist arthrodesis can help with symptom relief.

Preiser's Disease

1. Preiser's disease is idiopathic avascular necrosis of the scaphoid; it is a rare condition.

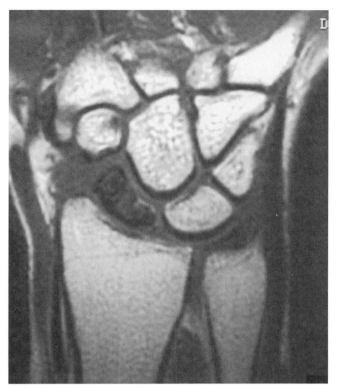

Figure 4-17 ❖ T1-weighted magnetic resonance image of a patient with Preiser's disease. Note diffuse loss of signal intensity of the scaphoid.

2. Sclerosis and fragmentation of the proximal pole are seen without evidence of fracture.
3. It usually affects patients older than 40 years.
4. The diagnosis is made with plain radiography, but magnetic resonance imaging can reveal the early stages of disease (Fig. 4-17).

TREATMENT

1. Observation with immobilization is effective in about 20% of patients.
2. Operative: drilling, revascularization, proximal row carpectomy, intercarpal fusion, and scaphoid excision have been described.

Capitate Head Avascular Necrosis

1. Idiopathic avascular necrosis of the capitate is a rare condition.
2. Sclerosis and fragmentation of the proximal pole of the capitate are seen.
3. The diagnosis is made with plain radiography, but magnetic resonance imaging can reveal the early stages of disease.
4. It can occur in post-traumatic cases (scaphocapitate syndrome) or postoperatively (after capitate shortening osteotomy).

TREATMENT

1. Observation with immobilization can be effective.
2. Excision of the avascular head with tendon interposition has been used with variable results.

Bibliography

Allan CH, Joshi A, Lichtman DM: Kienböck's disease: diagnosis and treatment. J Am Acad Orthop Surg 9:128–136, 2001.

Baratz ME, Divelbiss B: Kienböck's disease. J Am Soc Surg Hand 1:61–72, 2001.

Baratz ME, Watson AD, Imbriglia JE: Orthopaedic Surgery: The Essentials. New York, Thieme, 1999.

Buerger L: Thromboangiitis obliterans: a study of the vascular lesions leading to presenile spontaneous gangrene. Am J Med Sci 136:567–580, 1908.

Coleman SS, Anson BJ: Arterial patterns in the hand based upon a study of 650 specimens. Surg Gynecol Obstet 113:409–424, 1961.

Flatt AE: Digital artery sympathectomy. J Hand Surg Am 5:550–556, 1980.

Gelberman RH, Bauman TD, Menon J, Akeson WH: The vascularity of the lunate bone and Kienböck's disease. J Hand Surg Am 5:272–278, 1980.

Gelberman RH, Blasingame JP: The timed Allen test. J Trauma 21:477–479, 1981.

Gellman H, Nichols D: Reflex sympathetic dystrophy in the upper extremity. J Am Acad Orthop Surg 5:313–322, 1997.

Green DP, Hotchkiss RM, Pederson WC: Green's Operative Hand Surgery, 4th ed. New York, Churchill Livingstone, 1998.

Hanel DP, Hunt TR: Capitate shortening osteotomy. Atlas Hand Clin 4:45–57, 1999.

Holder LE, Merne DS, Yang A: Nuclear medicine, contrast angiography, and magnetic resonance imaging for evaluation of vascular problems in the hand. Hand Clin 9:85–114, 1993.

Hoppenfeld S, deBoer P: Surgical Exposures in Orthopaedics: The Anatomic Approach, 2nd ed. Philadelphia, JB Lippincott, 1994.

Horii E, Garcia-Elias M, An KN, et al: Effects on force transmission across the carpus in procedures used to treat Kienböck's disease. J Hand Surg Am 15:393–400, 1990.

Hunt TR, Bozentka DJ: Kienböck's disease. Atlas Hand Clin 4:2, 1999.

Jensen CH: Intraosseous pressure in Kienböck's disease. J Hand Surg Am 18:355–359, 1993.

Jones NF: Ischemia of the hand in ischemic disease: the potential role of microsurgical revascularization and digital sympathectomy. Clin Plast Surg 16:547–556, 1989.

Jones NF: Acute and chronic ischemia of the hand: pathophysiology, treatment, and prognosis. J Hand Surg Am 16:1074–1083, 1991.

Koman LA, Urbaniak JR: Ulnar artery insufficiency—a guide to treatment. J Hand Surg Am 6:16–24, 1981.

Koman LA, Urbaniak JR: Ulnar artery thrombosis. Hand Clin 1:311–325, 1989.

Kristenssen SS, Thomassen E, Christensen F: Kienböck's disease: late results by non-surgical treatment. A follow-up study. J Hand Surg Br 11:422–425, 1986.

Levin LS, Moore RS, Aponte R: Vascular injuries of the wrist and hand. In Baratz ME, Watson AD, Imbriglia JE: Orthopaedic Surgery: The Essentials. New York, Thieme, 1999.

Phillips CS, Murphy MS: Vascular problems of the upper extremity: a primer for the orthopaedic surgeon. J Am Acad Orthop Surg 10:401–408, 2002.

Miller LM, Morgan RF: Vasospastic disorders: etiology, recognition, and treatment. Hand Clin 9:171–187, 1993.

Miller MD: Review of Orthopaedics, 3rd ed. Philadelphia, WB Saunders, 2000.

Ruch DS, Koman LA, Smith TL: Chronic vascular disorders of the upper extremity. J Am Soc Surg Hand 1:73–80, 2001.

Schilenwolf M, Martini AK, Mau HC, et al: Further investigations of the intraosseous pressure characteristics in necrotic lunates (Kienböck's disease). J Hand Surg Am 21:754–758, 1996.

Sheetz KK, Bishop AT, Berger RA: The arterial blood supply of the distal radius and ulna and its potential use in vascularized pedicle bone grafts. J Hand Surg Am 20:902–914, 1995.

Shin AY, Bishop AT: Treatment of Kienböck's disease with dorsal distal radius pedicled vascularized bone grafts. Atlas Hand Clin 4:91–118, 1999.

Trumble T, Glisson RR, Seaber AV, et al: A biomechanical comparison of methods for treating Kienböck's disease. J Hand Surg Am 11:88–93, 1986.

Weiss AP, Weiland AJ, Moore JR, et al: Radial shortening for Kienböck's disease. J Bone Joint Surg Am 73:384–391, 1991.

✧ Ranjan Gupta, MD

NERVE

Peripheral Nerve Anatomy and Physiology

General Organization

The peripheral nervous system provides the mechanism for relay of information between the central nervous system (CNS) and the environment. It is composed of several different cell types including neurons and glial cells. Neurons are composed of a cell body, dendrite, axon, and presynaptic terminal. The axon arises from an axon hillock that generates the action potential. Nerves are bundles of axons enclosed in specialized connective sheaths. Within the nerve, there are several different satellite cells known as glial cells.

The two main types of glial cells are microglia and macroglia. Microglia are macrophages or phagocytes that are mobilized after injury, infection, or disease. Macroglia include astrocytes, oligodendrocytes, and Schwann cells. Astrocytes, a CNS cell type, support and provide structure to the brain and spinal cord. Oligodendrocytes and Schwann cells form the myelin sheath that helps increase the speed of conduction of the nerve impulse. Myelin is composed of lipid (70%) and protein (30%). Oligodendrocytes are located in the CNS. Schwann cells are located in the peripheral nervous system and myelinate a segment of one axon. Each axon may be myelinated by as many as 500 Schwann cells. The intervals between each myelinated region (where the myelinated sheath is discontinuous) are known as the nodes of Ranvier (Fig. 5-1).

CONNECTIVE TISSUE SHEATHS (Fig. 5-2)

Epineurium

The external epineurium is the outer layer of the peripheral nerve that provides a supportive and protective framework for the axon. The internal epineurium surrounds individual fascicles, serves as a cushion against external pressure, and allows longitudinal excursion. It has a well-developed vascular plexus with channels feeding the endoneurial plexus. Along the nerve path, there are larger amounts of this layer at the level of joints.

Perineurium

The perineurium is a thin sheath that surrounds each fascicle and acts as the blood-nerve barrier. This barrier provides a bidirectional barrier to diffusion. It is composed of up to 10 layers of flattened mesothelial cells with tight junctions. It provides elasticity and high tensile strength that resists up to 750 mm Hg.

Endoneurium

The endoneurium is a loose collagenous matrix that surrounds individual nerve fibers.

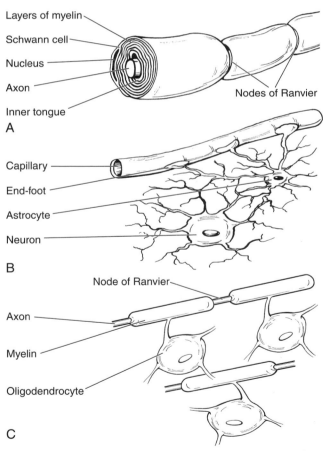

Figure 5-1 ✧ **A,** The Schwann cells wrap around the peripheral axons and provide the myelin sheath. **B,** Astrocytes are located in the central nervous system and provide support to the neurons. **C,** Oligodendrocytes in the white matter provide a myelin sheath to the axons, and support the neurons in the grey matter. *(From Simon SR, ed: Orthopaedic Basic Science, 2nd ed. Rosemont, Ill, American Academy of Orthopaedic Surgeons, 2000.)*

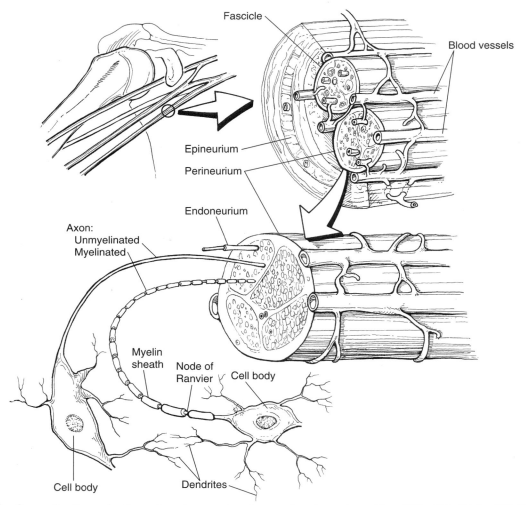

Figure 5-2 ◆ Connective tissue sheaths: epineurium, perineurium, and endoneurium. *(From Miller MD, Brinker MR: Fundamentals of Orthopaedics. Philadelphia, WB Saunders, 2000.)*

FASCICLES

Fascicles are groups of axons surrounded by endoneurial connective tissue. A fascicle is the smallest unit of nerve that can be surgically manipulated. It forms plexuses that possess a high degree of variability. The structure of each fascicle changes along the length of a major nerve.

BLOOD SUPPLY

The blood supply can be subdivided into extrinsic (surrounding the nerve trunk) and intrinsic (intraneural microvascular plexuses). The intraneural plexuses are located in the epineurium, perineurium, and endoneurium.

AXOPLASMIC AND AXONAL TRANSPORT

The neuron is a polarized cell with several intracellular transport systems that are dependent on adenosine triphosphate, calcium, and microtubules. Transport of molecules from the cell body toward the terminus is known as anterograde transport. Anterograde transport can be divided into fast and slow and is dependent

on the carrier protein kinesin. Transport of molecules from the terminus to the cell body is known as retrograde transport. Retrograde transport occurs at one-half to one-third the rate of fast anterograde transport and is primarily responsible for the recycling of proteins at the terminus. Retrograde transport relies on the carrier protein dynein.

Resting Membrane Potential and Action Potential

Transfer of information between the CNS and the periphery occurs through a series of electrical and chemical signals. There is an electric potential difference between the two sides of the cell membrane due to an unequal distribution of monovalent ions. The interior of the cell has a negative resting potential compared with the extracellular side, known as the resting membrane potential. This resting potential is maintained primarily by energy-dependent pumps that drive three sodium (Na^+) ions out of the cell and bring two potassium (K^+) ions into the cell to approximately −70 millivolts (mV). Furthermore, negatively charged

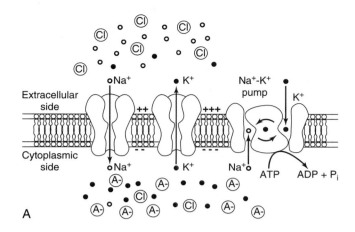

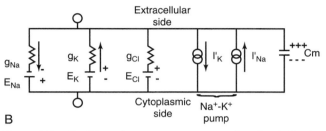

Figure 5-3 ◆ Electrolyte transport across cell walls. **A,** Passive fluxes of Na⁺ and K⁺ into and out of the cell are balanced by the energy-dependent sodium-potassium pump. **B,** Electrical circuit model of a neuron at rest. *(From Simon SR, ed: Orthopaedic Basic Science, 2nd ed. Rosemont, Ill, American Academy of Orthopaedic Surgeons, 2000.)*

protein molecules (A⁻) inside the cell contribute to the negative resting potential (Fig. 5-3).

Whereas the resting potential is negative at rest, the conduction of an electrical impulse is dependent on the depolarization of the cell membrane. When an electrical stimulus (e.g., electrical activity of a neighboring nerve cell) leads to depolarization of the cell membrane to a threshold level (usually −55 mV), the nerve cell will fire an action potential. During an action

potential, Na⁺ voltage-gated channels open, leading to an influx of Na⁺ ions into the cell to balance the concentration gradient maintained at rest by the Na⁺-K⁺ pump. This influx of Na⁺ ions leads to a complete depolarization of the nerve membrane and even to a positive potential (+30 mV) at the end of the Na⁺ influx. K⁺ voltage-gated channels are slower to open, but eventually an efflux of K⁺ ions from the cell tends to reverse the depolarization, and eventually the negative resting potential is restored (Fig. 5-4).

Sensory System

An axon is considered myelinated when the axonal diameter is greater than 1 to 2 μm. Axons can be classified by diameter and conduction velocity (Table 5-1). Sensory receptors transmit mechanical, pain, and thermal stimuli through the dorsal root ganglion to spinal cord or brainstem. Sensory axons have the cell body in the dorsal root ganglion. Pacinian corpuscles detect vibration, Meissner's receptors detect moving two-point discrimination, Merkel cells detect static two-point discrimination, naked endings of A delta fibers detect sharp pain, and naked endings of C fibers detect burning pain. Nociceptive information is mediated by small myelinated (A delta) and unmyelinated (C) fibers.

Motor System

The motor system consists of spinal cord, brainstem and reticular formation, motor cortex, and premotor cortical areas (basal ganglia and cerebellum). The spinal cord extends from the foramen magnum to L1 and is composed of white matter (columns of ascending and descending tracts with myelinated and nonmyelinated fibers) and gray matter. The gray matter is divided into dorsal horn, intermediate zone, and ventral horn. The motor unit includes the motor neuron, motor axon, and muscle fibers that it innervates. Muscle membrane depolarization at the motor end plate leading to a muscle action potential is created by Na⁺ influx across the cell membrane.

◆ Table 5-1			
CLASSIFICATION OF NERVE FIBERS			
Group	Function (Examples)	Average Fiber Diameter (μm)	Average CV*(ms)
Erlanger-Gasser classification			
Aα	Primary muscle spindle afferents, motor axons to muscle	15	100
Aβ	Cutaneous touch and pressure afferents	8	50
Aγ	Motor axons to muscle spindle	5	20
Aδ	Cutaneous temperature and pain afferents	3	15
B	Sympathetic preganglionic	3	7
C	Cutaneous pain afferents, sympathetic postganglionic	0.5	1
Lloyd-Hunt classification			
I	Primary muscle spindle afferents and afferents from tendon organs	13	75
II	Mechanoreceptors	9	55
III	Deep pressure sensors in muscle	3	11
IV	Unmyelinated pain afferents	0.5	1

*CV, conduction velocity.
From Simon SR, ed: Orthopaedic Basic Science, 2nd ed. Rosemont, III, American Academy of Orthopaedic Surgeons, 2000, p 629.

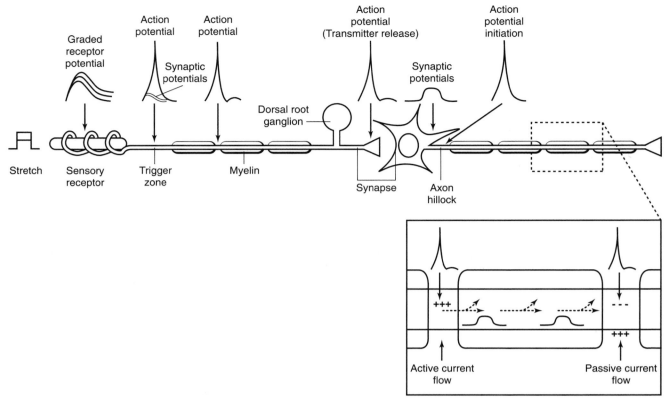

Figure 5-4 ◆ Propagation of action potential and passive current flow. Graded stretching of a muscle produces graded potentials in the terminal fibers of the sensory neuron. This potential spreads passively to the trigger zone, and if the potential is large enough, it will trigger an action potential that is actively propagated without change along the axon to the terminal region. At the terminal of the afferent fiber, the action potential triggers the release of transmitter that diffuses across the synaptic cleft and interacts with the membrane of the motoneuron to initiate a synaptic potential in the motoneuron. The synaptic potential passively spreads to the axon hillock, where an action potential is initiated if the membrane potential is above threshold. Action potential propagation results from the spread of local passive depolarizing currents between the nodes of Ranvier. At the nodes, voltage-gated channels open, producing an action potential. *(From Simon SR, ed: Orthopaedic Basic Science, 2nd ed. Rosemont, Ill, American Academy of Orthopaedic Surgeons, 2000.)*

Spinal cord reflexes can be monosynaptic or polysynaptic. The stretch reflex is a monosynaptic reflex initiated by afferent discharge from stretch spindles to alpha motor neurons innervating the muscle of origin. In general, it is strongest in the physiologic extensors that oppose gravity. This includes the flexors in the upper extremity and the extensors in the lower extremity.

Compression Neuropathies

Basic Science

A compression neuropathy occurs when a segment of peripheral nerve is contained within a constrained environment for a time, leading to a series of histopathologic changes. Initially, epineurial blood flow is slowed and axonal transport is slowed. Axonal transport is inhibited at 30 mm Hg. With either increased pressure or sustained compression, localized endoneurial pressure increases, epineurial edema occurs, and complete axonal block results. Persistent endoneurial edema induces fibroblast proliferation and endoneurial fibrosis. Progressive intraneural ischemia (pressures greater than 60 mm Hg in the acute setting) produces a sensory

blockade followed by motor blockade. Prolonged pressure leads to demyelination. When the myelin sheath is restituted, the distance between each node of Ranvier is diminished, leading to slowing of conduction of the nerve impulse. Animal studies have shown localized nodal displacement with invagination of compressed areas toward the uncompressed segments.

Epidemiology

Risk factors include female sex, pregnancy, diabetes, hypothyroidism, and rheumatoid arthritis. Other factors include middle age, gout, infection, alcoholism, obesity, and mucopolysaccharidosis or mucolipidosis. The role of occupational and repetitive activities in the development of compression neuropathies remains controversial.

Physical Examination

MOTOR

Muscle strength is graded on a scale of 1 to 5 (5 = full strength). Mild nerve compression does not result in measurable motor dysfunction. Moderate compression produces muscle weakness. Severe compression results in denervation and muscle wasting.

Sensory

Sensory examination can be divided into threshold and innervation density testing. Threshold tests evaluate a single nerve fiber innervating a receptor or group of receptors and are useful in evaluation of subtle changes that occur in a compression neuropathy. Changes in threshold are the earliest sensory changes in a compression neuropathy. These tests include Semmes-Weinstein monofilaments (slowly adapting fibers) and vibrometry (quickly adapting fibers). Innervation density tests evaluate multiple overlapping fields of sensory receptors. These tests include static two-point discrimination (slowly adapting fibers) and moving two-point discrimination (quickly adapting fibers). Two-point discrimination of greater than 5 mm on the volar aspect of the hand is considered abnormal. Abnormalities in two-point discrimination do not occur until the neuropathy reaches the severe stages. Threshold tests are more sensitive than the innervation density tests for the assessment of compression neuropathies. Semmes-Weinstein testing has the highest rate of interobserver reliability of all sensibility tests. Innervation density tests are useful in assessing the degree of functional nerve regeneration after repair (Table 5-2).

Electrical Testing

Nerve conduction studies (NCS) and electromyography (EMG) are used to evaluate function of skeletal muscle and of motor and sensory nerves. These are helpful in identifying involved muscles to determine level and degree of dysfunction. Electrical activity may be recorded extracellularly from muscle or nerve by use of surface electrodes.

Motor Nerve Conduction

Motor nerves are supramaximally stimulated at a superficial location with distal response from a muscle.
1. Compound muscle action potentials represent the muscle response after stimulation of the motor nerve. Compound muscle action potentials display the evoked motor response as a sum of the action potentials of the individual muscle fibers (Fig. 5-5). Amplitude of compound muscle action potentials is directly proportional to the number of muscle fibers depolarized and provides an estimate of the amount of functioning axons and muscle fibers.
2. Latency denotes the time from the application of the stimulus to the initial deflection from muscle contraction.
3. Conduction velocity for motor nerves is influenced by temperature, age, myelin sheath thickness, and internode distance. Edema, tremor, and wrinkled skin can also affect true measurements. These values at birth are 50% of adult values. They increase to 75% by 12 months and to 100% by 4 to 5 years of age. Limb surface temperature below 34°C results in a progressive increase in latency and decrease in conduction velocity. Conduction velocity in the upper extremity is 10% to 15% faster than in the lower extremity (45 m/s), and proximal segments are 5% to 10% greater than distal segments.
4. F waves represent delayed muscle stimulation that results from the initial motor nerve stimulation. In addition to the anterograde (orthodromic) transmission of the nerve impulse that leads to muscle contraction, there is also some retrograde (antidromic) transmission of the electrical impulse. This antidromic impulse conduction can stimulate the neuron in the spinal cord, sending a recurrent orthodromic nerve impulse that results in a second, delayed muscle contraction. F wave measurements reflect conduction along the entire nerve and are useful in the study of general polyneuropathy and Guillain-Barré syndrome.

Sensory Nerve Conduction

Sensory potentials are unaffected by lesions proximal to the dorsal root ganglion. They are useful to detect pathologic changes distal (brachial plexus or peripheral nerve) to the dorsal root ganglion. The amplitudes are much smaller than those in motor conduction studies because the recordings are carried out on the nerve itself. The stimulation recording and conduction velocity

---

◆ **Table 5-2**

SPECIFIC SENSORY TESTS OF FUNDAMENTAL DIFFERENCES BETWEEN NERVE FIBER POPULATIONS AND RECEPTOR SYSTEMS

Clinical Test	Sensation	Fiber Type and Size	Fiber Population	Receptor	Type of Test
Weber two-point discrimination	Constant touch	A beta, 15–20 μm	Slowly adapting	Merkel cell–neurite complex	Innervation density
Moving two-point discrimination	Moving touch	A beta, 15–20 μm	Quickly adapting	Meissner corpuscle	Innervation density
Tuning fork (256 cps)	256 cps vibration	A beta, 15–20 μm	Quickly adapting	Pacinian corpuscle	Threshold
Von Frey hair or Semmes-Weinstein monofilament	Constant touch	A beta, 15–20 μm	Slowly adapting	Merkel cell–neurite complex	Threshold

From Gelberman RH: Operative Nerve Repair and Reconstruction. Philadelphia, JB Lippincott, 1991, p 877.

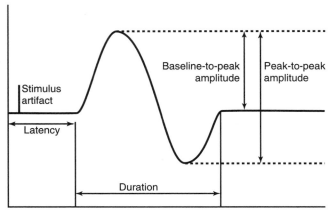

Figure 5-5 ❖ Measured parameters of a compound motor action potential. *(From Sethi RK, Thompson LL: The Electromyographer's Handbook, 2nd ed. Boston, Little, Brown, 1989.)*

calculation can be performed in both the orthodromic and antidromic directions.

1. The sensory nerve under study is stimulated with a surface electrode, which will result in the production of a measurable sensory nerve action potential.
2. Latency denotes the time from the application of the stimulus to the initial deflection on the recording electrode.
3. Conduction velocity is calculated by dividing the length of the nerve segment from the stimulus point to the recording point by the latency.
4. The amplitude is proportional to the total number of nerve fibers activated.

EMG

EMG is used to study the electrical activity of individual muscle fibers and motor units. It can be helpful in differentiating between primary nerve and muscle dysfunction and partial and complete nerve dysfunction.

1. Insertional activity: burst of muscle activity when the needle is inserted into muscle due to mechanical stimulation. Insertional activity is increased in nerve compression syndromes, nerve injury, and polymyositis. It is decreased in prolonged denervation due to loss of muscle fibers.
2. Rest activity: muscle is normally silent during rest. Denervated muscle fibers can become spontaneously active and produce fibrillations (action potentials that arise from single muscle fibers) and positive sharp waves. Spontaneous activity may not be seen until 3 to 5 weeks after nerve injury. It may also be seen in primary muscle disorders. Fasciculations result from spontaneous activity of groups of muscle fibers and are common in amyotrophic lateral sclerosis. Other electrodiagnostic findings in amyotrophic lateral sclerosis include fibrillations, increased amplitude of motor unit action potentials, and minimal delay in motor velocity.
3. As the contraction is increased to maximal levels, the number of muscle fibers generating action potentials of varying rates and amplitude are increased, generating an interference pattern.

Double Crush Syndrome

Entrapment at one level can be associated with symptoms of compression at a different level. Endoneurial edema at a proximal site can alter axonal transport and is believed to decrease the delivery of cytoskeletal proteins and nutrients distally. This disruption in neuronal transport can lower the threshold for the occurrence of nerve compression symptoms at a different site on the same nerve.

Median Nerve

CARPAL TUNNEL SYNDROME

Carpal tunnel syndrome (CTS), caused by median nerve compression at the wrist, is the most common compression neuropathy.

Anatomy

The carpal canal is defined by the scaphoid tubercle and trapezium radially, the hook of the hamate and pisiform ulnarly, and the transverse carpal ligament palmarly (the roof). It contains nine flexor tendons: flexor pollicis longus (FPL), flexor digitorum superficialis (FDS), and flexor digitorum profundus (FDP). Many anatomic variations of the median nerve have been described. The motor branch of the median nerve is most commonly extraligamentous, arising from the radial side of the nerve (Fig. 5-6). The lowest carpal pressure is 2.5 mm Hg at rest (wrist in neutral and fingers in full extension), which can increase to 30 mm Hg with wrist flexion. Patients with CTS on average will have canal pressures of 30 mm Hg at rest and 90 mm Hg with wrist flexion.

Etiology

Synovial biopsy of the carpal canal in idiopathic CTS shows fibrous tissue and edema with scattered lymphocytes. Potential causes include the following:

1. Anatomic abnormalities, such as congenital anomalies, persistent median artery, and proximal lumbrical muscles.
2. Associated medical conditions (in decreasing order of incidence): cervical spine and wrist degenerative joint disease, rheumatoid arthritis, thyroid disease, and diabetes.
3. Inflammatory factors, such as rheumatoid arthritis, gout, and infection.
4. Fluid balance abnormalities, including hemodialysis and pregnancy. There is a high correlation between the side of hemodialysis access and the side affected by CTS.
5. Traumatic factors, such as hematoma and fractures of the distal radius.
6. Positional factors: full flexion and extension of the wrist decrease the size of the carpal canal, leading to increased carpal canal pressure.

Clinical Assessment

Patients present with pain and paresthesias of the palmar aspect of the radial 3½ digits. Pain can also radiate to the palmar forearm proximally. Feelings of clumsiness, weakness, night pain, and hypesthesia are also common. Long-standing disease will lead to thenar atrophy. Sensation along the radial aspect of the palm

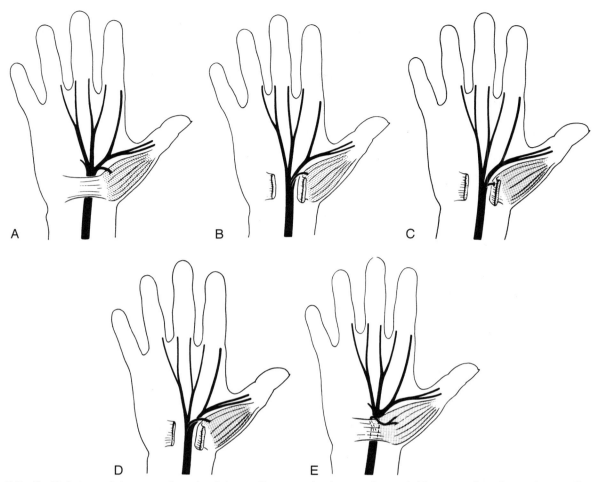

Figure 5-6 ❖ Variations of the motor branch of the median nerve in the carpal tunnel. The motor branch may be extraligamentous (**A,** 46% to 90%), subligamentous (**B,** 31%), or transligamentous (**C,** 23%). Less commonly, the motor branch may lie ulnar to the median nerve in the carpal tunnel (**D**) or lie on top of the transverse carpal ligament (**E**). *(From Green DP, Hotchkiss RN, Pederson WC, eds: Operative Hand Surgery, 4th ed. New York, Churchill Livingstone, 1999.)*

should be normal because the palmar cutaneous branch of the median nerve does not travel within the carpal canal. Classic provocative maneuvers include Tinel's sign (percussion over the nerve, which produces electrical sensation distally in the distribution of the nerve), Phalen's maneuver (wrist flexion with the elbow in extension for 60 seconds, which produces paresthesias), and the carpal compression test. The most sensitive maneuver is the carpal compression test in which direct compression is applied over the volar aspect of the forearm at the level of or slightly proximal to the wrist crease for 60 seconds and distal paresthesias in the median distribution are elicited. This is considered the most reliable and valid provocative maneuver for the diagnosis of CTS. The sensitivity and specificity of other maneuvers are given in Table 5-3.

EMG/NCS
EMG and NCS represent the "gold standard" for the diagnosis of CTS. The changes consistent with CTS on EMG and NCS include a distal motor latency greater than 4.0 msec or asymmetry of 1.0 msec between hands and a distal sensory latency greater than 3.5 msec or asymmetry of 0.5 msec between hands. Fibrillation potentials and positive sharp waves in the thenar muscles are noted in severe CTS.

Treatment
Treatment of mild CTS includes nonsteroidal anti-inflammatory drugs and a static splint to maintain the wrist in neutral. Steroid injections can also provide relief. Lack of improvement after a corticosteroid injection is a poor prognostic factor. If the symptoms progress immediately after a corticosteroid injection, one must consider that the injection was intraneural and consider urgent débridement.

Surgical treatment is considered for patients with persistent or progressive symptoms despite nonoperative treatment. Surgical treatment is performed more expeditiously for patients with severe CTS because nonoperative modalities are typically unsuccessful for the severe stages. Surgery can be open or endoscopic. Potential benefits of endoscopic treatment include less postoperative pain, earlier return of grip strength, and earlier return to work. A shortcoming of endoscopic treatment is the increased incidence of complications

◆ **Table 5-3**

DIAGNOSTIC TESTS FOR CARPAL TUNNEL SYNDROME

Name of Test	How Performed	Condition Measured	Positive Result	Interpretation of Positive Result
Phalen's test	Patient places elbows on table, forearms vertical, wrists flexed	Paresthesias in response to position	Numbness or tingling on radial side of digits within 60 seconds	Probable CTS (sensitivity 0.75, specificity 0.47)
Percussion test (Tinel's)	Examiner lightly taps along median nerve, at the wrist, proximal to distal	Site of nerve lesion	Tingling response in fingers at site of compression	Probable CTS if response is at the wrist (sensitivity 0.60, specificity 0.67)
Carpal tunnel compression test	Direct compression of median nerve by examiner	Paresthesias in response to pressure	Paresthesias within 30 seconds	Probable CTS (sensitivity 0.87, specificity 0.90)
Hand diagram	Patient marks sites of pain or altered sensation on the outline diagram of the hand	Patient's perception of site of nerve deficit	Signs on palmar side of radial digits without signs in the palm	Probable CTS (sensitivity 0.96, specificity 0.73), negative predictive value of a negative test = 0.91
Hand volume stress test	Measures hand volume, by water displacement, repeated after 7-minute stress test and 10-minute rest	Hand volume	Hand volume increased by 10 mL or more	Probable dynamic carpal tunnel syndrome
Direct measurement of carpal tunnel pressure	Wick or infusion catheter is placed in carpal tunnel; pressure measured	Hydrostatic pressure: resting and in response to position or stress	Resting pressure 25 mm Hg or more (this number is variable and may not be valid in and of itself)	Hydrostatic compression at wrist is cause of probable CTS
Static two-point discrimination	Determines minimum separation of two points perceived as distinct when lightly touched to palmar surface of digit	Innervation density of slowly adapting fibers	Failure to discriminate points more than 6 mm apart	Advanced nerve dysfunction
Moving two-point discrimination	As above, but with points moving	Innervation density of quickly adapting fibers	Failure to discriminate points more than 5 mm apart	Advanced nerve dysfunction
Vibrometry	Vibrometer head is placed on palmar side of digit; amplitude at 120 Hz increased to threshold of perception; compare median, ulnar nerves, both hands	Threshold of quickly adapting fibers	Asymmetry with contralateral hand or radial vs. ulnar	Probable CTS (sensitivity 0.87)
Semmes-Weinstein monofilaments	Monofilaments of increasing diameter touched to palmar side of digit until patient can tell which digit is touched	Threshold of slowly adapting fibers	Value greater than 2.83 in radial digits	Median nerve impairment (sensitivity 0.83)
Distal sensory latency and conduction velocity	Orthodromic stimulus and recording across wrist	Latency, conduction velocity of sensory fibers	Latency greater than 3.5 msec or asymmetry of conduction velocity greater than 0.5 m/s vs. contralateral hand	Probable CTS
Distal motor latency and conduction velocity	Orthodromic stimulus and recording across wrist	Latency, conduction velocity of motor fibers of median nerve	Latency greater than 4.5 msec or asymmetry of conduction velocity greater than 1.0 m/s	Probable CTS
EMGs	Needle electrodes placed in muscle	Denervation of thenar muscles	Fibrillation potentials, sharp waves, increased insertional activity	Very advanced motor median nerve compression

From Szabo RM: Hand Surgery Update. Rosemont, Ill, American Academy of Orthopaedic Surgeons, 1996, p 223.

(superficial arch injury and nerve injury including the median, ulnar, and common digital nerves). The incidence of pillar pain is similar and time to return to work is similar for patients receiving workers' compensation. Incomplete release of the transverse carpal ligament is the most common reason for persistent symptoms after surgery, especially with endoscopic carpal tunnel release. Success after carpal tunnel release is most correlated with improved pain and numbness. The electrodiagnostic study values often do not return to normal after surgical release, and the amount of postoperative improvement is dependent on preoperative EMG dysfunction. Repeated surgical release for CTS is uncommon, and failure rates after reoperation are 25% to 40%. Acute CTS presents with progressive neurologic deterioration after a distal radius or carpal bone fracture. Emergent carpal tunnel release is indicated in these cases. Internal median nerve neurolysis is of no benefit.

PRONATOR SYNDROME

Anatomy

Potential sites of compression include the lacertus fibrosus, the origin of the pronator teres, the ligament of Struthers (which connects the supracondylar process of the distal humerus with the medial epicondyle), and the origin of the FDS (Figs. 5-7 and 5-8). Motor interconnections from the median to the ulnar nerve in the forearm are termed Martin-Gruber anastomoses. Interconnections from the median to the ulnar nerve in the hand are termed Riche-Cannieu anastomoses.

Clinical Assessment

Patients present with pain and paresthesias of the palmar aspect of the radial 3½ digits. The numbness can extend to the proximal palm, in the distribution of the palmar cutaneous branch of the nerve. Pain can also radiate to the palmar forearm proximally. Night pain is seldom a complaint. Provocative maneuvers include Tinel's sign over the proximal forearm, resisted elbow flexion with the forearm in supination (entrapment by lacertus fibrosus), resisted forearm pronation with the elbow in extension (entrapment by pronator teres), and resisted flexion of the proximal interphalangeal joint of the long finger (entrapment by FDS). Manual palpation for the presence of a supracondylar process should be performed.

EMG/NCS

EMG and NCS are misleading in the diagnosis of pronator syndrome. NCS is generally inaccurate. Fibrillation potentials and positive sharp waves in the pronator quadratus and FPL muscles can aid in diagnosis.

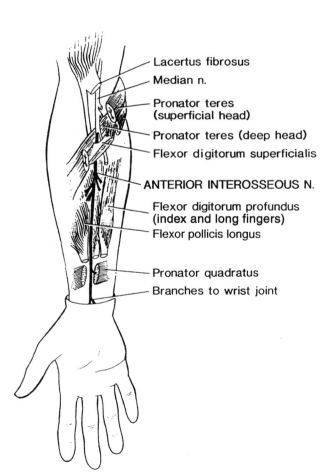

Figure 5-7 ◆ Schematic anatomy of the anterior interosseous nerve. (*From Chidgey LK, Szabo RM: Anterior interosseous nerve compression syndrome. In Szabo RM, ed: Nerve Compression Syndrome—Diagnosis and Treatment. Thorofare, NJ, Slack, 1989.*)

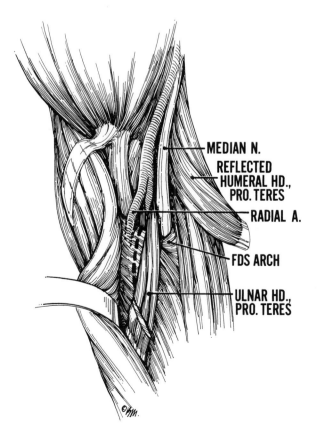

Figure 5-8 ◆ Exposure of the median nerve at the elbow. (*From Green DP, Hotchkiss RN, Pederson WC, eds: Operative Hand Surgery, 4th ed. New York, Churchill Livingstone, 1999.*)

Treatment

Treatment includes activity modification, specifically of activities involving repetitive flexion and pronation. Splinting and anti-inflammatory medication can be helpful. Surgery to release all four potential sites of compression yields good results.

ANTERIOR INTEROSSEOUS NERVE SYNDROME

Anatomy

The anterior interosseous nerve is primarily a motor nerve that branches from the median nerve 4 to 6 cm distal to the elbow. It supplies the radial half of the FDP, FPL, and pronator quadratus. The nerve may be compressed by the deep head of the pronator teres, origin of the FDS, flexor carpi radialis, accessory muscles that connect the FDS to the FDP, and Gantzer's muscle (accessory head of the FPL).

Clinical Assessment

Anterior interosseous nerve syndrome may occur spontaneously or after repetitive motion. Signs and symptoms include ill-defined forearm pain and inability to flex the thumb interphalangeal joint and index finger distal interphalangeal joint because of weakness of FPL and FDP index, respectively (often termed the "O" sign because the patient is unable to make a circle with index finger and thumb). Pronator quadratus weakness is evaluated by testing forearm pronation with the elbow in flexion. In cases with bilateral involvement, Parsonage-Turner syndrome should be considered. Tendon rupture should be ruled out as well.

EMG/NCS

EMG and NCS are valuable in substantiating the diagnosis.

Treatment

Treatment is surgical if motor function does not recover after 3 to 6 months of observation. Treatment includes release of superficial arch of FDS, lacertus fibrosus, and superficial head of pronator teres. In chronic cases, tendon transfers can be effective in restoring function.

Ulnar Nerve

CUBITAL TUNNEL SYNDROME

The cubital tunnel is the most common site of compression of the ulnar nerve.

Anatomy

The ulnar nerve (C8-T1) originates from the medial cord of the brachial plexus. Potential sites of compression include the arcade of Struthers (medial intermuscular septum), medial epicondyle, roof of cubital tunnel (arcuate ligament), Osborne's fascia (proximal fascial band between the two heads of the flexor carpi ulnaris), and proximal flexor profundus arch. The most common sites of compression are the epicondylar groove and the two heads of the flexor carpi ulnaris (Fig. 5-9). The volume of the canal is maximum in extension and decreases by 50% with flexion as the canal changes from oval to a slit shape. Maximum strain in the ulnar nerve occurs at the medial epicondyle with the elbow held in flexion. The normal excursion of the nerve is 1 cm above and 6 cm below the elbow joint.

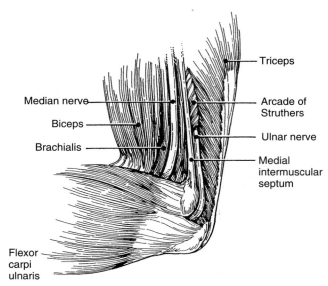

Figure 5-9 ◆ Potential sites of compression of the ulnar nerve at the elbow. *(From Gelberman RH: Operative Nerve Repair and Reconstruction. Philadelphia, JB Lippincott, 1991.)*

Clinical Assessment

Signs and symptoms include paresthesias in the volar and dorsal aspect of the small finger and ulnar half of the ring finger. In addition, common complaints are medial elbow pain, night pain, and symptoms exacerbated with elbow flexion. Possible causes are repetitive use of vibrating tools, playing musical instruments, tourniquet use, intraoperative malpositioning, cubitus varus and valgus deformity, adhesions, burns, heterotopic ossification, space-occupying lesions (ganglion, lipoma, osteochondroma), and arthritis. Clawing of the ulnar two digits is a late finding. Clawing of all fingers is seen in combined ulnar and median nerve dysfunction. Provocative tests include Tinel's sign over the cubital tunnel and the elbow flexion test (reproduction of symptoms with the elbow in maximal flexion). Another finding on examination is Froment's sign (weakness in thumb adduction with compensatory FPL flexion during pinch). An abducted small finger related to an ulnar nerve injury proximal to the wrist (Wartenberg's sign) is due to weakness of the third palmar interosseous muscle and unopposed pull of the extensor digiti minimi. Differential diagnosis includes C8 or T1 radiculopathy, thoracic outlet syndrome, Pancoast's tumor, and double crush syndrome.

EMG/NCS

NCS may show slowing across the elbow and low amplitudes of sensory nerve action potentials and compound muscle action potentials. A conduction velocity differential of 10 m/s above and below the elbow is considered abnormal.

Treatment

Treatment includes nonsteroidal anti-inflammatory drugs and night elbow extension splinting at 45 degrees of flexion and neutral rotation. A lumbrical bar splint (anticlaw splint) may be used to block hyperextension of the metacarpophalangeal joints of the ring and small fingers, limiting the claw deformity. Poor prognosis after surgical intervention is closely correlated with intrinsic atrophy. Surgery may be one of the following procedures:

1. In situ decompression of the ulnar nerve limits disruption of nerve vascularity that may occur with the other procedures. Vascular supply to the nerve after transposition is likely to be due to intraneural circulation. Decompression involves the release of Osborne's ligament and the aponeurosis of the FCU.
2. Medial epicondylectomy.
3. Anterior transposition procedures, including subcutaneous, submuscular, and intramuscular transposition. The medial intermuscular septum is excised at the time of the procedure so that it does not become a site of ulnar nerve compression after transposition. The medial antebrachial cutaneous nerve is most at risk during anterior transposition. Progressive or continued symptoms after transposition and Tinel's sign proximal to the medial epicondyle are usually secondary to inadequate resection of the medial intermuscular septum.

Ulnar Tunnel Syndrome

Anatomy

Entrapment of the ulnar nerve at the wrist occurs at Guyon's canal. This canal is defined by the flexor retinaculum and the muscles of the hypothenar eminence as the floor of the canal, the pisiform and abductor digiti minimi muscle as the ulnar boundary, the hook of the hamate as the radial border of the canal, and the volar carpal ligament and palmaris brevis as the roof. The ulnar nerve divides into the superficial sensory and the deep motor branches within the canal. The area is divided into three zones: zone I is the area proximal to the bifurcation of the nerve; zone II includes the deep motor branch to just beyond the fibrous arch of the hypothenar muscles; zone III involves only the superficial branch or the sensory component. The motor branch supplies all the intrinsic muscles in the hand (including the deep head of the flexor pollicis brevis) except the remaining thenar muscles and the radial two lumbricals (Fig. 5-10).

Clinical Assessment

In contrast to patients with cubital tunnel syndrome, patients with ulnar tunnel syndrome will not have a sensory deficit on the dorsal ulnar aspect of the hand (dorsal ulnar sensory nerve distribution). Ganglion cysts are the most common source of ulnar nerve compression at the wrist. Other etiologic factors include lipomas, ulnar artery thrombosis or aneurysm, hook of the hamate fracture, pisiform dislocation, inflammatory arthritis, fibrous band, congenital bands, and bone anomalies. It may be due to repetitive trauma in patients who use a walker or bicyclists. Allen tests and Doppler studies are helpful for diagnosis of arterial thrombosis; computed tomographic scans are helpful in evaluation for fractures of the hook of the hamate. Magnetic resonance imaging is helpful in detecting cysts or other compressive masses. Symptoms of an ulnar neuropathy at Guyon's canal vary according to the location of compression. Compression at zone I is

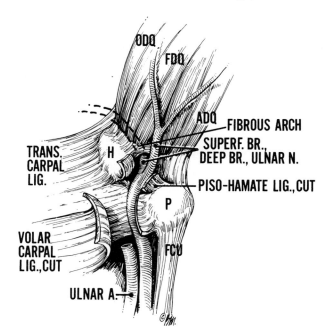

Figure 5-10 ❖ Anatomic relationships of the ulnar nerve at Guyon's canal. The ulnar nerve travels superficial to the transverse carpal ligament and deep to the volar carpal ligament. H, hamate, P, pisiform. *(From Green DP, Hotchkiss RN, Pederson WC, eds: Operative Hand Surgery, 4th ed. New York, Churchill Livingstone, 1999.)*

manifested by sensory symptoms of the ring and small fingers as well as by motor weakness of the ulnarly innervated intrinsic muscles. In zone II, only motor symptoms are noted, whereas compression at zone III causes sensory symptoms only. Thrombosis of the ulnar artery is the most common source of problems in zone III. Grip strength is decreased by half in patients with low ulnar nerve palsy.

EMG/NCS

EMG and NCS are valuable in substantiating the diagnosis.

Treatment

Treatment includes wearing padded gloves, avoidance of offending provocative actions, splinting, and nonsteroidal anti-inflammatory drugs. Surgery includes nerve decompression, release of the hypothenar muscle origin, and removal of any space-occupying lesions.

Radial Nerve

Radial Nerve Compression in the Arm

Radial nerve compression in the arm is caused by humerus fracture, tourniquet palsy, or prolonged postural compression. Patients present with weakness of wrist, finger, or thumb extension. Recovery is usually spontaneous. If no recovery has occurred by 3 to 4 months, consider neurolysis, nerve grafting, or tendon transfers. In patients with open fractures of the humerus with associated nerve palsy, exploration of the radial nerve is indicated at the time of fracture fixation.

POSTERIOR INTEROSSEOUS NERVE SYNDROME

Anatomy

The radial nerve (C5-8) supplies triceps, brachioradialis, extensor carpi radialis longus (ECRL), anconeus, and half of brachialis. The nerve supplies branches proximal to the elbow to the ECRL, brachioradialis, and occasionally extensor carpi radialis brevis (ECRB). The nerve divides into a superficial sensory branch and the posterior interosseous nerve. The posterior interosseous nerve supplies the supinator, ECRB, extensor digitorum communis, extensor carpi ulnaris, extensor digiti minimi, abductor pollicis longus, extensor pollicis brevis, extensor indicis proprius, and extensor pollicis longus. Offending anatomic structures include the **F**ibrous bands anterior to the radial head, **R**adial recurrent vessels (leash of Henry), fibrous edge of **E**CRB, **A**rcade of Frohse (proximal edge of the supinator, most common site of compression), and distal edge of the **S**upinator (**FREAS**). Most patients present with wrist and digit extension weakness and pain.

Clinical Assessment

Posterior interosseous neuropathy may be related to repetitive forearm motion, Monteggia's fracture-dislocation, radial head fracture-dislocations, blunt trauma, and space-occupying lesions (lipoma or ganglions) or can be idiopathic. No sensory changes occur because the posterior interosseous nerve is mostly a motor nerve. Patients with posterior interosseous nerve palsy will have difficulty extending the digits at the metacarpophalangeal joints in addition to the thumb interphalangeal joint. Interphalangeal joint extension of the fingers will be intact through interossei muscle innervation by the ulnar nerve. Wrist extension occurs with radial deviation because of loss of extensor carpi ulnaris function. ECRL will continue to function through innervation by the radial nerve proximally. One must differentiate between a posterior interosseous nerve palsy and tendon rupture in patients with rheumatoid disease. Patients with extensor tendon ruptures will have lost the tenodesis effect, and the digits will not extend passively as the wrist is placed in flexion.

Treatment

Initial treatment includes activity modification and splinting. Surgical treatment involves release of all involved structures. Patients may continue to improve for up to 18 months after surgery.

RADIAL TUNNEL SYNDROME

This is primarily a pain syndrome not associated with motor or sensory deficits (unlike posterior interosseous nerve syndrome, which is characterized by weakness).

Anatomy

The offending structures in radial tunnel syndrome are similar to those in posterior interosseous nerve syndrome. The most common site of nerve compression in radial tunnel syndrome is the arcade of Frohse.

Clinical Assessment

The signs and symptoms of radial tunnel syndrome include deep, aching pain in the dorsal-radial forearm in the radial neck region that radiates from the lateral elbow to the dorsal aspect of the wrist. Physical examination reveals tenderness in the mobile wad over the supinator arch, pain with resistive supination with the elbow and wrist in extension, and pain with passive pronation of the forearm with the wrist in flexion. Although the primary differential diagnosis is lateral epicondylitis, these two conditions may often coexist.

EMG/NCS

Findings on EMG and NCS are typically normal. One objective test involves relief of symptoms after an injection of anesthetic about the radial nerve in the radial tunnel region. Relief of symptoms in addition to a wrist drop (due to motor paralysis from the anesthetic) is diagnostic.

Treatment

The treatment of radial tunnel syndrome is similar to the treatment of posterior interosseous nerve syndrome (Fig. 5-11).

LATERAL ANTEBRACHIAL CUTANEOUS NERVE COMPRESSION

Lateral antebrachial cutaneous nerve compression occurs as the nerve enters the superficial forearm between the brachioradialis and the biceps tendon. Patients complain of pain in the forearm while performing activities with the elbow in extension. Diagnostic anesthetic injections may temporarily relieve the pain.

SENSORY RADIAL NERVE COMPRESSION (WARTENBERG'S SYNDROME, CHEIRALGIA PARESTHETICA)

Anatomy

Scissor-like action of the brachioradialis and ECRL tendons over the dorsal forearm may compress the nerve. The nerve may also arise between slips of brachioradialis tendon. Diagnostic wrist block may temporarily relieve the pain.

Clinical Assessment

Symptoms include paresthesias in the dorsal-radial aspect of the hand with ill-defined pain in the radial forearm and wrist. Repetitive wrist flexion and ulnar deviation may exacerbate the symptoms. It can result from a direct blow, handcuffs, tight cast, external fixator pins, or tight watch band. Provocative tests including Tinel's sign and symptom development after forceful forearm pronation are helpful. Diagnostic wrist block may temporarily relieve the pain. It must be differentiated from de Quervain's tenosynovitis.

Treatment

Treatment includes wrist splinting, avoidance of offending activities, and rarely surgery. If surgery is performed, a longitudinal incision is used with neurolysis and release of fascia between the brachioradialis and the ECRL.

Thoracic Outlet Syndrome

Anatomy

The cervicothoracobrachial passage consists of an interscalene triangle, costoclavicular space, and coracopectoral tunnel.

and first rib malunion, repetitive shoulder use, and athletic activities (weightlifting, rowing, and swimming). Thoracic outlet syndrome more often affects women. The clinical diagnosis is made with positive results of provocative tests, including Adson's, Wright's, hyperabduction, and costoclavicular maneuvers. These maneuvers have low specificity. Noninvasive vascular studies and angiography identify the vascular form of thoracic outlet syndrome. Pancoast's tumor should be ruled out.

EMG/NCS
Findings on EMG and NCS are usually equivocal.

Treatment
Initial treatment includes activity modification and physical therapy to strengthen the shoulder girdle muscles. If there is intractable pain, neurologic deficit, or persistent vascular insufficiency, surgery is an option. Procedures include scalenotomy, scalenectomy, and excision of cervical or first rib (through the transaxillary approach).

Compression Neuropathies of the Shoulder

SUPRASCAPULAR NERVE ENTRAPMENT

1. The suprascapular nerve (C5-6) takes almost a direct course across the posterior triangle of the neck to supply the supraspinatus and infraspinatus muscles. Pathologic change may result from fractures, blunt trauma, traction lesions, repetitive motion with resistive exercise, or encroachment from space-occupying lesions at either the suprascapular notch or the spinoglenoid notch.
2. The suprascapular nerve passes through the suprascapular notch below the superior transverse scapular ligament; the suprascapular artery (branch of the thyrocervical trunk of the subclavian artery) passes above the ligament. The transverse scapular ligament at the suprascapular notch is the most common offending structure in chronic suprascapular nerve compression. If the nerve is entrapped at the spinoglenoid notch, the infraspinatus only is affected.
3. Signs and symptoms include posterior lateral shoulder pain, suprascapular notch tenderness, and muscle weakness of shoulder external rotation.
4. Nonsurgical treatment includes muscle strengthening. Ganglion cysts originating from the glenohumeral joint commonly result in compression of the nerve in the suprascapular notch. Surgery involves release of the suprascapular notch from a posterior approach and enlargement of the bone notch.

MUSCULOCUTANEOUS NERVE COMPRESSION

1. The musculocutaneous nerve (C5-7) originates from the lateral cord and supplies the coracobrachialis, biceps brachii, and half of the brachialis and the sensory aspect of the lateral antebrachial cutaneous nerve.
2. It may be compressed within the substance of the coracobrachialis secondary to shoulder dislocation and rarely distally as the nerve emerges from the biceps tendon. The nerve is most frequently injured during shoulder surgery.

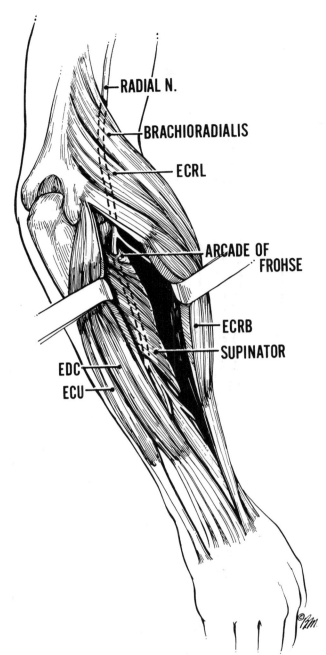

RADIAL N.
BRACHIORADIALIS
ECRL
ARCADE OF FROHSE
ECRB
SUPINATOR
EDC
ECU

Figure 5-11 ◆ Release of the radial nerve through a posterior muscle-splitting approach. *(From Green DP, Hotchkiss RN, Pederson WC, eds: Operative Hand Surgery, 4th ed. New York, Churchill Livingstone, 1999.)*

Clinical Assessment
There are two types: neurologic and vascular. Neurologic symptoms include sensory and motor dysfunction. The upper plexus syndrome involves C5-7 and is localized to the lateral arm, occiput, and scapula. The lower plexus C8-T1 syndrome is localized to scapular, axillary, medial arm, and forearm areas. Vascular symptoms include arterial ischemia, venous congestion, and Raynaud's phenomenon. Possible causes are cervical rib, vertebral transverse process, anomalous insertion of the scalenes, fibromuscular bands, clavicular

3. Signs and symptoms include weakness of elbow flexion, tenderness over the musculocutaneous nerve, and lateral forearm hypesthesias.
4. Treatment is conservative. Surgery to release the nerve is rarely necessary.

LONG THORACIC NERVE ENTRAPMENT

1. The long thoracic nerve (C5-7) is susceptible to traction injuries with shoulder depression, a direct blow, and prolonged hyperabduction of the arms with flexed elbows. The nerve supplies the serratus anterior to maintain scapula position and assists the trapezius with shoulder elevation.
2. Patients present with dull shoulder pain, weakness, scapular winging when arms push against resistance, and pain with arm elevation.
3. This entrapment usually recovers spontaneously with bracing. Rarely is a pectoralis major transfer required.

SPINAL ACCESSORY NERVE ENTRAPMENT

1. This cranial nerve supplies the sternocleidomastoid and the trapezius muscles. Injury may be due to a direct blow, wrestling accident, acromioclavicular dislocations, iatrogenic injury after radical neck dissection, and heavy loads applied to the shoulder.
2. Signs and symptoms include a sensation of heaviness in the arms, dull shoulder pain, trapezius muscle atrophy, drooping shoulder girdle, and lateral displacement of the scapula.
3. The palsy usually resolves spontaneously unless it occurs after surgery. Surgical treatment may require neurolysis, nerve repair, or grafting. If the palsy has been present for an extended time, the scapula may be stabilized with fascia lata to the ribs or spinal processes or transfer of the rhomboids and levator muscles laterally into the scapula.

AXILLARY NERVE ENTRAPMENT

1. Axillary nerve entrapment is also known as quadrilateral space syndrome. This syndrome involves compression of axillary nerve and posterior circumflex humeral artery. The axillary nerve supplies the teres minor and deltoid muscles.
2. The cause may be idiopathic or traumatic (most commonly after shoulder dislocation), or it may occur in throwing athletes. It may present as shoulder pain and paresthesias in the arm. There is point tenderness over the quadrilateral space and provocative pain and paresthesias with shoulder abduction, elevation, and external rotation for 1 minute. Angiography demonstrates arterial occlusion when the shoulder is abducted beyond 60 degrees.
3. Treatment includes avoidance of provocative maneuvers and surgical release of the teres minor and transverse fibrous bands.

Nerve Injury

Classification of Nerve Injuries

Nerve injury classification was initially described by Seddon and modified by Sunderland (Fig. 5-12).

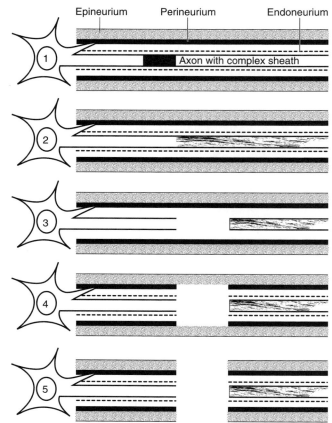

Figure 5-12 ❖ Diagram illustrating the five degrees of nerve injury. 1, Conduction block. 2, The lesion confined to the axon within an intact endoneurial sheath and resulting in wallerian degeneration. 3, Loss of nerve fiber continuity (axon and endoneural sheath) inside an intact perineurium. 4, Loss of fascicular continuity with nerve trunk continuity depending solely on epineurial tissue. 5, Loss of continuity of the entire nerve trunk. *(Modified from Sunderland S: Nerve Injuries and Their Repair: A Critical Appraisal. New York, Churchill Livingstone, 1991.)*

TYPE I: NEURAPRAXIA

This is a localized lesion producing a conduction block with axon continuity preserved. There is no wallerian degeneration, so there are no fibrillation potentials or degenerative changes in the affected muscles. The process is reversible but may take 3 to 4 months. The order of nerve fiber failure is motor, proprioception, touch, temperature, and pain.

TYPE II: AXONOTMESIS

This type involves axonal damage but with an intact endoneurial sheath and basal lamina of Schwann cells. Complete recovery is observed, but at a slower pace than with type I lesions. Distal to the site of injury, EMG and NCS demonstrate fibrillation potentials and slowing of conduction velocity. Slowing of the conduction velocity distal to the site of injury is the earliest finding that helps differentiate axonotmesis from neurapraxia.

TYPE III

Nerve fiber continuity is lost with disruption of Schwann cells, axons, and endoneurium, but perineurium is intact.

There is complete motor and sensory loss with delayed recovery and inappropriate reinnervation. "Pure" sensory or motor nerves have better outcomes than do mixed nerves. Endoneurial scarring leads to variable recovery.

TYPE IV

Nerve fiber continuity is lost, with only epineurium intact, so there is more severe retrograde degeneration with associated axonal loss. There is extensive intraneural scarring that may require excision and surgical repair.

TYPE V: NEUROTMESIS

Complete nerve transection is most likely to result in a neuroma at the proximal stump. EMG and NCS reveal fibrillation potentials and positive sharp waves 2 to 5 weeks after injury. Surgical repair is required for functional recovery in adults.

Wallerian Degeneration

After an axon is transected, the distal stump undergoes wallerian degeneration to clear axon and myelin debris and to create an environment hospitable for regeneration. The axonal degeneration extends distally to the somatosensory receptor (Fig. 5-13). The breakdown of axoplasm and cytoskeleton is triggered by increased axoplasmic calcium.

1. Schwann cell response. Normally, Schwann cells do not divide. Distal segment Schwann cells divide within 24 hours of injury with peak response by 72 hours.

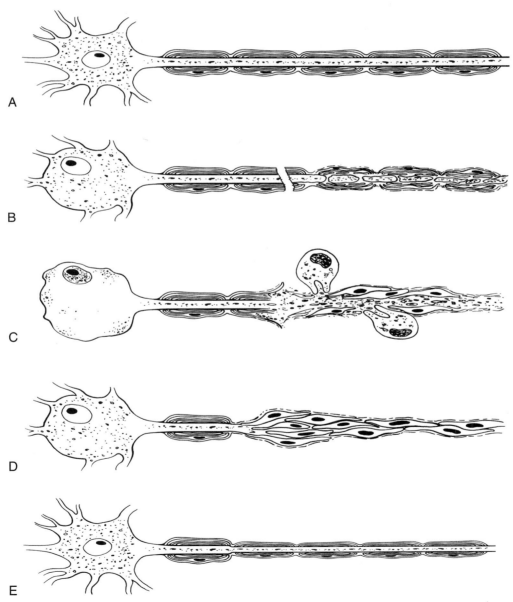

Figure 5-13 ◈ Degeneration and regeneration of myelinated fiber. **A,** Normal appearance. **B,** Nerve fiber transection causes fragmentation of the distal segment, and proximal nerve degeneration occurs to at least the nearest node of Ranvier. **C,** The distal segment Schwann cells proliferate. **D,** Axonal sprouting occurs from the proximal segment, and the advancing sprouts are embedded in the Schwann cell cytoplasm. **E,** Axonal connection and maturation of the nerve fibers. *(From Lundborg G: Nerve Injury and Repair. New York, Churchill Livingstone, 1988.)*

2. Macrophage response. This cell line is the primary phagocyte of myelin and accumulates by 72 hours after injury. Early in the process, macrophages are not phagocytic. Later, as macrophages penetrate basal lamina, they change their phenotypic expression and become phagocytic. They produce cytokines and stimulate Schwann cells to produce nerve growth factor.

3. Nerve cell body response. Metabolic priority is significantly altered because there is a decrease of neurotransmitter and an increase in protein (tubulin, actin, and growth-associated cytokines) production.

4. Proximal segment response. The proximal segment will degenerate if the cell body dies, but it will regenerate if the cell body survives. Early in the postinjury timeline, there is a decrease in myelin thickness and axon diameter. Eventually, there is an increase in myelin thickness and axon diameter, but it will remain smaller than originally. Conduction velocity does not return to normal. Collateral sprouts arise from nodes of Ranvier and terminal sprouts from the tips of remaining axons. Axonal regeneration across the zone of injury is limited by scar tissue between the stumps that is obstructive to axonal advancement and decreases the number of axons to the end organ, delays elongation, and causes misdirection of axons. There is an axonal growth of 1 to 2 mm/day with decreased rate in distal regions.

5. Axonal regeneration. Guidance across gaps is aided by nerve tubes and axonal guidance channels (arteries, veins, muscle, collagen, and silicone). Contact guidance is important in early axonal regeneration, with extracellular matrix proteins (collagen, laminin, fibronectin) playing a role in cell-cell recognition. Neurotropic factors, such as nerve growth factor, promote neurite survival.

Neuroma Formation

1. After nerve injury, axonal regeneration is stimulated by target-derived trophic factors, which may lead to successful reinnervation if the distal endoneurial tube is reached.

2. If there is no distal connection, a collection of neuronal tissue, fibroblasts, and connective tissue develops at the site of injury and is known as a neuroma.

3. A neuroma-in-continuity forms with an incomplete nerve injury in which some of the axons may not reach the distal site.

4. Neuromas may produce pain, cold sensitivity, dystrophic symptoms, and impaired function.

5. Treatment
   a. Nonsurgical treatment includes oral medications, desensitization, transcutaneous nerve stimulation, and local or regional injections.
   b. Surgical options include (1) alteration of the proximal nerve segment, (2) repositioning of the neuroma's host environment (implantation into muscle, bone, or fat versus muscle or skin flap), and (3) alteration of the neuronal environment with direct neurorrhaphy versus nerve to vein or nerve graft or nerve stimulators.

6. Bowler's thumb: pseudoneuroma of the ulnar digital nerve of the thumb due to chronic pressure. Treatment is by modification of bowling technique and equipment.

Nerve Repair

The objectives of surgical nerve repair are to maximize the number of axons regenerating across the injury site and to maximize the accuracy of reinnervation. Younger patients usually have better functional outcome, and age is considered the most important factor in nerve function recovery (Fig. 5-14). Primary repair is defined as immediate repair or repair within several hours of injury. Primary repair is indicated for sharp nerve transections. Delayed primary repair is performed within 5 to 7 days from injury and is best for avulsive-type injuries in which the zone of injury is initially not clear. A secondary repair is performed more than 7 days from the time of injury.

PRINCIPLES OF NERVE REPAIR

Quantitative preoperative and postoperative clinical assessment of both motor and sensory systems should include an assessment of pinch and grip strength. Microsurgical technique should be employed, including microscope, loupes, microsurgical instruments, and appropriate sutures. The repair must be tension free. An interposition nerve graft should be considered if a tension-free repair is not possible. An epineurial repair should be performed in nerves without well-defined fascicle groups. A grouped fascicular repair can be attempted when a fascicle is recognized as mediating a specific function. The most important factor affecting recovery after injury is the age of the patient. The recovery rate of nerve function after a gunshot wound is about 70%. Motor and sensory re-education is required postoperatively.

TYPES OF REPAIR

Epineurial

The fascicular or vascular landmarks are identified with the epineurial sleeves joined to oppose the contents in the correct orientation. After the nerve ends are trimmed, the axons should be aligned if possible. Tension is uniform, with additional sutures used sparingly.

Grouped Fascicular

Higher magnification is needed for a grouped fascicular repair. The nerve ends are inspected to determine alignment of fascicles so that fascicular groups are matched, trimmed, and repaired. Superiority of this technique has not been proved. The potential benefits of fascicular repair may be lost because of the increased surgical manipulation and repair of inappropriate fascicles. Fascicle matching techniques include intraoperative nerve stimulation and histochemical identification (acetylcholinesterase [for motor fibers], carbonic anhydrase [for sensory fibers]).

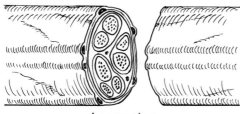

Laceration

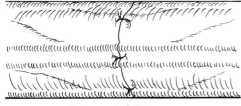

Epineurial Suture

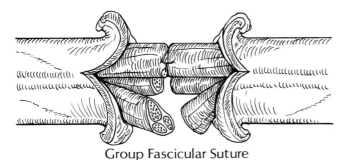

Group Fascicular Suture

Individual Fascicular Suture

Figure 5-14 ◆ Types of nerve suture techniques. *(From Green DP, Hotchkiss RN, Pederson WC, eds: Operative Hand Surgery, 4th ed. New York, Churchill Livingstone, 1999.)*

Nerve Grafts

PRINCIPLES OF NERVE GRAFTING

1. The nerve defect is the actual amount of tissue lost; nerve gap refers to the distance between proximal and distal nerve ends.
2. A nerve graft should be performed when an end-to-end repair cannot be performed without undue tension.
3. An ideal graft has large fascicles, little connective tissue, separate parallel fascicles, and large diameter.

In addition, it should have large-caliber axons, be in an accessible location, and have little variability and branching.
4. The functional outcome of the graft decreases as the length of the graft increases.
5. Donor nerves include sural, anterior branch of the medial antebrachial cutaneous, lateral antebrachial cutaneous, and terminal branch of the posterior interosseous nerve.
6. The Schwann cells in a nonvascularized intercalary nerve graft survive and later are replaced by Schwann cells migrating from the grafted nerve.
7. The role of vascularized nerve grafts has not been established, but potential indications include large nerve gaps, very proximal injuries, compromised tissue beds (irradiated tissue), and large-caliber donor nerve grafts.
8. Early tendon transfers should be considered for an extensive nerve gap that has a poor prognosis for functional recovery despite nerve grafting.
9. Autogenous vein conduits can also be used to bridge gaps of up to 3 cm in length.

Nerve Regeneration

1. Without specificity of reinnervation, there is a lack of functional recovery with axonal misdirection. Lack of functional recovery 6 months after repair is correlated with axonal misdirection at the site of injury. Mechanical alignment after surgery improves both contact recognition and neurotropic cues.
2. Neurotropism: diffusion of factors released from distal targets that guide axons to appropriate targets.
3. Neurotrophism: axons will grow randomly, but only axons entering the correct pathway or target will receive trophic factors allowing continued regeneration and myelination.
4. Muscle alterations contribute to the lack of motor recovery because of the loss of motor fiber units and the inability of muscle fibers to increase in size and to reverse atrophy. Long-term denervation results in loss of muscle fibers. Early tendon transfers should be considered if long-term denervation has occurred.

Brachial Plexus

Anatomy (Fig. 5-15)

1. The ventral primary rami of nerve roots C5 to T1 form a complex, predictable pattern of connections as the nerve roots travel from the spinal cord to the distal aspects of the upper extremity.
2. The brachial plexus is organized into roots, trunks, divisions, cords, and branches. If the C4 nerve root is included, the plexus is called prefixed. If the T2 nerve root is included, the plexus is called postfixed.
3. The plexus lies between the scalenus anterior and medius and deep to the clavicle. The axillary artery runs between the medial and lateral cords. An axillary block injection to best obtain anesthesia in the

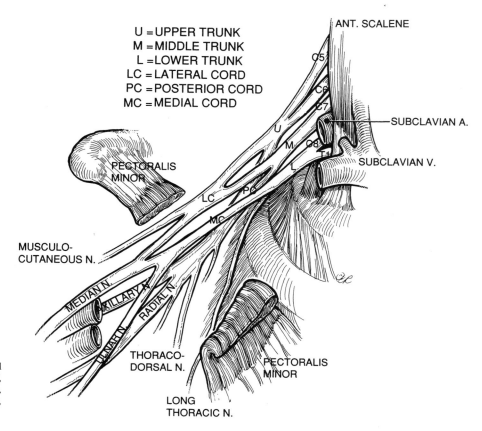

U = UPPER TRUNK
M = MIDDLE TRUNK
L = LOWER TRUNK
LC = LATERAL CORD
PC = POSTERIOR CORD
MC = MEDIAL CORD

ANT. SCALENE

SUBCLAVIAN A.

SUBCLAVIAN V.

PECTORALIS MINOR

MUSCULO-CUTANEOUS N.

MEDIAN N.

AXILLARY N.

ULNAR N.

RADIAL N.

THORACO-DORSAL N.

PECTORALIS MINOR

LONG THORACIC N.

Figure 5-15 ◆ Anatomy of the brachial plexus. *(From Green DP, Hotchkiss RN, Pederson WC, eds: Operative Hand Surgery, 4th ed. New York, Churchill Livingstone, 1999.)*

median distribution should be directed lateral to the artery.

4. There are three trunks (upper, middle, and lower), six divisions (anterior and posterior for each trunk), and three cords (medial, lateral, and posterior, named relative to the axillary artery).

5. There are four preclavicular branches from the roots and upper trunks: the dorsal scapular nerve (C5), the long thoracic nerve (C5-7), the suprascapular nerve (C5-6), and the nerve to the subclavius.

Injury

Injuries are most commonly grade V lesions. The low-energy injuries are more likely to be reversible injuries; high-energy injuries result in avulsion of nerve roots from spinal cord (Fig. 5-16).

CLINICAL ASSESSMENT

A thorough neurovascular examination of the extremity is essential.

1. Horner's sign indicates a severe injury to C8 and T1 nerve roots and is strongly correlated with root avulsions. It usually presents 3 to 4 days after injury as ptosis, meiosis, and anhidrosis. Horner's syndrome results from involvement of the preganglionic sympathetic fibers.

2. Supraganglionic injuries (root avulsions) have a worse prognosis than infraganglionic lesions do. Root avulsions are differentiated from infraganglionic lesions by the presence of Horner's syndrome,

denervation of muscles innervated by intradural nerve roots (paravertebral muscles, serratus anterior, rhomboids), and loss of motor and sensory nerve conduction (supraganglionic lesions may have intact sensory nerve conductions). The presence of Tinel's sign over the supraclavicular area is an indicator of a root avulsion. Severe pain with an anesthetic limb and a flail arm are also strong signs of a root avulsion.

RADIOGRAPHIC ASSESSMENT

1. Computed tomographic myelography is considered the current standard for imaging root avulsions. The presence of a pseudomeningocele is strongly correlated with root avulsion at a given level.

2. Magnetic resonance imaging may show the pseudomeningocele as increased signal intensity on T2-weighted images at the affected level because of increased water content. T1-weighted images highlight the fat content of the brachial plexus and may allow the detection of "empty sleeves" at the level of the cervical roots. In addition, magnetic resonance imaging may detect spinal cord edema.

3. Plain radiographs of the cervical spine should be obtained to rule out bone injury. Disruption of transverse processes of the cervical spine is indicative of root avulsions. Chest radiographs may reveal diaphragm paralysis due to phrenic nerve dysfunction, indicative of a severe injury to the upper roots of the plexus.

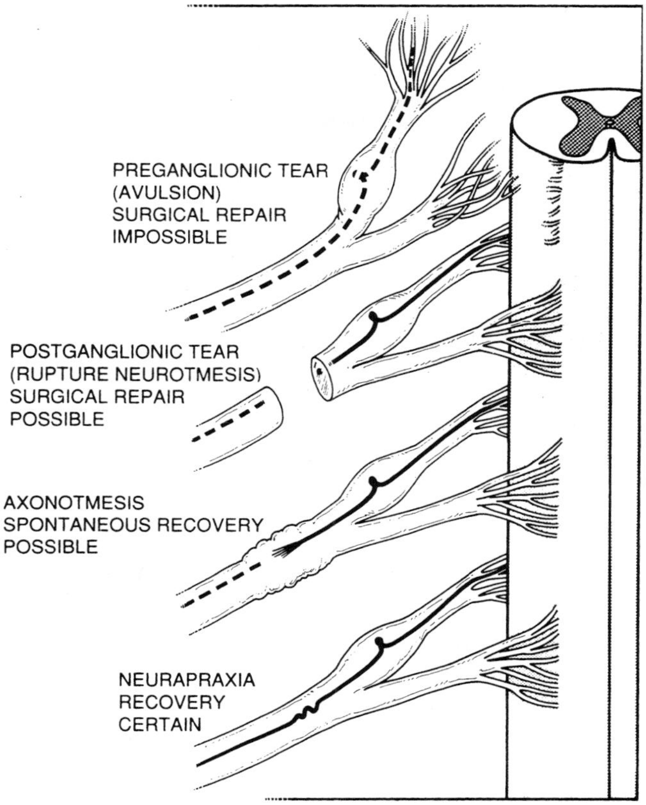
PREGANGLIONIC TEAR
(AVULSION)
SURGICAL REPAIR
IMPOSSIBLE
POSTGANGLIONIC TEAR
(RUPTURE NEUROTMESIS)
SURGICAL REPAIR
POSSIBLE
AXONOTMESIS
SPONTANEOUS RECOVERY
POSSIBLE
NEURAPRAXIA
RECOVERY
CERTAIN

Figure 5-16 ◈ Varying severity of brachial plexus traction injuries. The injury may involve avulsion of the nerve root from the spinal cord (not repairable), extraforaminal rupture of the root or trunk (surgically repairable), and intraneural rupture of fascicles (some spontaneous recovery possible). *(From Green DP, Hotchkiss RN, Pederson WC, eds: Operative Hand Surgery, 4th ed. New York, Churchill Livingstone, 1999.)*

Electrodiagnostic Studies

1. Sensory evoked potentials, corticosensory evoked potentials, and spinograms are more helpful than EMG and NCS and should be performed 3 to 6 weeks after injury to allow time for wallerian degeneration and spontaneous fibrillation potentials to occur.
2. Stimulation over Erb's point and signal recording of the cortex from scalp electrodes can provide evidence of root continuity. Positive recordings can demonstrate that the root is intact; negative recordings cannot discriminate avulsion from rupture. Spinograms detect level of innervation of paraspinous muscles. Because these muscles are innervated by posterior primary rami of the brachial plexus, this test is helpful in detecting proximal injury. None of these tests is usually conclusive.

Surgical Treatment

Timing of Surgery

1. Immediate intervention is considered in cases of penetrating or iatrogenic injury.
2. Early surgery (3 weeks to 3 months) is indicated if there is total or nearly total palsy or a high-energy injury. The patient should be evaluated regularly, and exploration is undertaken if recovery plateaus or Tinel's sign is not advancing. Advancement of Tinel's sign is the best indication of nerve function recovery.
3. Late surgery (3 to 6 months after injury) should be performed in patients who have not been showing continued improvement with their low-energy insult or who have an upper trunk lesion.
4. Chronic injuries in patients presenting 12 to 18 months from injury are usually not amenable to nerve repair or reconstructive procedures. Tendon transfers and functioning free tissue transfers in combination with shoulder or wrist fusion are the reconstructive options of choice.
5. Surgical intervention for an adult with a C8-T1 palsy is controversial because patients rarely recover intrinsic function. Therefore, early tendon transfer has been recommended for these patients.

Priorities for Repair or Reconstruction

1. Provision for elbow flexion by biceps or brachialis muscle is the main reconstructive priority. This can be achieved by neurotization of the musculocutaneous nerve, bipolar latissimus dorsi transfer, or Steindler flexoplasty.
2. Shoulder stabilization, abduction, and external rotation with axillary or suprascapular nerve reinnervation.
3. Arm adduction to chest with lateral pectoral nerve reinnervation.
4. Sensation below the elbow with reinnervation of lateral cord (C6-7 distribution).
5. Wrist extension and finger flexion by reinnervation of the lateral and posterior cords.

Donor Nerve Grafts

Donor nerve grafts include sural, medial brachial, antebrachial cutaneous nerves, and posterior interosseous nerve. Results are better with shorter distances to graft. Autologous fibrinogen may be used as nerve glue. A vascularized nerve graft can be considered for injuries including C8-T1 nerve root avulsion with large proximal stumps, with the ulnar nerve as the donor nerve based on the superior ulnar collateral artery.

Nerve Transfers

Extraplexal sources, such as spinal accessory nerve (1700 axons), intercostal nerves (1300 axons each), motor branches from C3 to C6 (3400 to 4000 axons), contralateral lateral pectoral nerve (400 to 600 axons), and contralateral C7 nerve root, can be used for neurotization of distal branches. Other experimental sources include the ulnar nerve and pectoral branches transferred into the musculocutaneous nerve. Nerve transfers can also be considered in the treatment of peripheral nerve injuries with significant gapping (>6 cm).

Results

Surgical repair or reconstruction does improve function. Infraclavicular lesions have a better prognosis than do supraclavicular injuries, and supraclavicular lesions do better with at least two repairable roots.

Obstetric Brachial Plexus Palsy

1. Obstetric palsy is usually due to a traction injury during delivery with the upper roots usually ruptured extraforaminally and the lower roots avulsed. Spontaneous recovery is possible, and early recovery of biceps by the second month is a good prognostic sign. Microneural repair with grafting or neurotization is possible.
2. Obstetric brachial plexus palsy is associated with higher birth weight (4 kg), breech presentation, cephalopelvic disproportion, prolonged labor, shoulder dystocia, and forceps delivery.
3. Classification
   a. Erb-Duchenne palsy involves C5-6 levels, so the shoulder will lack normal external rotation and abduction because the deltoid, rotator cuff, elbow flexors, and wrist or hand dorsiflexors are affected. This type has the best prognosis.
   b. Klumpke's palsy involves C8-T1, so the wrist flexors and intrinsics are affected. Horner's sign is present, and prognosis is poor.
   c. Complete plexus palsy affects the entire plexus and produces a flaccid upper extremity. This palsy has the worst prognosis.
4. Physical examination can differentiate between a complete palsy (flail limb) and upper root palsy or Erb's palsy (extremity internally rotated and adducted, forearm pronation, and wrist flexion). Sensory examination provides limited information. Biceps muscle function is a reliable indicator of recovery. Biceps function at 1 to 2 months of age is a good prognostic sign.
5. Muscle grading system: M0, no contraction; M1, contraction without movement; M2, contraction with slight movement; M3, complete movement.
6. If at 1 month there is complete palsy with Horner's sign, early surgery should be recommended, given the incidence of poor spontaneous recovery. Surgical exploration should be recommended for patients without evidence of biceps contraction at 3 months post partum.
7. Late surgical interventions involve contracture release and muscle and tendon rerouting (Table 5-4).

Brachial Neuritis (Parsonage-Turner Syndrome)

1. Brachial neuritis presents acutely with severe brachialgia and weakness. Sensory symptoms may be noted but are minimal and usually resolve.
2. Weakness usually involves the shoulder girdle, but distal weakness may occur. Muscle weakness in decreasing frequency includes deltoid, supraspinatus, infraspinatus, serratus anterior, biceps, and triceps. Weakness of the anterior interosseous nerve–innervated muscles can occur. Brachial neuritis should be considered in patients with suspected bilateral anterior interosseous nerve syndrome.
3. Viral and immunologic etiology has been proposed. Antibody titers for IgM and IgG ganglioside proteins may be increased.
4. EMG and NCS will show evidence of denervation, with positive sharp waves and fibrillations.
5. Symptoms typically resolve with observation, although complete restoration of strength is not always achieved. Overall recovery may take several years.

Reflex Sympathetic Dystrophy

Definition

Reflex sympathetic dystrophy (RSD) is also known as complex regional pain syndrome. RSD requires the

---

◆ **Table 5-4**		
TREATMENT RECOMMENDATIONS FOR OBSTETRIC PALSY		
Ruptured/Avulsed Roots	**Recipient Site**	**Functional Goal**
C5, 6/0	Superior trunk	Shoulder, elbow, wrist control
C5, 6, 7/0	Superior trunk	Above plus
	Middle trunk	Finger extension
C5, 6, 7/C8, T1	Posterior cord	Shoulder control
	Lateral cord	Elbow control
	Medial cord	Finger flexion + ?intrinsics
C5, 6/C7, 8, T1	Lateral cord	Elbow control
	Medial cord	Finger flexion + ?intrinsics
	?Suprascapular n.	Shoulder control
C5/C6, 7, 8, T1	Musculocutaneous n.	Elbow control
	Suprascapular n.	Shoulder control
	Intercostal n. 2–5 to lateral cord	Sensation
0/C8, T1	Graft from C6 to medial cord	Finger flexion + ?intrinsics
0/C5, 6	Graft from medial pectoral n. to musculocutaneous n.	Elbow control

From Green DP, Hotchkiss RN, Pederson WC, eds: Operative Hand Surgery, 4th ed. New York, Churchill Livingstone, 1999, p 1281.

presence of regional pain after a noxious event. Type I corresponds to classic RSD without any definitive nerve injury; type II (causalgia) refers to post-traumatic pain that occurs after identifiable nerve injury. RSD may be mediated sympathetically. The syndrome refers to abnormally severe and inappropriately prolonged manifestation of normal postinjury responses that may produce significant changes in end-organ anatomy and function. Some believe that it results from sustained efferent sympathetic nerve activity continued within a reflex arc.

Clinical Presentation

1. Patients are often between 30 and 50 years old, smokers, and female and have identifiable nerve injury 50% of the time. The most common injury for type I is distal radius and ulna fracture. Most common injuries for type II include injury to palmar cutaneous branch of the median nerve, superficial branch of the radial nerve, and dorsal branch of the ulnar nerve.
2. Symptoms include burning pain and restlessness early, pain out of proportion to identifiable injury, joint stiffness, discoloration, vasomotor and autonomic dysfunction, and atrophy.
3. Other signs include allodynia, hyperpathia, changes in nail and skin texture, abnormal sweating, and piloerection.
4. Three stages
   a. Swelling, warmth, hyperhidrosis.
   b. Brawny edema and trophic changes.
   c. Glossy cool dry skin with stiffness.

Diagnosis

1. The diagnosis of RSD is based on the presence of pain, functional impairment, and autonomic nervous system dysfunction.
2. Objective tests include use of monofilaments, dolorimetry, and computer-controlled stimuli to quantify the pain thresholds.
3. Plain radiographs demonstrate patchy osteopenia, which is initially periarticular and then diffuse in the region of interest.
4. Triple-phase bone scan is usually considered specific but not sensitive for the diagnosis.
5. Response is positive to intravenous administration of phentolamine mesylate (a mixed α_1- and α_2-antagonist), stellate ganglion block, and peripheral or epidural block.
6. Other tests include evaluation of thermoregulatory and nutritional blood flow to the region of interest with temperature, laser Doppler fluxmetry, and vital capillaroscopy. Sudomotor activity is monitored with resting sweat output, galvanic skin response, and quantitative sudomotor axon reflex test.

Treatment

1. The most important variable for successful treatment is early diagnosis; 80% will show improvement if treated within the first year of injury, and less than 50% will show any improvement if treated 1 year after injury.
2. Treatment has several components and includes physical and occupational therapy, medications (calcium channel blockers, antidepressants, anticonvulsants, corticosteroids), surgical sympathectomy, continuous autonomic blockades, dorsal column and periventricular gray matter stimulators, and biofeedback.
3. Chronic pain related to compression neuropathy is best treated with decompression. Amputation is usually limited to those with infection, intractable pain, and physical impairment secondary to contractures or mass effect.

Miscellaneous

Clenched Fist or Psycho-Flexed Hand Syndrome

This is a factitious disorder in which posturing of digits occurs in positions not explainable anatomically.

Syrinx

1. A syrinx is a fluid-filled cavity in the spinal cord (syringomyelia) or brainstem (syringobulbia).
2. Most are associated with hindbrain abnormalities of the Chiari type. Additional etiologic factors include spine trauma and tumors.
3. Clinical findings may include weakness, sensory changes, and spasticity.
4. The most common cause of neuropathic joints (Charcot) in the upper extremity is syringomyelia. This should be considered in cases of failed arthrodeses.

Cervical Spinal Cord Injury

1. Upper extremity surgery is considered after return of maximal function and psychological adjustment, which is approximately 12 months after injury.
2. Tetraplegic patients may be classified according to the lowest nerve root functioning considered as a fair or grade 4 muscle strength.
3. Operative procedures and splints appropriate for each level are reviewed in Chapter 13.

Bibliography

Antoniou J, et al: Suprascapular neuropathy. Variability in the diagnosis, treatment and outcome. Clin Orthop 386:131–138, 2001.

Archer DR, Dahlin LB, McLean WG: Changes in slow axonal transport of tubulin induced by local application of colchicines to rabbit vagus nerve. Acta Physiol Scand 150:57–65, 1994.

Bodine S, Lieber R: Peripheral nerve physiology, anatomy and pathology in orthopaedic basic science biology and mechanics of the musculoskeletal system. In Buckwalter J, Einhorn T, Simon S, eds: Orthopaedic Basic Surgery, 2nd ed. Rosemont, Ill, American Academy of Orthopaedic Surgeons, 2000, pp 617–682.

Brand PW: Biomechanics of tendon transfers. Hand Clin 4:137–154, 1988.

Campion D: Electrodiagnostic testing in hand surgery. J Hand Surg Am 21:947–956, 1996.

Dahlin LB, McClean WG: Effects of graded experimental compresson on slow and fast axonal transport in rabbit vagus nerve. J Neurol Sci 72:19–30, 1986.

Dahlin LB, Archer DR, McLean WG: Axonal transport and morphological changes following nerve compression: an experimental study in the rabbit vagus nerve. J Hand Surg Br 18:106–110, 1993.

Dellon AL, et al: Intraneural ulnar nerve pressure changes related to operative techniques for cubital tunnel decompression. J Hand Surg Am 19:923–930, 1994.

Diao E, Vannuyen T: Techniques for primary nerve repair. Hand Clin 16:53–66, viii, 2000.

Eversmann WW Jr: Tendon transfers for combined nerve injuries. Hand Clin 4:187–199, 1988.

Eversmann WW: Proximal median nerve compression. Hand Clin 8:307–315, 1992.

Gassmann M, Lemke G: Neuregulins and neuregulin receptors in neural development. Curr Opin Neurobiol 7:87–92, 1997.

Gelberman RH, et al: Results of treatment of severe carpal tunnel syndrome without internal neurolysis of the median nerve. J Bone Joint Surg Am 69:896–903, 1987.

Gilbert A, Brockman R, Carlioz H: Surgical treatment of brachial plexus birth palsy. Clin Orthop 264:39–47, 1991.

Gupta R, Villablanca PJ, Jones NF: Evaluation of an acute nerve compression injury with magnetic resonance neurography. J Hand Surg Am 26:1093–1099, 2001.

Kandel E, Schwartz J, Jessel T: Principles of Neural Science, 4th ed. McGraw-Hill, 2000, pp 243–252.

Lee SK, Wolfe SW: Peripheral nerve injury and repair. J Am Acad Orthop Surg 8:243–252, 2000.

Leffert RD: Thoracic outlet syndrome. J Am Acad Orthop Surg 2:317–325, 1994.

Lundborg G, et al: Trophism, tropism and specificity in nerve regeneration. J Reconstr Microsurg 10:345–354, 1994.

Lundborg G, Dahlin LB: Anatomy, function and pathophysiology of peripheral nerves and nerve compression. Hand Clin 12:185–193, 1996.

Millesi H, Meissl G, Berger A: Further experience with interfascicular grafting of the median, ulnar and radial nerves. J Bone Joint Surg Am 58:209–218, 1976.

Rempel D, Dahlin L, Lundborg G: Pathophysiology of nerve compression syndromes: response of peripheral nerves to loading. J Bone Joint Surg Am 81:1600–1610, 1999.

Seddon H: Three types of nerve injury. Brain 66:237–288, 1943.

Shum C, et al: The role of flexor tenosynovectomy in the operative treatment of carpal tunnel syndrome. J Bone Joint Surg Am 84A:221–225, 2002.

Stoll G, et al: Wallerian degeneration in the peripheral nervous system: participation of both Schwann cells and macrophages in myelin degradation. J Neurocytol 18:671–683, 1989.

Sunderland S: A classification of peripheral nerve injuries producing loss of function. Brain 74:491–516, 1951.

Syroid DE, et al: Cell death in the Schwann cell lineage and its regulations by neuregulin. Proc Natl Acad Sci USA 93:9229–9234, 1996.

Syroid DE, et al: Induction of postnatal Schwann cell death by the low-affinity neurotrophin reception in vitro and after axotomy. J Neurosci 20:5741–5747, 2000.

Trumble TE, McCallister WV: Repair of peripheral nerve defects in the upper extremity. Hand Clin 16:37–52, 2000.

Upton AR, McComas AJ: The double crush in nerve entrapment syndromes. Lancet 2(7825):359–362, 1973.

6

✧ Kent H. Chou, MD   ✧ Ioannis Sarris, MD, PhD

✧ Nikolaos G. Papadimitriou, MD, PhD   ✧ Dean G. Sotereanos, MD

FRACTURES OF THE HAND, WRIST, AND FOREARM AXIS

General Considerations

1. Initial evaluation of these injuries should include a history pertaining to the mechanism of injury, symptoms of sensory or motor dysfunction, and a history of previous injury. Information is obtained about handedness, occupation, medical history, and tetanus vaccination status in the case of open injuries.

2. On physical examination, the presence of intact sensation to light touch does not preclude subtle neurologic impairment, and two-point discrimination, normally 5 mm or less, should be routinely measured. Circulation is best documented by capillary refill time in the distal digit or nail bed; a time of less than 2 seconds is normal. The integrity of the adjacent flexor and extensor tendon structures is confirmed. Alignment of the digits in relation to each other is also assessed; in flexion, digital overlap should be minimal, and comparison to the contralateral side is helpful. Careful assessment of hand and forearm compartments should be routine. Skin integrity to rule out open fractures is also essential.

Open Fractures

1. Open fractures are treated with irrigation and débridement of necrotic tissue as well as bone stabilization when indicated.

2. In comparison to open fractures of the long bones, open fractures distal to the carpus are known to have a low risk of infection and thus mandate less aggressive operative intervention. In open fractures with limited soft tissue injury, irrigation and débridement can usually be performed under local anesthetic in the emergency department.

3. Open fractures can be graded according to the Gustilo classification of open fractures (Table 6-1).

4. Open injuries distal to the carpus that exhibit significant contamination or soft tissue devitalization and open fractures of the carpus, distal radius, and forearm are treated with emergent, formal operative irrigation and débridement and bone stabilization.

   a. Tetanus prophylaxis is administered when indicated (see Chapter 11).

   b. Appropriate antibiotic treatment is as follows:

      i. Grade I: first-generation cephalosporin.

      ii. Grade II: first-generation cephalosporin.

      iii. Grade IIIA, IIIB: first-generation cephalosporin and gentamycin.

      iv. Grade IIIC: first-generation cephalosporin, gentamycin, and penicillin.

5. Risk of infection after open fractures of the hand is increased as the magnitude of the overlying soft tissue injury increases. Other factors that lead to infection include systemic illness, severe wound contamination, and delay in treatment of more than 24 hours.

6. Poor outcomes after open injuries are most closely correlated with associated soft tissue injuries.

Compartment Syndrome

1. Compartment syndrome in forearm fractures can be seen in the setting of open fractures, gunshot wounds, vascular injuries, and coagulopathy.

2. Compartment syndrome occurs when the end-capillary perfusion pressure is less than the pressure within the compartment.

✧ **Table 6-1**

OPEN FRACTURE CLASSIFICATION
Gustilo Classification

I		Wound less than 1 cm
II		Wound greater than 1 cm with moderate soft tissue damage
		High-energy wound greater than 10 cm with extensive soft tissue damage
III	IIIA	Adequate soft tissue coverage
	IIIB	Inadequate soft tissue coverage
	IIIC	Associated with arterial injury; farm injuries

3. The diagnosis of compartment syndrome is made clinically. Patients affected have pain out of proportion to the injury; pain on passive finger extension is the most sensitive finding. The compartments are typically tense to palpation. Other findings include pallor, paresthesias, and paralysis. In addition, intrinsic muscle tightness may develop. Pulselessness rarely occurs.

4. Measurement of compartment pressures is used as an adjuvant to diagnosis, particularly in obtunded or unresponsive patients. Pressures in excess of 30 to 40 mm Hg are indicative of a compartment syndrome. A lower pressure threshold for release should be applied for hypotensive patients.

5. Emergent surgical treatment in the form of fasciotomies of all affected compartments is critical.

   a. There are three main compartments in the forearm—volar, dorsal, and mobile wad compartments. In addition, a pronator quadratus compartment has been described. Treatment includes release of all compartments, and there is evidence that release of the volar compartment leads to pressure reduction in the other compartments.

   b. There are 10 separate compartments in the hand—dorsal interossei (n = 4), volar interossei (n = 3), thenar, hypothenar, and thumb adductor. The carpal tunnel, although not a true muscle compartment, should also be released routinely.

   c. Wound closure is delayed until pressures are normalized. Skin grafting may be necessary to achieve wound closure.

6. In addition to soft tissue or bone trauma, compartment syndrome can occur after high-voltage electrical injuries and snake (pit viper) bites. Surgical management of the compartment syndrome in these patients is similar.

Splinting

Splinting of hand fractures should generally be in the position of function: 20 degrees of extension at the wrist, 60 to 70 degrees of flexion at the metacarpophalangeal (MP) joints, and full extension at the proximal interphalangeal (PIP) and distal interphalangeal (DIP) joints. When necessary, the thumb MP joint is immobilized in palmar abduction.

Distal Phalanx Fractures

1. The distal phalanx is the most commonly fractured bone in the hand.

2. These fractures are often the result of a crushing injury and may be accompanied by significant soft tissue disruption (Fig. 6-1).

   a. The presence of subungual hematoma suggests nail bed disruption, which may require repair (see Chapter 3).

   b. Subungual hematoma formation is common and can be decompressed if the pressure in the subungual space is severely painful.

   c. If necessary, the nail bed can be repaired and the nail bed irrigated, inspected, and repaired with 6-0 or 7-0 suture under digital or wrist block anesthesia. The nail is washed and replaced to act as a biologic splint after nail bed repair.

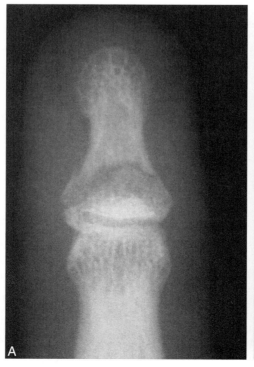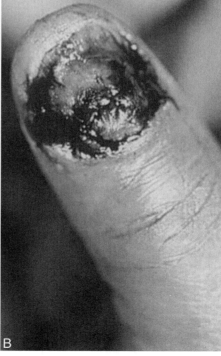

Figure 6-1 ◆ **A,** Fracture of the distal phalanx after a crush injury to the fingertip. **B,** Clinical appearance of the digit after removal of the nail plate revealing a significant nail bed injury.

Piercing the removed nail with a large-gauge needle one or more times before replacement can prevent recurrence of hematoma. The proximal portion of the nail should be reinserted into the nail fold to prevent premature scarring of the eponychium to the germinal matrix. In the absence of a salvageable nail, reinforced silicone sheeting, a piece of nonadherent gauze, or a commercial nail substitute may be placed temporarily into the nail fold.

3. Most distal phalanx tuft fractures do not require manipulation or fixation. Treatment generally consists of digital splinting for 3 to 4 weeks, allowing interphalangeal joint motion to prevent stiffness. Grossly displaced and unstable shaft fractures can be treated with closed reduction and percutaneous pinning. Open fractures of the distal phalanx are treated with irrigation and débridement.

4. Radiographic evidence of healing can be slow and may take months to occur. Even in the absence of bone bridging, most tuft fractures go on to asymptomatic fibrous union that does not require treatment.

5. Common complications include cold intolerance, altered sensibility, and nail plate deformity.

6. Articular fractures often involve extensor or flexor tendon disruption (see Chapter 2).

   a. Fractures involving the dorsal aspect of the articular surface are often extensor tendon avulsion fractures. Most of these injuries can be treated with DIP extension splinting (mallet splint) for 6 weeks. Consideration should be given to fracture fixation if there is DIP joint subluxation or if the fracture fragment is more than 50% of the articular surface.

   b. Fractures involving the volar aspect of the articular surface are often flexor digitorum profundus avulsion fractures. These are treated with bone or tendon reattachment to the distal phalanx.

Middle and Proximal Phalanx Fractures

Phalangeal Base Fractures

Fractures at the base of the proximal and middle phalanges can be either extra-articular or intra-articular (Fig. 6-2).

EXTRA-ARTICULAR FRACTURES

1. Nondisplaced or minimally displaced fractures can be treated with closed reduction and splint or cast immobilization. Adequate reduction is important because imbalance of the extensor mechanism can lead to a symptomatic extensor lag.

2. Displaced, unstable fractures can be treated with closed reduction and percutaneous pinning. Open reduction and internal fixation (ORIF) should be considered for irreducible and combined injuries (e.g., fractures with associated tendon muscle, skin, and/or neurovascular injuries) to allow early motion.

INTRA-ARTICULAR FRACTURES

1. Fractures of the base of the middle phalanx can be nondisplaced, volar or dorsal lip fractures

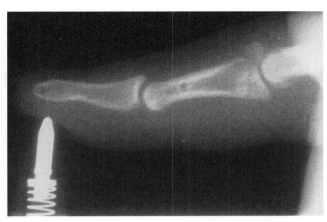

Figure 6-2 ◈ Lateral radiograph of an intra-articular fracture of the base of the middle phalanx.

associated with PIP joint instability, or comminuted (pilon fractures).

   a. Nondisplaced or minimally displaced fractures may be treated with buddy taping and early range of motion.

   b. Articular fractures associated with PIP joint instability are discussed in Chapter 7.

   c. Pilon fractures are comminuted and often the result of axial injuries. These can be technically difficult to reconstruct. Surgical options include ORIF with miniplates and screws and static and dynamic spanning external fixators (Fig. 6-3). Depressed intra-articular fractures may also require elevation of the articular surface and bone grafting.

2. Fractures of the base of the proximal phalanx can be nondisplaced, collateral ligament avulsion fractures, T or Y displaced, or comminuted (pilon fractures).

   a. Nondisplaced or minimally displaced fractures may be treated with buddy taping and early range of motion.

   b. Collateral ligament avulsion fractures that are displaced more than 1 to 2 mm are candidates for surgical repair with percutaneous pinning or ORIF with a minifragment screw.

   c. Displaced articular and comminuted fractures typically require surgical fixation in the form of pinning or ORIF to restore congruity to the articular surface. In addition to ORIF, surgical options include static or dynamic joint-spanning external fixators. These depressed intra-articular fractures may also require bone grafting.

Phalangeal Shaft Fractures

1. The location of the fracture, by virtue of the site of tendinous attachments, determines the angulation of the fracture in the sagittal plane.

   a. Fractures of the proximal phalanx tend to assume an *apex volar* angulation because of a flexion force of the proximal fragment exerted by the insertion of the interossei muscles and

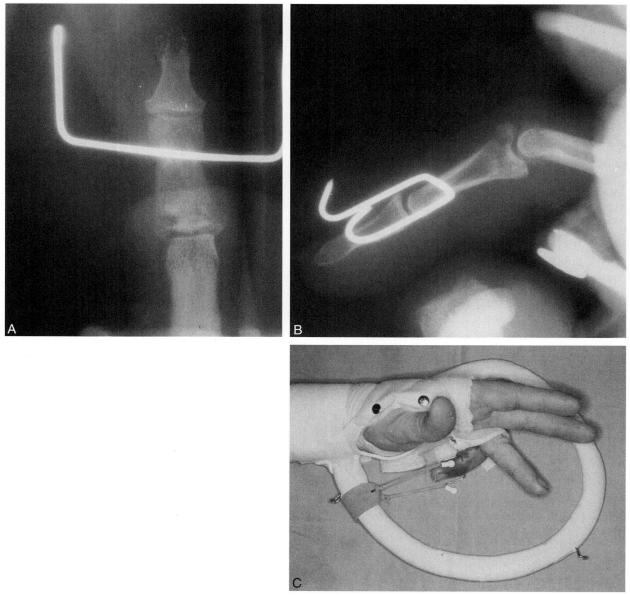

Figure 6-3 ◆ Fracture in Figure 6-2 after treatment with an assembled dynamic traction apparatus; anteroposterior **(A)** and lateral **(B)** radiographs of the digit in traction and photograph **(C)** of the traction apparatus.

an extension force of the distal fragment by the central slip insertion into the dorsum of the middle phalanx.

b. Fractures of the middle phalanx proximal to or at the flexor digitorum superficialis (FDS) insertion tend to assume an *apex dorsal* angulation because of an extension force of the proximal fragment exerted by the insertion of the central slip into the proximal aspect of the middle phalanx and a flexion force of the distal fragment by the insertion of the FDS.

c. Fractures of the middle phalanx distal to the FDS insertion tend to assume an *apex volar* angulation because of a flexion force of the proximal fragment exerted by the insertion of the FDS and an extension force of the distal fragment by the terminal tendon insertion into the dorsum of the distal phalanx.

2. The assessment of digital rotation (particularly with the fingers in flexion) is critical after these injuries because any degree of malrotation can lead to digital overlap and significant functional disability (Fig. 6-4).

3. These fractures can be classified with regard to degree of displacement and according to fracture pattern as transverse, oblique, spiral, or comminuted.

NONOPERATIVE TREATMENT

a. Nondisplaced or minimally displaced fractures can be treated with casting or buddy taping and progressive range-of-motion exercises as long as

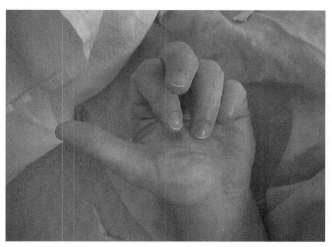

Figure 6-4 ❖ Digital overlap in a patient with a middle phalanx malunion of the long finger.

they are observed radiographically to determine displacement in the healing period.

b. Displaced fractures that can be closed reduced and are stable after reduction are treated with cast immobilization for 3 to 4 weeks. Adequate reduction implies no rotational deformity and no more than 10 degrees of angulation in the sagittal plane; greater angulation can interfere with flexor and extensor tendon balance and function.

OPERATIVE FIXATION

Oblique, spiral, and comminuted fractures tend to be unstable and in spite of an adequate reduction initially have a high propensity for displacement (Fig. 6-5). Unstable fractures require operative fixation in the form of percutaneous pinning, ORIF, or external fixation.

1. Percutaneous pinning after closed reduction can be achieved with crossed or intramedullary K-wires. Intramedullary fixation is most appropriate for transverse fractures (Fig. 6-6).
2. ORIF can be performed through a dorsal or a midaxial approach. The dorsal approach may be further subdivided into the central or tendon-splitting approach and the parasagittal approach, which uses the interval between the central tendon and lateral band. Techniques of internal fixation include use of minifragment screws and plates, K-wire fixation, and interosseous wiring.
   a. Interfragmentary compression screws provide the best resistance to torsion and cantilever bending in spiral and long oblique fractures compared with K-wires and plates.
      i. The length of the fracture should be at least the same as two diameters of the bone.
      ii. Screws placed at 90 degrees perpendicular to the long axis of the bone help resist longitudinal forces; screws placed at 90 degrees perpendicular to the

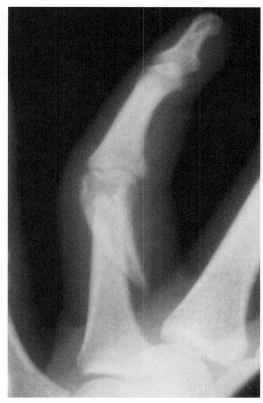

Figure 6-5 ❖ Anteroposterior radiograph of an unstable, long oblique, proximal phalangeal shaft fracture.

help resist torsional forces. For this reason, actual screw placement should be somewhere in between the two.
      iii. At least two screws should be placed for each fracture.
      iv. Screws should be placed at least two screw diameters from the edge of the fracture to prevent fracture propagation.

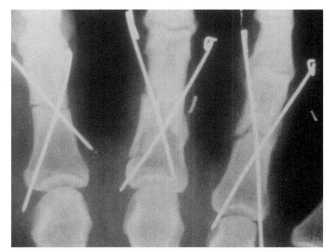

Figure 6-6 ❖ Anteroposterior radiograph of multiple phalangeal shaft fractures treated with crossed K-wires.

v. Self-tapping miniscrews have been developed. There are no disadvantages to their use, and they provide ease of insertion.
b. The bending strength of a plate is proportional to the cube of its thickness and inversely proportional to the cube of its length.
c. If rigid fixation is obtained, an early postoperative motion protocol can be established.
3. External fixation is indicated when there is severe soft tissue injury, excessive contamination, or segmental bone loss.

Phalangeal Neck Fractures

Neck fractures are uncommon in adults but tend to be more unstable than their diaphyseal counterparts. Surgical fixation in the form of crossed or intramedullary pinning is often needed to maintain reduction. Mini condylar plating and interosseous wiring may also be appropriate, depending on the nature of the fracture.

Phalangeal Condylar Fractures

1. Of all phalangeal fractures, condylar fractures carry the worst prognosis, with flexion contracture and post-traumatic arthritis being the most common complications. Regardless of the form of treatment, anatomic reduction of the fracture is critical.
2. Phalangeal condylar fractures are classified as type I (unicondylar, nondisplaced), type II (unicondylar, displaced), and type III (bicondylar).
   a. Unicondylar fractures (types I and II) can be subclassified according to the plane of the fracture line (volar, sagittal, and coronal).
3. Minimally displaced condylar fractures may be treated closed with digital splinting for 7 to 10 days, followed by buddy taping and early motion. Close radiographic follow-up is essential.
4. Displaced fractures require ORIF to allow anatomic reduction and to permit early motion.
   a. Unicondylar fractures tend to be rotationally unstable because of the pull of the collateral ligament on the condylar fragment. Secure fixation may be provided by two 0.035 K-wires or minifragment screws through both condyles (Fig. 6-7).
   b. The problem of lateral and rotational displacement is compounded in bicondylar fractures, making closed reduction extremely difficult. These fractures can be fixed with one or two minifragment plates placed laterally so as not to interfere with the extensor mechanism. Mini condylar plates can also be useful in this setting.

Metacarpal Fractures

Metacarpal Base Fractures

Thumb

1. The affected patient is usually young and male. The mechanism of injury involves an axial load on a partially flexed thumb.

2. A true lateral radiograph as well as a Robert's or true anteroposterior view of the thumb taken with the forearm in maximum pronation is essential for adequate characterization of the fracture and to rule out carpometacarpal (CMC) subluxation or dislocation.
3. Two major types of thumb metacarpal base fractures are described: extra-articular, or epibasal, and intra-articular. Intra-articular fractures can be subclassified as Bennett's and Rolando's fractures, depending on the articular fracture pattern. Fractures with severe intra-articular comminution are sometimes considered separately.

Extra-articular Fractures
Extra-articular fractures carry the best prognosis and can usually be treated with closed reduction and immobilization in a thumb spica cast for 3 to 4 weeks. Percutaneous pinning or ORIF is reserved for widely displaced or unstable oblique fractures. As much as 30 degrees of angulation and 3 to 4 mm of shortening can be acceptable, given the substantial mobility of the thumb CMC joint.

Intra-articular Fractures
1. Bennett's fracture represents an intra-articular fracture-dislocation of the CMC joint of the thumb (Fig. 6-8).
   a. A fragment of variable size of the volar and ulnar aspect of the metacarpal articular surface remains attached to the anterior oblique or beak ligament and stays in its normal position. Because this ligament is the primary stabilizer of the CMC joint, the rest of the metacarpal and thumb become subluxated from the trapezium.
   b. Deforming forces include adductor pollicis and abductor pollicis longus. These two combine to supinate, adduct, and flex the metacarpal shaft.
   c. Surgical treatment of the fracture in the form of closed reduction and percutaneous pinning is generally sufficient. The pins can be placed across the fracture site into the trapezium or the index metacarpal.
   d. If adequate reduction cannot be achieved with closed manipulation of the fracture, ORIF with K-wires or minifragment screws and plates can be used. Rupture of the collateral ligaments of the MP joints can also be seen in association with this injury.
   e. After surgical fixation, the relationship between joint congruence and subsequent degenerative change is unclear. Unlike in other articular fractures, joint surface displacement appears to be tolerated, probably owing to the lack of constraint of the joint architecture.
2. Rolando's fracture is characterized by a Y- or T-shaped fracture-dislocation of the CMC joint of the thumb.
   a. Like Bennett's variant, there is a volar fragment remaining attached to the trapezium by the anterior oblique ligament.
   b. Fixation of this and other comminuted thumb metacarpal base fractures is difficult and may

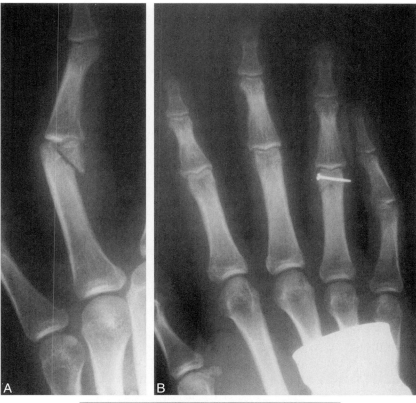

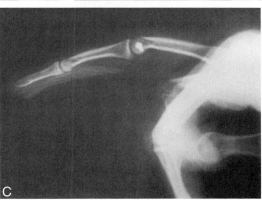

Figure 6-7 ◈ **A,** Anteroposterior radiograph of a unicondylar, unstable fracture of the proximal phalanx. **B** and **C,** Anteroposterior and lateral radiographs of the fracture treated by miniscrew fixation with restoration of the articular surface.

consist of variable combinations of ORIF, percutaneous pinning, external fixation, traction, and bone grafting, depending on the size and geometry of the fracture fragments.

SMALL FINGER

See Chapter 7.
1. Metacarpal base fracture-dislocations of the small finger CMC joint are not uncommon and typically are the result of indirect trauma. A "reversed Bennett's" fracture pattern most commonly occurs with a volar-radial articular fragment left in situ with dorsal dislocation of the remainder of the metacarpal in continuity with the majority of the articular surface.
2. Diagnosis can be difficult, and a 30-degree pronated radiograph can help in diagnosis.

3. Treatment can most often be achieved with closed reduction and percutaneous pinning and ORIF for comminuted fractures.

Metacarpal Shaft Fractures

1. These fractures can be classified with regard to degree of displacement and according to fracture pattern as transverse, oblique, spiral, or comminuted.
2. Nondisplaced or minimally displaced fractures can be treated with casting for 4 to 5 weeks in a short-arm cast. Functional casting with the digits free is also acceptable and allows earlier return to work and activity.
3. Unstable or displaced fractures can be treated with closed reduction and casting, percutaneous pinning, ORIF, or external fixation.

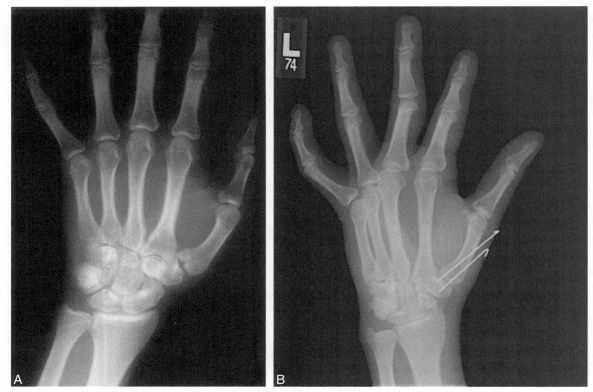

Figure 6-8 ❖ **A,** Anteroposterior radiograph of an articular fracture of the base of the thumb metacarpal (Bennett's fracture). **B,** Treatment with K-wire fixation.

a. Fractures that should be considered for reduction are those with
   i. rotational deformities leading to digital overlap on attempted finger flexion; 5 degrees of malrotation can result in 1.5 cm of digital overlap in flexion.
   ii. shortening of more than 4 to 5 mm because it can lead to imbalance between the intrinsic and extrinsic tendon systems.
   iii. more than 20 degrees of angulation on the sagittal plane (30 degrees for the ring and small fingers because of increased mobility at the CMC joints). Excessive volar angulation can result in prominence of the metacarpal head in the palm, disturbing grip. In addition, excessive angulation results in weakened grip, hyperextension of the MP joint, loss of extension at the PIP joint, and cosmetic deformity.
b. Oblique, spiral, and comminuted fractures tend to be unstable and in spite of an adequate reduction initially have a high propensity for displacement and should have close radiographic follow-up after closed reduction. Displacement is typically secondary to the proximal and volar pull of the intrinsics, and thus most displace with apex dorsal angulation.
c. Non-border (long and ring fingers) fractures tend to be more stable than their border counterparts because of the stabilizing effects of the adjacent

metacarpals, investing interossei and lumbrical muscles, and intermetacarpal ligaments.
d. Radiographic evaluation should include a 30-degree pronated lateral view for index and long metacarpal fractures and a 30-degree supinated lateral view for the ring and small metacarpals. The long and ring metacarpals tend to shorten less because of the tethering effect of the deep transverse intermetacarpal ligaments.
4. Indications for ORIF include displaced fractures not adequately reduced by closed manipulation, open fractures, and multiple metacarpal fractures. Operative approach for ORIF is usually through dorsal, longitudinal incisions between the metacarpal shafts. The juncturae tendinum can be divided for exposure and tagged for later repair. The incision can be curved proximally toward a CMC joint of interest. Exposure of the metacarpal heads is accomplished by splitting the extensor mechanism in the midline or through the radial sagittal band because the radial side offers slightly better exposure than the ulnar side.
a. Interfragmentary screws should be less than one-third the width of the fracture spike to avoid iatrogenic comminution.
b. Plate fixation alone with a minifragment plate generally requires four cortices of fixation on either side of the fracture and is appropriate only when the overlying soft tissue envelope is intact (Fig. 6-9).

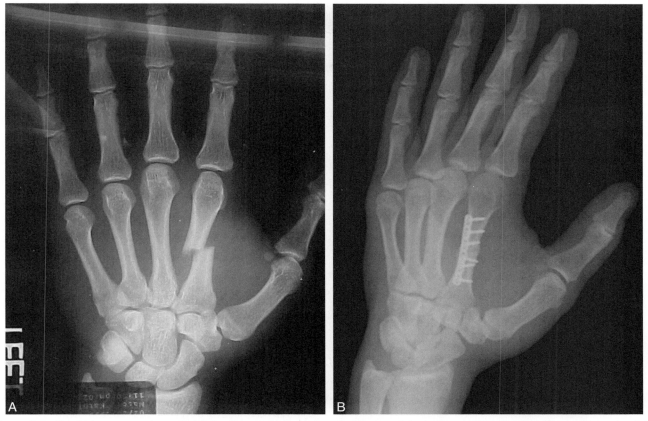

Figure 6-9 ❖ **A,** Anteroposterior radiograph of an unstable, transverse fracture of the index metacarpal. **B,** Oblique radiograph of the fracture treated by ORIF with a miniplate and screws. The fracture is healed.

c. Dorsally placed plates act as a tension band in the presence of an intact volar cortex but may interfere with gliding of the overlying extensor tendon.

d. If rigid fixation is obtained, an early postoperative motion protocol can be established.

5. External fixation can be considered if the surrounding soft tissue is severely compromised, as in crush or burn injuries, and in fractures with segmental bone loss.

6. Bone grafting may be required in any fracture configuration if there is comminution or bone loss.

7. Rotational malunions that are symptomatic should be treated with derotational osteotomies.

Metacarpal Neck Fractures

1. The fifth and fourth metacarpals are most commonly affected; this fracture is commonly known as boxer's fracture and almost always results from axial loading of a clenched fist (Fig. 6-10).

2. Apex dorsal angulation is the usual deformity due to the force of the intrinsic muscles.

3. The amount of angulation that can be tolerated increases from the index to the small finger because of increased mobility at the CMC joints of the ulnar digits.

a. Acceptable angulation: index, 10 degrees; long, 20 degrees; ring, 30 degrees; small, 40 degrees.

b. There is some controversy in the literature as to how much angulation is acceptable, probably due to the poor reliability of measuring angulation on the lateral radiograph. Digital malrotation is commonly an indication for surgical treatment of these injuries.

c. Excessive angulation may result in prominence of the metacarpal head in the palm, affecting power grip.

d. Rotational deformity as assessed by digital overlap with digit flexion can occur.

4. Most of these injuries can be treated with closed reduction and casting for 3 to 4 weeks. The reduction maneuver is performed by first flexing the MP joint to 90 degrees to relax the intrinsics and to tighten the collateral ligaments, then exerting dorsal pressure on the distal metacarpal through the flexed proximal phalanx while simultaneously exerting volar pressure at the fracture site.

5. Displaced or unstable fractures can be treated with reduction and percutaneous pinning or ORIF.

6. Open fractures should be presumed to be the result of a human bite and are treated with aggressive irrigation and débridement and adequate

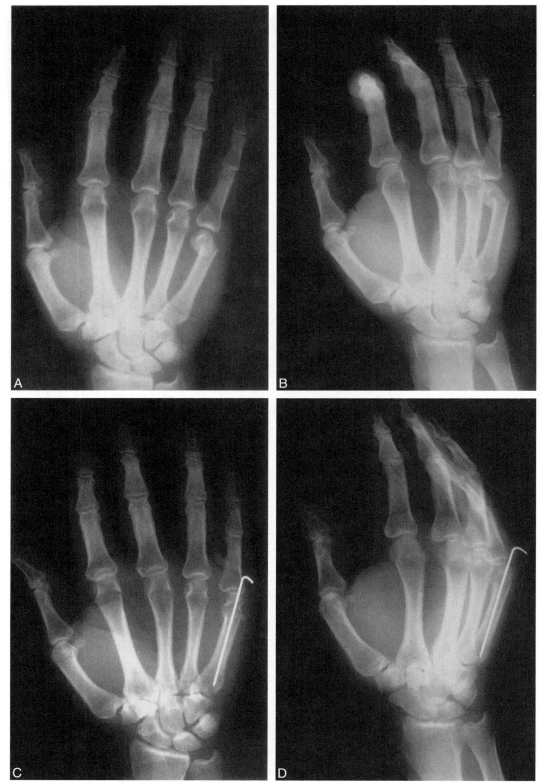

Figure 6-10 ◈ **A** and **B,** Anteroposterior and oblique radiographs of an angulated small metacarpal neck fracture (boxer's fracture). **C** and **D,** Anteroposterior and oblique radiographs after closed reduction and pinning with a single K-wire.

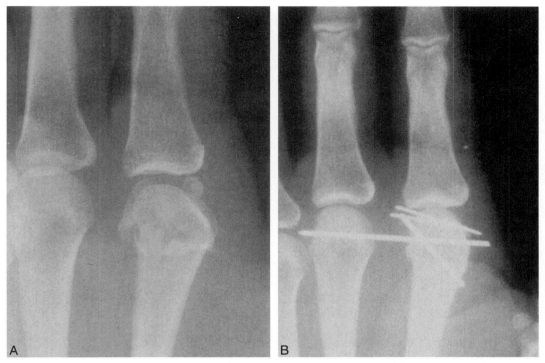

Figure 6-11 ❖ **A** and **B,** Anteroposterior radiographs of a metacarpal head fracture treated by ORIF with multiple K-wires.

intravenous antibiotics (see Chapter 11), followed by wound care, repeated irrigation and débridement, and surgical fixation if indicated.

Metacarpal Head Fractures

1. Fractures of the metacarpal head are rare but difficult to treat; some element of MP stiffness is almost inevitable regardless of treatment modality.
2. In addition to the standard posteroanterior, lateral, and oblique views, radiographic evaluation should include a Brewerton view, taken with the MP joints flexed 60 to 70 degrees, the dorsal surfaces of the digits placed flat on the x-ray cassette, and the beam angled 15 degrees radial, to rule out collateral ligament avulsion fractures. A skyline view may help delineate the articular surface of the metacarpal head. Computed tomographic (CT) scans may also be obtained if the degree of intra-articular incongruity is questionable.
3. As with other intra-articular fractures, the goal of surgical treatment is restoration of articular congruity with sufficient rigidity to permit early mobilization.
4. Open reduction to restore articular congruity followed by K-wire or plate and screw fixation is typically necessary (Fig. 6-11). Small conventional screws recessed beneath the articular surface or headless compression screws should also be considered. Fractures too comminuted for rigid fixation may be treated with joint-spanning external fixation, silicone arthroplasty in carefully selected patients, MP joint arthrodesis, or early motion alone.

5. Open fractures of the metacarpal head are treated with irrigation and débridement, followed by staged internal fixation if necessary.
6. Associated injuries include base fractures of the proximal phalanx and dorsal MP joint dislocations. In addition to stiffness, focal or global avascular necrosis (AVN) of the metacarpal head can compromise final outcomes, especially in young adults.

Carpal Fractures

Scaphoid Fractures

1. Scaphoid fractures classically follow a fall onto an outstretched hand and present with anatomic snuffbox tenderness on physical examination.
2. Fractures of the waist or middle third are by far the most common in adults; distal third fractures are more common in children (Fig. 6-12). Associated injuries may include fractures of the distal radius, radial head, first metacarpal base, and trapezium.
3. Scaphoid fractures may also be present in perilunate injury patterns (see Chapter 7).
4. Radiographic evaluation includes posteroanterior, lateral, and ulnar deviation (scaphoid) views of the wrist centered on the scaphoid.
   a. The sensitivity of fracture detection with the standard radiographic series in the acute setting is moderate at best.
   b. The 45-degree pronation and supination oblique views may increase sensitivity.

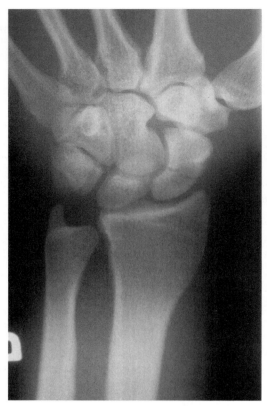

Figure 6-12 ◆ Posteroanterior radiograph of the wrist revealing a nondisplaced waist fracture of the scaphoid.

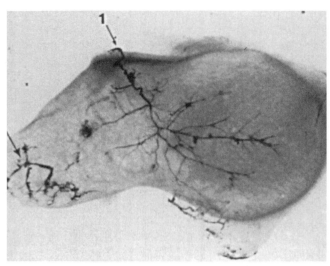

Figure 6-13 ◆ Vascular anatomy of the scaphoid. Sagittal section of the scaphoid (proximal pole on the left) reveals dorsal (1, dorsal scaphoid branch of the radial artery) and volar (2) osseous branches to the scaphoid. *(From Gelberman RH, Menon J: The vascularity of the scaphoid bone. J Hand Surg Am 5:508-513, 1980.)*

    c. Patients with suggestive findings on history and clinical examination but with normal radiographs are treated empirically in a thumb spica splint or cast, followed by repeated radiographs in 7 to 14 days.

    d. If follow-up films are also normal, further studies, such as bone scan, CT scan, or magnetic resonance imaging (MRI), should be obtained.

5. Scaphoid fractures are commonly classified by location and chronicity because both have significant implications with regard to prognosis. Nonunion and AVN are more common in proximal pole fractures, given the predominantly retrograde blood supply of the scaphoid.

    a. The dorsal scaphoid branches of the radial artery enter through the nonarticular dorsal ridge and the distal tubercle, supplying 70% to 80% of the bone, including the proximal pole.

    b. A second group of vessels arising from the volar scaphoid branches of the radial artery enters through the scaphoid tubercle to supply the distal 20% to 30% of the bone (Fig. 6-13).

6. Fracture pattern also has prognostic significance. Oblique or vertical fractures are known to be more difficult to treat than their horizontal counterparts.

7. Instability in scaphoid fractures is defined by the following:

    a. Fracture displacement greater than 1 mm (Fig. 6-14).

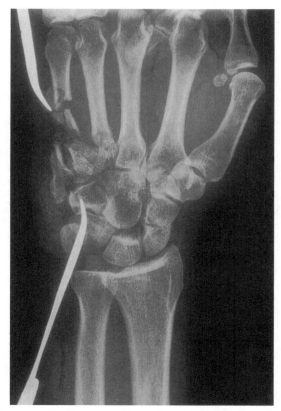

Figure 6-14 ◆ Posteroanterior radiograph of the wrist and hand revealing a displaced (>1 mm) waist fracture of the scaphoid. Note associated small metacarpal fracture.

b. Fracture angulation: scapholunate angle greater than 60 degrees (normally 30 to 60 degrees), or radiolunate or capitolunate angle greater than 15 degrees (normally 0 to ±15 degrees).

TREATMENT

Nondisplaced Fractures

1. Stable distal pole fractures are immobilized in a short- or long-arm thumb spica cast for 8 to 12 weeks.
2. Stable waist fractures can be managed in a long-arm thumb spica cast for 6 weeks followed by short-arm thumb spica casting for another 6 weeks or until union is achieved. The long-arm cast prevents forearm rotation that is known to create motion at the fracture site and decreases time to bony union.
3. Proximal pole fractures are notoriously difficult to treat closed and may require as long as 20 weeks to heal without operative intervention.
4. Stable fractures in which the diagnosis has been delayed should still be treated with a trial of cast immobilization.
5. Splints and casts are applied with the wrist in mild flexion and radial deviation to relax the radial collateral ligament of the wrist and aid in fracture reduction.

Unstable or Displaced Fractures

Unstable or displaced fractures require surgical fixation.

1. Surgical options include closed reduction and percutaneous pinning, closed reduction and percutaneous compression screw insertion, and ORIF with a compression screw.

a. Distal pole fractures are best approached volarly; proximal pole and waist fractures are best approached dorsally.
b. Union is most predictably achieved with a single compression screw placed beneath the articular surface (Fig. 6-15). Closed, arthroscopic, or open reduction may be required, depending on displacement and comminution.
c. Primary bone grafting should be considered in comminuted fractures.
d. Central screw placement results in improved mechanical properties of the fracture.
2. Surgical fixation should be considered for fractures not healed after 20 weeks of closed treatment.

FRACTURE HEALING

1. Assessment of fracture healing can be difficult. CT scans are a valuable adjunct obtained before the discontinuation of immobilization if union is in question.
2. With proper management, nearly 100% of distal pole fractures, 80% to 90% of waist fractures, and 60% to 70% of proximal pole fractures go on to bone union.
   a. Delay in diagnosis by more than 28 days is associated with a much higher incidence of nonunion.

SCAPHOID NONUNION

1. Ununited fractures are characterized radiographically by sclerosis, cyst formation, flexion (humpback) deformity of the scaphoid due to the flexed

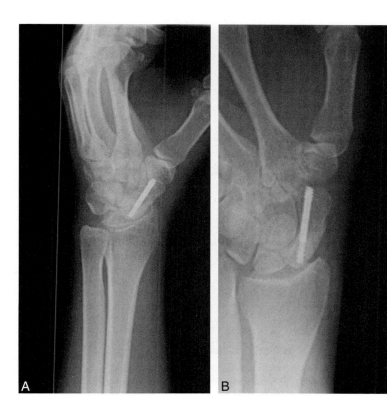

Figure 6-15 ◈ Oblique **(A)** and scaphoid **(B)** view radiographs of a waist fracture of the scaphoid treated by ORIF with a Herbert compression screw. The fracture is healed.

posture of the distal fragment, and dorsal intercalated segment instability deformity of the wrist.

2. This change in carpal mechanics as a result of scaphoid nonunion leads to a recognizable pattern of instability and articular degeneration of the wrist joint termed the SNAC (scaphoid nonunion advanced collapse) wrist (see Chapter 9).

Treatment

Fracture nonunions can be treated with cancellous, corticocancellous, or vascularized bone grafting in conjunction with internal fixation (compression screw).

1. Nondisplaced nonunions can be treated with cancellous grafting from a volar approach (Russe technique).
2. Displaced nonunions with a humpback deformity require the placement of a corticocancellous volar wedge graft from a volar approach to correct the humpback deformity.
3. For proximal fractures or those in which the proximal fragment has developed AVN, volar grafting techniques are contraindicated.
   a. Proximal pole AVN can be difficult to establish preoperatively.
   b. Vascularity of the proximal pole can be assessed preoperatively with MRI scans or intraoperatively by assessing the presence of punctate bleeding from the proximal pole (more accurate).
   c. In the absence of fragmentation and presence of structural integrity of the proximal pole at the time of surgery, reconstruction in the form of ORIF and bone grafting should be attempted. With the use of ORIF and conventional bone grafts, only 55% of scaphoid nonunions with proximal pole AVN will go on to heal.

4. Local vascularized bone grafts are used for the treatment of scaphoid nonunions complicated by AVN (Fig. 6-16). The distal radius vascularized bone graft based on the 1,2 intercompartmental supraretinacular artery is most commonly used for the treatment of scaphoid nonunion.
   a. Other grafts that have been described include a vascular pedicle originating from the second dorsal intermetacarpal vascular bundle, which is directly implanted into the nonunion site; vascularized bone grafts from the distal radius based on a pronator quadratus pedicle; grafts from the second metacarpal pedicled on the superficial dorsal interosseus artery; volar radial grafts based on the volar carpal artery; and volar grafts from the distal ulna based on the ulnar artery.
   b. In the presence of fragmentation and absence of structural integrity of the proximal pole at the time of surgery, salvage procedures such as fragment excision, intercarpal arthrodeses, and proximal row carpectomy are recommended.
   c. Radiographically apparent nonunions that appear healed at the time of surgery have a 50% nonunion rate, and therefore all should be treated with ORIF and bone grafting.

Lunate Fractures

1. Acute fractures are rare, and most are seen in association with AVN of the lunate (Kienböck's disease) (see Chapter 4).

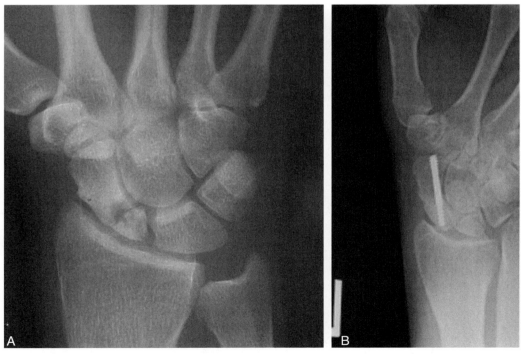

Figure 6-16 ❖ **A,** Posteroanterior radiograph of the wrist revealing nonunion of a proximal pole scaphoid fracture. The patient was treated with internal fixation and dorsal radius vascularized bone grafting. **B,** Posteroanterior radiograph of the wrist 2 years after the surgical procedure suggests healing of the nonunion.

2. Mechanism of injury typically involves a fall on an extended wrist, and associated carpal or distal radius fractures are seen in about 50% of patients.
3. Lunate fractures have been classified according to fracture pattern:
   a. Type I: fracture of the volar pole (most common).
   b. Type II: small, marginal chip fractures.
   c. Type III: fracture of the dorsal pole.
   d. Type IV: lunate body fractures on the sagittal plane (longitudinal).
   e. Type V: lunate body fractures on the coronal plane (transverse).
4. Fracture diagnosis with plain radiographs can be difficult, and CT or MRI scans are valuable adjuncts.
5. Nondisplaced fractures can be treated with cast immobilization for 4 to 6 weeks.
6. Displaced fractures should be treated with ORIF to achieve anatomic reduction of the fragments.

Triquetrum Fractures

1. Fractures of the triquetrum are second in occurrence behind the scaphoid and lunate.
2. Dorsal chip fractures secondary to impingement on the ulnar styloid on the proximal aspect of the bone can follow hyperextension injuries of the wrist.
   a. These injuries can be treated with 3 to 4 weeks of splint immobilization or with fragment excision for refractory cases.
3. Triquetral body fractures are less common.
   a. If nondisplaced, these fractures can be treated with 4 to 6 weeks of cast immobilization.
   b. Pinning or ORIF may be necessary for displaced or unstable body fractures.

Hamate Fractures

These fractures are predominantly of two types—hamate hook and hamate body fractures.

HAMATE HOOK FRACTURES

1. Fractures of the hook of the hamate typically occur after direct trauma to the proximal aspect of the palm and can also be seen in golfers, baseball players, and racquet-sport players.
2. Patients present with point tenderness on the proximal aspect of the palm directly over the hamate hook. Some may complain of associated ulnar nerve irritation.
3. Assessment with plain radiographs alone can be difficult. Radiographic evaluation includes a 45-degree supination oblique and a carpal tunnel view. If the clinical presentation is consistent with this fracture, evaluation of the injury with CT or MRI scans can aid in diagnosis if radiographs are normal.
   a. CT scan is the most sensitive diagnostic tool to assess hook of the hamate fracture or nonunion and can help distinguish an os hamulus proprius from an acute fracture due to well-corticated edges around the accessory ossicle.
4. Injuries diagnosed acutely may be treated with cast immobilization for 6 weeks.

5. Unrecognized fractures typically go on to nonunion, probably because of disruption of the vascular supply that originates from the hamate body alone in 70% of cases.
   a. Patients present with chronic ulnar-sided wrist pain, particularly with weight bearing on the palm of the hand.
   b. Associated symptoms can include flexor tendinopathy, tendon rupture due to attritional wear of the tendon as it rubs on the area of nonunion (most common), and ulnar neuropathy.
   c. As in acute fractures, assessment of nonunion with plain radiographs alone can be difficult, and CT is an invaluable adjunct for diagnosis.
   d. Treatment of symptomatic nonunion involves excision of the symptomatic fragment. ORIF and bone grafting have been advocated for large fragments.

HAMATE BODY FRACTURES

Hamate body fractures are less common and may be associated with fourth and fifth CMC joint fracture-dislocations.
1. Undisplaced fractures may be treated closed.
2. Displaced or unstable fractures, particularly those in the coronal plane, are treated with closed reduction and percutaneous pinning or with ORIF.

Capitate Fractures

1. Fractures of the capitate are rare, except when they occur in association with perilunate fracture-dislocations, also termed scaphocapitate syndrome (see Chapter 7).
2. The vascular supply to the capitate head is retrograde, and thus displaced fractures can lead to AVN.
3. Cast treatment may be considered if the capitate fracture is undisplaced; displaced fractures require ORIF. Symptomatic nonunions and AVN are treated with limited midcarpal arthrodesis, capitate excision and tendon interpositional arthroplasty, or vascularized bone grafting.

Trapezium Fractures

1. Fractures of the trapezium are rare but may be seen in association with CMC joint dislocations and Bennett's fractures of the thumb.
2. The fracture can sometimes be visualized on oblique, ulnar deviation anteroposterior or posteroanterior views or on carpal tunnel views. A CT scan may be obtained if the diagnosis is in question.
3. Fractures can occur either in the body or along the trapezial ridge.
   a. Body fractures tend to be either vertical or comminuted. ORIF is required if intra-articular displacement is present.
   b. Ridge fractures can follow either a direct blow or a fall onto an outstretched palm; forced flattening of the transverse carpal arch in either scenario results in avulsion of the flexor retinaculum from its insertion onto the trapezial ridge.

Type 1 fractures involve the base of the ridge and may be treated conservatively, although many go on to painful nonunion. Type 2 fractures involve the tip of the ridge and may be treated in a cast with the first ray in abduction for 4 to 6 weeks. Painful nonunions of either type respond well to excision.

Pisiform Fractures

1. Pisiform fractures are rare and may occur in association with fractures of the distal radius, hamate, or triquetrum.
2. Mechanism of injury is typically a direct blow. Radiographic evaluation includes a 30-degree supination oblique and a carpal tunnel view. A CT scan should be obtained if the diagnosis is in question (Fig. 6-17).
3. Treatment includes cast immobilization with the wrist in ulnar deviation and 30 degrees of flexion.
4. Pisiform excision can be performed if symptomatic nonunion occurs or if degeneration of the pisotriquetral joint becomes symptomatic.

Trapezoid Fractures

1. Fractures of the trapezoid are extremely rare but may be seen in association with other carpal or CMC joint injuries.

2. CT scan is typically required for definitive diagnosis.
3. Most injuries can be treated with casting. Large, displaced fragments are best treated with ORIF to prevent late CMC instability.

Distal Radius Fractures

1. Distal radius fractures are among the most common of all skeletal injuries and occur in all age groups, with a higher incidence among the elderly and children.
2. Women are affected more commonly than are men, given the increased incidence of osteoporosis in women.
3. Physeal injuries of the distal radius can occur in young female gymnasts, a problem that can lead to growth arrest due to repetitive axial loading.
4. Several eponyms are used to describe fractures of the distal radius:
   a. Colles' fracture represents a dorsally angulated (apex volar), extra-articular fracture (Fig. 6-18).
   b. Smith's fracture is a volarly angulated (apex dorsal) extra-articular fracture (Fig. 6-19).
   c. Barton's fracture represents an articular shear fracture. These can be dorsal or volar.
   d. Chauffeur's fracture is a fracture of the radial styloid (Fig. 6-20).
5. Fractures of the distal radius are most clearly characterized in terms of their degree of articular

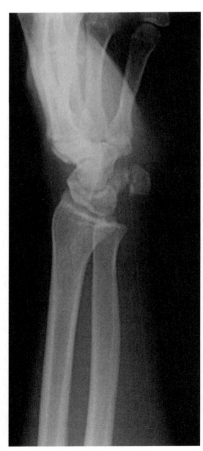

Figure 6-17 ◆ External rotation view of the wrist revealing a fracture of the pisiform.

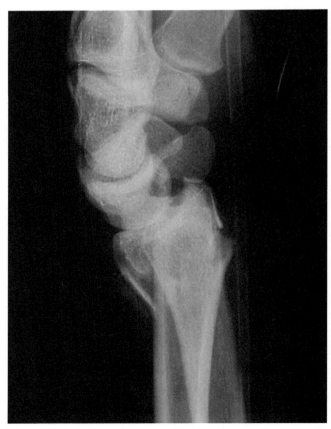

Figure 6-18 ◆ Lateral radiograph of the wrist revealing a dorsally angulated fracture of the distal radius (Colles' fracture).

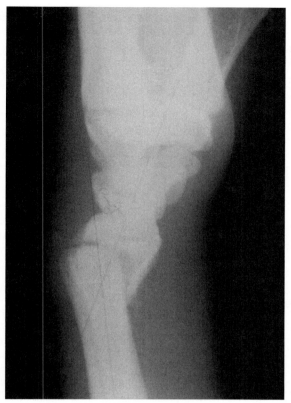

Figure 6-19 ❖ Lateral radiograph of the wrist revealing a volarly angulated fracture of the distal radius (Smith's fracture).

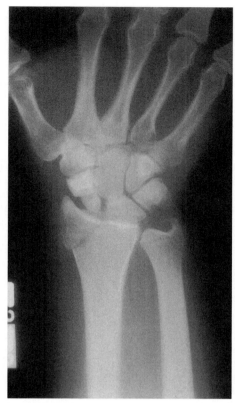

Figure 6-20 ❖ Posteroanterior radiograph of the wrist revealing radial styloid fracture (chauffeur's fracture). Note the associated scaphoid fracture.

involvement, comminution, displacement, and angulation and with various parameters including tilt, length, and angle.

Anatomy

OSTEOLOGY

1. The distal radius is composed of the metaphysis with the articulations for the radiocarpal joint and distal radioulnar joint (DRUJ). The metaphysis contains rich trabecular bone with a thin dorsal cortical surface.
2. The articulation at the radiocarpal joint includes the scaphoid facet, which is triangular and separated from the lunate facet by the interfacet ridge (Fig. 6-21).
3. The lunate fossa is a concave hemispherical surface that accommodates the proximal aspect of the lunate.
4. The third concave surface on the distal aspect of the radius is the sigmoid notch. The sigmoid notch accommodates the head of the ulna to form the DRUJ and serves as the radial site of attachment of the triangular fibrocartilage (TFC). The sigmoid notch is variable in depth and angular inclination. The articular surfaces of the sigmoid notch and ulnar head are not congruous because of different arcs.
5. On the lateral view, the volar cortex of the radius is concave. This needs to be appreciated in contouring plates for fixation of the volar distal radius.

LIGAMENTS

1. The major stabilizers of the radiocarpal joint originate from the volar aspect of the radius. The ligaments that contribute to the stability are as follows (from radial to ulnar): radioscaphocapitate, long radiolunate, radioscapholunate (Testut)

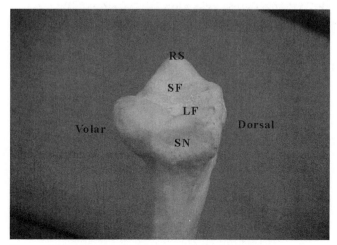

Figure 6-21 ❖ Osseous anatomy of the distal radius. The distal radius is seen from an ulnar perspective. SN, sigmoid notch; LF, lunate fossa; SF, scaphoid fossa; RS, radial styloid.

(mostly a neurovascular conduit), and the short radiolunate ligament.

2. The primary stabilizing structures on the dorsum of the radiocarpal joint are the dorsal radiocarpal ligament (composed of the radioscaphoid and radiotriquetral ligaments) and the dorsal intercarpal ligament. The dorsal structures provide little stability to the radiocarpal joint (see Chapters 1 and 7).

3. The dorsal and volar distal radioulnar ligaments arise from the dorsal and volar rim of the sigmoid notch. The distal aspect of the sigmoid notch serves as the site of radial attachment of the TFC as well as of the volar and dorsal radioulnar ligaments. These ligaments originate at the base of the radial styloid and insert on the dorsal and most volar aspects of the sigmoid notch. These radioulnar ligaments are thought to be the primary stabilizers of the DRUJ (see Chapters 1 and 7).

Evaluation

1. Evaluation of these injuries should always include assessment of the forearm and hand compartments and the DRUJ.

2. Assessment of the elbow joint and carpal bones, particularly the scaphoid, is important to rule out associated injuries.

3. Careful neurovascular examination with particular attention to the median nerve is performed and documented.
   a. Median nerve injury is the most common acute complication of distal radius fractures.
   b. Careful assessment and documentation of median nerve function are performed at the time of initial evaluation and after closed or open reduction. Dysfunction at the time of presentation may partially or totally resolve with fracture reduction.
   c. Progressive neurologic deterioration of median nerve function in spite of fracture reduction suggests the possibility of acute carpal tunnel syndrome, requiring emergent decompression. The first step in treatment is release of tight dressings, cast removal, and placement of the wrist in a neutral position.
   d. If acute median nerve symptoms fail to resolve, carpal tunnel decompression is performed.

4. Initial radiographic evaluation includes posteroanterior and lateral views of the wrist and forearm.
   a. Important radiographic parameters are radial length (normal, 11 mm), radial inclination (normal, 22 degrees), volar tilt (normal, 11 degrees), and ulnar variance (variable, should be compared with the contralateral side) (Fig. 6-22).
   b. Oblique, partially supinated views delineate the dorsal lip of the lunate fossa; oblique, partially pronated views provide good visualization of the radial styloid.
   c. CT scanning is clearly superior in assessment and measurement of articular surface (radiocarpal and DRUJ) disruption (gapping and step-off).

◆ Table 6-2

AO CLASSIFICATION		
A Extra-articular	A1	Isolated ulna
	A2	Simple radial fracture
	A3	Radial fracture with metaphysis impaction
B Intra-articular (one cortex intact)	B1	Radial styloid
	B2	Dorsal cortex
	B3	Volar cortex
C Intra-articular (no cortex intact)	C1	Joint congruity preserved
	C2	Articular displacement
	C3	Diaphyseal extension

   d. MRI can be helpful in determining associated soft tissue injury, such as scapholunate interosseous ligament and TFC complex tears.
   e. Fracture classification: several classification schemes have been described and are outlined in Tables 6-2 to 6-4.

Treatment (Fig. 6-23)

1. The treatment of distal radius fractures depends on a variety of factors including fracture pattern, age of the patient, and functional requirements. Elderly patients with a lower demand of the wrist are more tolerant of fracture displacement. Patients with a higher functional demand of the wrist tend to have a better result with a more anatomic alignment.

2. Fractures healing with displacement increase the risk of stiffness, instability of the DRUJ, midcarpal instability, and post-traumatic arthrosis.
   a. Biomechanical studies have shown that shortening of the distal radius by 2.5 mm or residual dorsal tilt will increase load transmission through the ulnar shaft and incongruity at the DRUJ.
   b. Increased dorsal tilt of the distal fragment leads to a smaller contact area for articulation at the radiocarpal joint, which potentially leads to post-traumatic arthritis.
   c. Some radiographic studies have reported a high incidence of post-traumatic arthrosis in young patients with fractures that healed with more than 1 to 2 mm of intra-articular incongruity.

3. Fractures associated with instability demonstrate the following:
   a. Articular displacement.
   b. More than 20 degrees of dorsal angulation.
   c. Displacement or shortening of more than 5 mm.
   d. Comminution.
   e. An associated ulnar fracture or DRUJ dislocation.
   f. Associated radiocarpal instability.

◆ Table 6-3

FRYKMAN CLASSIFICATION		
Distal Ulna Fracture	No	Yes
Extra-articular	I	II
Intra-articular into radiocarpal (RC) joint	III	IV
Intra-articular into radioulnar (RU) joint	V	VI
Intra-articular into RC + RU joints	VII	VIII

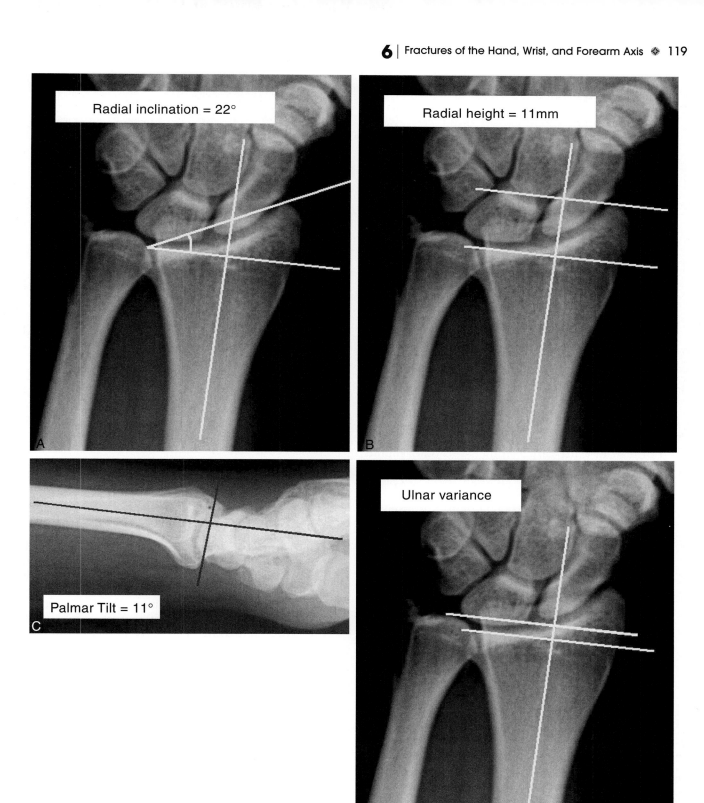

Figure 6-22 ❖ Radiographic parameters of the distal radius. **A,** Radial inclination. **B,** Radial height. **C,** Palmar tilt. **D,** Ulnar variance.

◆ Table 6-4	
MELONE CLASSIFICATION	
I	Minimally displaced
II	Comminuted/stable
	Displaced medial complex
	Dorsal: die-punch, Barton
III	Displaced medial complex as a unit
	Displaced radial shaft fragments
IV	Wide separation or rotation of medial fragments
	Extensive soft tissue and periarticular damage

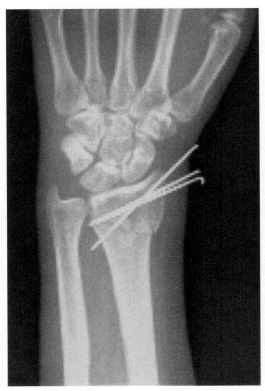

Figure 6-24 ◆ Posteroanterior radiograph of the wrist revealing a fracture of the distal radius treated with closed reduction and percutaneous pinning.

CLOSED REDUCTION AND CASTING

1. Closed reduction is considered acceptable if change in volar tilt is less than 10 degrees, change in radial length is less than 2 mm, change in radial inclination is less than 5 degrees, and articular step-off is less than 1 to 2 mm.
2. After immobilization, patients are placed in a sugar tong splint until swelling decreases. The splint is then changed to a long-arm cast in slight wrist flexion and ulnar deviation for 2 to 3 weeks, followed by short-arm casting for an additional 3 to 4 weeks.
3. Placement of the wrist in excessive flexion, which can lead to acute carpal tunnel syndrome, should be avoided.
4. Restoration of relatively normal alignment after closed reduction may not reflect final outcome, and close follow-up of unstable injuries is essential to prevent malunion.

CLOSED REDUCTION AND PERCUTANEOUS PINNING

1. Displaced extra-articular distal radius fractures with dorsal comminution are most amenable to percutaneous pinning. These unstable fractures are likely to heal in a nonanatomic alignment with treatment by cast immobilization.
2. Several pinning techniques have been described. After pinning, patients are typically placed in a

short-arm cast for 4 to 6 weeks. The pins are removed after fracture healing (Fig. 6-24).
3. Another technique of percutaneous pinning is interfocal pinning as described by Kapandji. The technique involves placement of Kirschner wires within the fracture site to act as a buttress limiting dorsal tilt and loss of radial height. This minimally invasive procedure is best used for the unstable distal radius fracture without intra-articular extension.

OPEN REDUCTION AND INTERNAL FIXATION

1. The goal of ORIF is anatomic reconstruction of the distal radius. The use of stable internal fixation allows early mobilization protocols. The indications for open reduction and plate fixation include the following:
   a. Unstable articular fractures, such as the volar shearing injury (volar Barton's).
   b. Impacted articular fractures.
   c. Open fractures.
   d. Radiocarpal fracture-dislocations.
   e. Complex fractures.
   f. Failed closed reduction.
2. The open reduction of fracture is complemented by internal fixation in the form of plating and, if necessary, K-wire fixation. Both dorsal and volar approaches to the distal radius have been described. Each approach is indicated according to

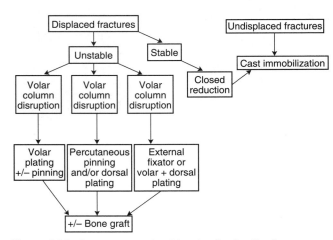

Figure 6-23 ◆ Treatment algorithm for distal radius fractures.

the location of major fracture fragments and the direction of their displacement.

a. Volar approach. A longitudinal incision is made along the flexor carpi radialis tendon. The radial artery is identified and retracted radially; the flexor carpi radialis is retracted ulnarly. The pronator quadratus is identified and incised along the border of the radius. The dissection is taken subperiosteally while the pronator quadratus is elevated and the volar surface of the distal radius is exposed (Fig. 6-25).

b. Dorsal approach. A longitudinal incision is made on the dorsal aspect of the radius just ulnar to Lister's tubercle. The extensor retinaculum is identified and incised along the line of the incision directly over the third dorsal compartment, which contains the extensor pollicis longus tendon. The deep layer of the retinaculum (which is confluent with the periosteum of the radius) is elevated sharply off the radius radially and ulnarly with care not to enter the other extensor compartments in the process. The purpose of maintaining the deep layer of the retinaculum intact is to avoid direct contact of the extensor tendons with the plate. The distal radius can be exposed from the sigmoid notch ulnarly to the radial styloid radially (Fig. 6-26).

3. Elevation of the joint surface and primary bone grafting should be considered when there is significant articular depression, as in lunate "die-punch" fractures.

4. Dorsal plating can lead to extensor tendon irritation which may lead to tendon rupture and may necesitate hardware removal.

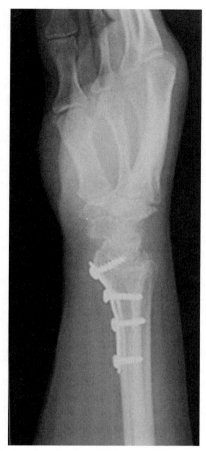

Figure 6-25 ❖ Lateral radiograph of the wrist revealing a fracture of the distal radius treated by ORIF through a volar approach.

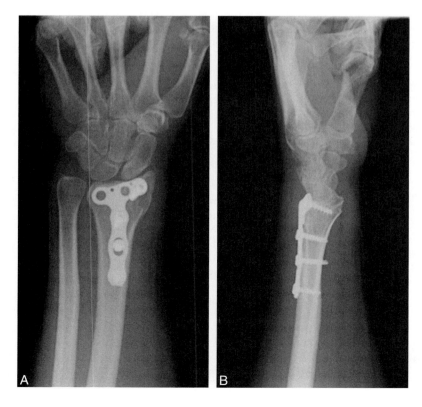

A   B

Figure 6-26 ❖ Posteroanterior (**A**) and lateral (**B**) radiographs of the wrist revealing a fracture of the distal radius treated by ORIF through a dorsal approach.

EXTERNAL FIXATION

1. The indications for external fixation of distal radius fractures include severely unstable and comminuted fractures, which because of fracture pattern are not amenable to ORIF. Open fractures or those involving significant soft tissue injury can also benefit from external fixation.
2. Reduction is performed by ligamentotaxis. Longitudinal traction alone will not reconstitute the volar tilt of the distal fragment and may in fact worsen the dorsal tilt because of the pull of the volar extrinsic ligaments. Distraction in combination with volar translation of the fracture will effect a reduction in the dorsally displaced fracture.
3. In the majority of cases, adjuvant K-wire fixation should be considered. K-wires add to the stability of the construct such that it approaches levels of plate fixation.
4. The rate of complications with external fixation is high, however; these can include pin track infections, pin loosening, radial sensory nerve injury, stiffness, and reflex sympathetic dystrophy. These complications may be prevented to some degree by avoiding carpal overdistraction, excessive wrist flexion, and prolonged fixator treatment.
5. External fixators should generally be removed at 4 to 6 weeks; pins may be left up to 8 weeks in the absence of pin track problems.

WRIST ARTHROSCOPY

Wrist arthroscopy may be a useful adjunct in the treatment of displaced intra-articular fractures to confirm adequacy of reduction.

ULNAR STYLOID FRACTURE

Ulnar styloid fractures are present in at least 50% of distal radius fractures. Nonunion is common but rarely symptomatic.

1. Painful nonunions can be treated with excision or ORIF with a small screw or tension band.
2. Injury to the TFC complex should be suspected even in the absence of an ulnar styloid fracture if initial fracture angulation exceeds 25 degrees.
3. Some authors recommend fixation of large fragments with a tension band construct to restablish the competency of the TFC complex and DRUJ stability.

BONE GRAFTING

Bone grafting is indicated in cases of severe comminution, bone loss, or articular impaction.

1. Autologous bone graft is osteoinductive and osteoconductive and has remodeling capabilities.
2. Autografts, fresh and frozen allografts, and demineralized bone matrix have residual organic material. Coralline hydroxyapatite does not.

Complications

1. In addition to median nerve dysfunction, other complications seen in the acute setting include ulnar nerve injury, instability of the DRUJ, and compartment syndrome.

2. Late complications may include post-traumatic arthritis of the radiocarpal joint or DRUJ, ulno-carpal abutment syndrome, rupture of the extensor pollicis longus, tendon adhesion formation, stiffness, chronic median nerve compression, reflex sympathetic dystrophy, malunion, and nonunion.
   a. Rupture of the extensor pollicis longus is generally attributed to ischemia due to pressure exerted by hematoma trapped beneath the extensor retinaculum. It may also be related to mechanical irritation and should be treated with transfer of the extensor indicis proprius.
   b. Flexor tendon adhesion formation is largely preventable but can be extremely problematic once it has occurred. Regardless of treatment modality, therefore, digital range of motion is emphasized during and after the treatment period.
   c. Fracture malunion with incongruity of the DRUJ is also difficult to treat and may require a complex biplanar distal radial osteotomy or hemiresection arthroplasty of the DRUJ. Dorsally angulated malunions will lead to dorsal intercalated segment instability (DISI) of the proximal carpal row.
   d. Attritional tendon rupture has been observed in about 15% of patients treated by ORIF with dorsal plates. This incidence may be lowered with the use of newer low profile plates.
3. Functional outcomes correlate best with fracture comminution and associated carpal bone injuries.
   a. Functional outcome of intra-articular fractures appears to be least affected by palmar or radial tilt. There is a strong correlation between increasing degree of injury, more than four fragments, postoperative articular gap or step-off, articular comminution, and postoperative radial shortening and poor functional outcomes.
   b. Lunate facet depression is predictive of poor long-term outcome.

Forearm Fractures

Ulnar Shaft Fractures

1. Isolated fractures of the ulnar shaft typically result from a direct blow and are commonly referred to as "nightstick" fractures.
2. Nonoperative treatment is indicated for middle and distal third fractures angulated less than 10 degrees and displaced less than 50%. Greater displacement may be associated with instability of the radial head or DRUJ.
3. A long-arm splint or cast is applied initially, but it may be converted to functional bracing after 7 to 10 days.
4. Proximal third fractures, displaced fractures, and fractures failing closed treatment are treated by ORIF with a 3.5-mm dynamic compression plate.

Radial Shaft Fractures

1. Radial shaft fractures are seldom stable or nondisplaced.
2. Most of these injuries are treated by ORIF with a 3.5-mm dynamic compression plate.
3. For isolated shaft fractures, careful assessment of DRUJ stability is performed and documented.

Radius and Ulna (Both Bones) Fractures

1. Closed treatment of these extremely unstable fractures is rarely successful in the adult population, and ORIF is performed with a 3.5-mm dynamic compression plate for each bone.
2. During fixation, seven cortices, including an interfragmentary lag screw if possible, are required on either side of a noncomminuted fracture. If the comminution involves greater than one third of the diaphyseal cortex, primary bone grafting is recommended by some authors (Fig. 6-27).
3. The radius and ulna are approached separately to decrease the incidence of radioulnar synostosis. In general, the Henry or volar approach is preferred for distal third radius fractures, whereas the dorsal or Thompson approach is preferred for middle third radius fractures. Proximal third fractures may be approached either dorsally or volarly.
4. Intramedullary fixation, although satisfactory in the pediatric population, is often complicated by delayed union in adults.

5. Restoration of forearm rotation is dependent on anatomic reduction of the fractures.

Proximal Ulna Fractures Associated with Radiocapitellar Dislocations (Monteggia's Fracture-Dislocations)

1. Monteggia's fracture or fracture-dislocation consists of an ulnar shaft fracture in conjunction with a dislocation of the radial head.
2. Classification (Bado)
   a. Type 1 injuries account for the majority of Monteggia's fractures and are characterized by anterior dislocation of the radial head and apex anterior fracture of the proximal ulna. Anterior interosseous nerve injuries can be seen in type 1 injuries.
   b. Type 2 injuries are characterized by posterior dislocation of the radial head and apex posterior angulation of the proximal ulna. They can be associated with posterior interosseous nerve injury, which is the most common neuropathy associated with Monteggia's fractures (Fig. 6-28).
   c. Type 3 injuries are characterized by lateral dislocation of the radial head in addition to a fracture of the proximal ulnar metaphysis.
   d. Type 4 injuries consist of proximal fractures of both bones in addition to an anterior radial head dislocation.
3. Treatment in all cases includes ORIF of the ulna and anatomic reduction of the radiocapitellar joint.

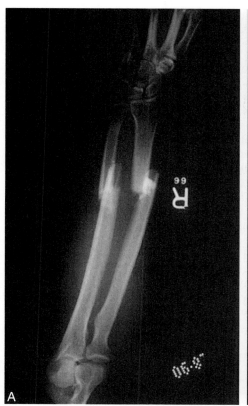
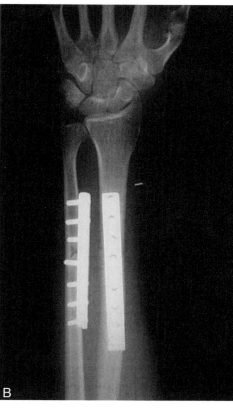

Figure 6-27 ◆ Posteroanterior (**A**) and lateral (**B**) radiographs of the forearm revealing a fracture of both bones of the forearm treated by ORIF.

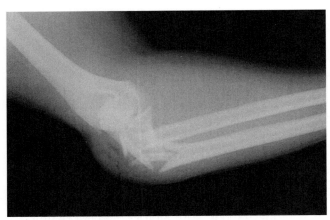

Figure 6-28 ◆ Lateral radiograph of the elbow in a patient with a proximal ulna fracture in combination with a posterior radial head dislocation (Monteggia's fracture-dislocation, Bado 2).

In most cases, the radial head will reduce with anatomic fixation of the ulna. If concentric reduction of the radiocapitellar joint is not achieved by closed means, despite anatomic reduction of the ulna, an open reduction is necessary.

4. As with most forearm fractures, short-term immobilization is followed by early motion.

Middle to Distal Third Radius Fracture Associated with DRUJ Instability (Galeazzi's Fracture-Dislocation)

1. Mechanism of injury may be a fall or a direct blow.
2. Deforming forces on the fracture include the pronator quadratus, which tends to rotate and flex the distal fragment, and the brachioradialis, which tends to pull it proximally.
3. Clinical assessment of radial shaft fractures should include evaluation of DRUJ instability.
4. The presence of an ulnar styloid fracture, widening of the DRUJ on the anteroposterior radiograph, dislocation of the DRUJ on the lateral radiograph, and 5 mm or more of radial shortening are suggestive of a DRUJ injury.
5. Other associated injuries include tears of the TFC complex.
6. Treatment in all cases includes ORIF of the radius and anatomic reduction of the DRUJ. In most cases, the DRUJ will reduce with anatomic fixation of the radius. Anatomic fixation of the radius is the most important factor in re-establishing DRUJ stability. If concentric reduction of the DRUJ is not achieved by closed means, interposition of the extensor carpi ulnaris tendon (most common) or pronator quadratus should be suspected, and an open reduction is performed.
   a. If a stable reduction of the DRUJ is achieved after fixation of the radius, immobilization of the forearm in supination for 4 to 6 weeks is adequate treatment of the DRUJ.
   b. Residual instability of the DRUJ after radius ORIF may be treated with DRUJ pinning for

4 weeks with the forearm in supination, ORIF of the ulnar styloid fracture, or open repair of the distal radioulnar ligaments.

7. Fractures of the distal third of the radial shaft are more likely to have residual DRUJ instability.

Radial Head Fracture Associated with Instability of the Forearm Axis (Essex-Lopresti Injury)

1. Essex-Lopresti lesion consists of a fracture of the radial head in conjunction with disruption of the interosseous membrane and DRUJ stabilizing ligaments.
2. Patients with radial head fractures should be evaluated for interosseous and DRUJ instability.
3. If this injury is recognized acutely, the radial head should not be excised. ORIF of the radial head or prosthetic replacement of a radial head in cases of unreconstructible fractures is necessary to prevent proximal migration of the radius relative to the ulna. Pinning of the DRUJ may be added if instability persists after fixation or replacement of the radial head.
4. Immobilization for 4 to 6 weeks follows operative treatment.
5. Chronic instability of the DRUJ may require reconstruction of the interosseous membrane or radioulnar arthrodesis.

Complications

1. Plate removal after ORIF of forearm fractures should not be performed routinely. The incidence of fracture after plate removal can be as high as 20%. Refracture rates drop considerably for plates removed after 15 to 24 months, but they may be higher in the case of large implants. Splint protection for 6 to 8 weeks should be considered after plate removal. Risk of refracture after plate removal is increased with the use of larger implants.
2. Synostosis occurs in approximately 3% of forearm fractures treated operatively; risk factors include fracture of both bones at the same level, high-energy injuries, concomitant closed head injuries, infection, single-incision approaches to both bones, bone graft or hardware placement in the vicinity of the interosseous membrane, and primary fixation after 2 weeks.
3. Hypertrophic nonunions are best treated with ORIF. Atrophic nonunions should be treated with ORIF and bone grafting.
4. Other complications associated with the treatment of forearm fractures include malunion, infection, instability, stiffness, and anterior or posterior interosseous nerve injury, especially in Monteggia's fractures.

Bibliography

Bado JL: The Monteggia lesion. Clin Orthop 50:71-86, 1967.

Bradway JK, Amadio PC, Cooney WP: Open reduction and internal fixation of displaced, comminuted intra-articular fractures of the distal end of the radius. J Bone Joint Surg Am 71:839-847, 1989.

Breen TF, Gelberman RH, Jupiter JB: Intra-articular fractures of the basilar joint of the thumb. Hand Clin 4:491-501, 1988.

Cain JE Jr, Shepler TR, Wilson MR: Hamatometacarpal fracture-dislocation: classification and treatment. J Hand Surg Am 12: 762-767, 1987.

Chan PS, Steinberg DR, Pepe MD, Beredjiklian PK: The significance of the three volar spaces in forearm compartment syndrome: a clinical and cadaveric correlation. J Hand Surg Am 23:1077-1081, 1998.

Chapman MW, Gordon JE, Zissimos AG: Compression-plate fixation of acute fractures of the diaphyses of the radius and ulna. J Bone Joint Surg Am 71:159-169, 1989.

DeLuca PA, Lindsey RW, Ruwe PA: Refracture of bones in the forearm after the removal of compression plates. J Bone Joint Surg Am 70:1372-1376, 1988.

Duncan RW, Freeland AE, Jabaley ME, Meydrech EF: Open hand fractures: an analysis of the recovery of active motion and of complications. J Hand Surg Am 18:387-394, 1993.

Firoozbakhsh KK, Moneim MS, Doherty W, et al: Internal fixation of oblique metacarpal fractures. A biomechanical evaluation by impact loading. Clin Orthop 325:296-301, 1996.

Geissler WB, Freeland AE, Savoie FH, et al: Intracarpal soft-tissue lesions associated with an intra-articular fracture of the distal end of the radius. J Bone Joint Surg Am 78:357-365, 1996.

Gelberman RH, Garfin SR, Hergenroeder PT, et al: Compartment syndromes of the forearm: diagnosis and treatment. Clin Orthop 161:252-261, 1981.

Gelberman RH, Menon J: The vascularity of the scaphoid bone. J Hand Surg Am 5:508-513, 1980.

Gelberman RH, Wolock BS, Siegel DB: Fractures and non-unions of the carpal scaphoid. J Bone Joint Surg Am 71:1560-1565, 1989.

Gonzales MH, Hall RF Jr: Intramedullary fixation of metacarpal and proximal phalangeal fractures of the hand. Clin Orthop 327:47-54, 1996.

Grace TG, Eversmann WW Jr: Forearm fractures: treatment by rigid fixation with early motion. J Bone Joint Surg Am 62:433-438, 1980.

Green DP: The effect of avascular necrosis on Russe bone grafting for scaphoid non-union. J Hand Surg Am 10:597-605, 1985.

Herbert TJ, Fisher WE: Management of the fractured scaphoid using a new bone screw. J Bone Joint Surg Br 66:114-123, 1984.

Hornbach EE, Cohen MS: Closed reduction and percutaneous pinning of fractures of the proximal phalanx. J Hand Surg Br 26:45-49, 2001.

Jupiter JB: Fractures of the distal end of the radius. J Bone Joint Surg Am 73:461-469, 1991.

Jupiter JB, Lipton H: The operative treatment of intraarticular fractures of the distal radius. Clin Orthop 292:48-61, 1993.

Jupiter JB, Masem M: Reconstruction of post-traumatic deformity of the distal radius and ulna. Hand Clin 4:377-390, 1988.

Knirk JL, Jupiter JB: Intra-articular fractures of the distal end of the radius in young adults. J Bone Joint Surg Am 68:647-659, 1986.

Leung YL, Beredjiklian PK, Monaghan BA, Bozentka DJ: Radiographic assessment of small finger metacarpal neck fractures. J Hand Surg Am 27:443-448, 2002.

Mack GR, Bosse MJ, Gelberman RH, et al: The natural history of scaphoid non-union. J Bone Joint Surg Am 66:504-509, 1984.

Melone CP Jr: Open treatment for displaced articular fractures of the distal radius. Clin Orthop 202:103-111, 1986.

Moed BR, Kellam JF, Foster RJ, et al: Immediate internal fixation of open fractures of the diaphysis of the forearm. J Bone Joint Surg Am 68:1008-1017, 1986.

Ouellette EA, Freeland AE: Use of the minicondylar plate in metacarpal and phalangeal fractures. Clin Orthop 327:38-46, 1996.

Ouellette EA, Kelly R: Compartment syndromes of the hand. J Bone Joint Surg Am 78:1515-1522, 1996.

Rawles JG Jr: Dislocations and fracture-dislocations at the carpometacarpal joints of the fingers. Hand Clin 4:103-112, 1988.

Rayhack JM, Bottke CA: Intraosseous compression wiring of displaced articular condylar fractures. J Hand Surg Am 15:370-373, 1990.

Rozental TD, Beredjiklian PK, Steinberg DR, Bozentka DJ: Open fractures of the distal radius. J Hand Surg Am 27:77-85, 2002.

Rozental TD, Beredjiklian PK, Bozentka DJ: Longitudinal radioulnar dissociation. J Am Acad Orthop Surg 11:68-73, 2003.

Schenck RR: Dynamic traction and early passive movement for fractures of the proximal interphalangeal joint. J Hand Surg Am 11:850-858, 1986.

Sochart DH, Paul AS: A simple external fixator for use in metacarpal and phalangeal fractures: a technique paper. J Orthop Trauma 9:333-335, 1995.

Stern PJ, Kastrup JJ: Complications and prognosis of treatment of mallet finger. J Hand Surg Am 13:329-334, 1988.

Vince KG, Miller JE: Cross union complicating fracture of the forearm. Part I: adults. J Bone Joint Surg Am 69:640-653, 1987.

✧ Philip E. Blazar, MD

DISLOCATIONS/ INSTABILITY

Finger Joints

Distal Interphalangeal Joint

ANATOMY

The distal interphalangeal joint (DIP) is an inherently stable joint with broad articular surfaces and a "box" ligament configuration that includes the radial and ulnar collateral ligaments and the volar plate (Fig. 7-1). Additional stability is from the terminal portions of the extensor tendon dorsally and the flexor digitorum profundus (FDP) tendon volarly, both of which are intimately approximated to the capsule. In contrast to the proximal interphalangeal (PIP) joint (and the hand in general), mobility of the DIP joint is functionally less important than stability. The DIP joint is less frequently injured than is the PIP joint.

COLLATERAL LIGAMENT INJURIES

Mechanism and Patterns of Injury

The short distal phalanx generates a small moment arm that in turn translates into fewer ligament injuries compared with the PIP joint. The ligaments usually fail at the proximal or distal attachments, and this may occur with small bone avulsions.

Evaluation

Examination typically demonstrates asymmetric swelling or tenderness. Active flexion-extension is present, but full range of motion is lacking. Careful examination is important to rule out extensor or flexor tendon avulsion injuries. Instability to varus-valgus stressing may be present and is more reliably demonstrated after digital block anesthesia. Isolated collateral injuries seldom result in joint dislocation. Posteroanterior and lateral radiographs are important to assess concentric reduction of the joint (especially on the true lateral film). If any radiographic signs of instability are present, the injury is unlikely to be an isolated collateral ligament disruption. Small avulsion fracture fragments may also be seen.

Treatment

These injuries can be treated with early active motion, compression wrapping, and symptomatic treatment. Manual laborers may require static splints for up to 3 weeks with the PIP joint free and intermittent splint removal for mobilization. Chronic instability is rare. Permanent loss of motion and swelling are not uncommon but rarely functionally limiting.

DISLOCATIONS

1. DIP joint dislocations involve disruption of supporting bone or soft tissue structures. Dislocations may be dorsal, volar, simple, or complex (irreducible) and can be open.
   a. Dorsal dislocations are the most common. Hyperextension of the DIP joint is the most

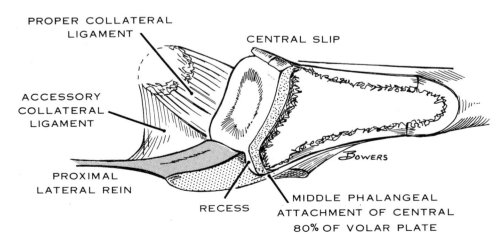

PROPER COLLATERAL LIGAMENT

CENTRAL SLIP

ACCESSORY COLLATERAL LIGAMENT

PROXIMAL LATERAL REIN

RECESS

MIDDLE PHALANGEAL ATTACHMENT OF CENTRAL 80% OF VOLAR PLATE

Figure 7-1 ✧ Hemisection of the bone and ligament anatomy of an interphalangeal joint. (*From Bowers WH: The anatomy of the interphalangeal joints. In The Hand and Upper Limb, vol 1. New York, Churchill Livingstone, 1987.*)

common mechanism of injury. This injury typically occurs with a ball's striking the extended or slightly flexed digit. Hyperextension ruptures the volar plate but leaves the collateral ligaments spared unless there is a concomitant varus or valgus force. The FDP insertion is typically spared, but the volar skin may be torn, leading to an open dislocation. Reduction with digital block anesthesia is performed with accentuation of the deformity followed by flexion with slight longitudinal traction. Postreduction stability through full flexion-extension and with gentle varus-valgus stress is assessed. Posteroanterior and true lateral radiographs after reduction are mandatory for evaluation of subtle subluxation. Immobilization of the DIP joint for 7 to 10 days after reduction for comfort and to reduce swelling is followed by protected active motion. Splinting is discontinued at about 1 month, depending on the patient's symptoms.

b. Volar dislocations are higher energy injuries with disruption of much of the ligamentous support and the extensor tendon. In addition to manual reduction, K-wire fixation across the DIP joint is typically required to maintain reduction. The wire is left in place for 6 weeks to protect the extensor repair. A slight extensor lag and moderate loss of motion are common.

c. Complex (irreducible) dislocations are unusual at the DIP joint. Interposed FDP, volar plate, and osteochondral fragments impeding joint reduction have all been described. The majority of these dislocations are open. The FDP tendon may be removed without further dissection to the deep structures, but collateral ligament release may be necessary to remove the volar plate if it is interposed. Volar plate or ligament repair is usually not indicated. For persistent instability after reduction, K-wire fixation with the joint in full extension is recommended. The wire is maintained in place for 3 weeks, followed by joint mobilization.

d. Treatment of open dislocations includes wound irrigation and débridement, intravenous antibiotics, and tetanus prophylaxis. Treatment is otherwise similar to that of the closed counterparts. Soft tissue injury is typically more extensive, which may necessitate K-wire fixation and compromise outcome (Fig. 7-2).

2. Pain and stiffness may persist for up to 6 months after DIP joint dislocation. Slight loss of motion and permanent swelling are common and proportional to the energy of injury.

FRACTURE-DISLOCATIONS

1. The mechanisms of injury involve axial loads, tendon avulsions, and more rarely crush injuries. Axial loads tend to produce articular comminution. Treatment of fractures associated with tendon avulsions is dependent on the amount of articular involvement, and consideration should be given to fracture fixation if there is DIP joint subluxation or

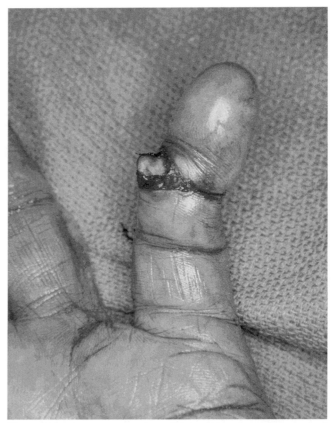

Figure 7-2 ❖ Open, complex DIP joint dislocation with interposed FDP tendon.

if the fracture fragment involves more than 50% of the articular surface (see Chapter 6).

a. Volar lip fractures of the distal phalanx associated with DIP joint dislocation are volar plate avulsion injuries that may or may not involve the FDP insertion. It is essential to document FDP function. Volar plate avulsion typically produces a stable joint after reduction. Treatment is identical to that of dislocations without fracture. Injuries with instability with extension can be treated with extension block splinting for 3 weeks. Radiographs in the splint confirming reduction are mandatory. If there is avulsion of the FDP tendon, surgical repair is necessary (see Chapter 2).

b. Comminuted fractures of the distal phalanx associated with DIP joint dislocation are often due to axial load injuries with significant bone comminution. Reduction of the articular surface can be technically challenging or impossible. If there are large fragments, open reduction to reapproximate the bone elements and to reattach the displaced tendon insertions can be attempted. External fixation, interfragmentary screws, sutures, wire loops, or K-wires can be used. Extensive articular destruction may necessitate primary or delayed arthrodesis. Some authors recommend initial nonsurgical management with splinting and early motion of these injuries. Fusion may then be performed electively if symptoms warrant after fracture union.

c. Post-traumatic instability is unusual if the joint is reduced adequately and immobilized with internal or external splinting. Residual subluxation does not preclude a clinically successful result, albeit with reduced motion. In symptomatic patients, DIP arthrodesis in slight flexion reduces symptoms of post-traumatic joint instability or arthrosis.

ATRAUMATIC INSTABILITY

Atraumatic instability is usually the result of end-stage inflammatory or degenerative arthritis or connective tissue disorders (e.g., Ehlers-Danlos syndrome). Digital dysfunction is high with DIP instability because the patient is unable to maintain the position of the tip in any forceful pinch or grasp. Splinting may be helpful in low-demand situations. DIP arthrodesis is the treatment of choice for patients with higher functional demands.

Proximal Interphalangeal Joint

ANATOMY

The bone configuration of the PIP joint (bicondylar with an intercondylar sulcus of proximal phalanx) makes the joint inherently stable (see Fig. 7-1). In addition to bony congruence, the soft tissue supports include the volar plate, the proper collateral ligaments, the accessory collateral ligaments, and the central slip of the extensor mechanism. The proper collateral ligaments are the primary restraint to varus-valgus instability in extension; the volar plate is the primary restraint to dorsal translation.

COLLATERAL LIGAMENT INJURIES

1. Lateral instability corresponds to disruption of the collateral ligaments. Injury to the radial side of the digits is more common. Injuries to the index finger are more common than are injuries to the ulnar three digits. The volar plate is a secondary restraint against varus-valgus instability and may avulse from the base of the middle phalanx, resulting in gross instability.
2. There is typically some degree of asymmetry on examination of swelling, tenderness, and stability. In vitro studies show that more than 20 degrees of lateral deviation corresponds to a disrupted collateral ligament. Three types of injury have been described.
   a. Type I: no instability on stress testing. These injuries are treated with 1 week of immobilization followed by active exercises and buddy taping for up to 3 to 4 weeks. Rehabilitation progresses to passive motion as needed at 6 weeks.
   b. Type II: less than 20 degrees of lateral instability on stress testing with a firm endpoint. The collateral ligaments may have ruptured, but secondary supports (volar plate) are intact. Treatment is controversial, but most surgeons treat with a short period of immobilization

(3 weeks) followed by mobilization as for type I.
   c. Type III: lateral instability greater than 20 degrees. The collateral ligaments and the volar plate are typically ruptured or may be avulsed with a small fragment off the lateral base of the proximal phalanx. Treatment may be conservative or surgical, although most authors report more rapid resolution of the symptoms of instability with surgical repair. Repair can be performed through a dorsal or midlateral approach by open reduction and internal fixation (ORIF) of bone fragments or anatomic repair of ligaments to bone (usually to the middle phalanx).

DISLOCATIONS

Dorsal Dislocation

1. The most common mechanism of injury is hyperextension. The volar plate typically fails distally, and small avulsion fractures are seen in up to one third of injuries. Dislocation in a purely dorsal direction may leave both collaterals intact, although any varus-valgus moment will result in rupture of one collateral ligament as well.
2. Radiographs are necessary to evaluate fracture of the volar lip of the middle phalanx and to confirm concentric reduction of the joint (Fig. 7-3). Reduction with digital block anesthesia is typically performed with post-reduction stress testing of the collaterals and the volar plate.
3. Irreducible dislocations are rare. Soft tissue interposition, which may be from the volar plate or flexor tendons, requires open reduction. Simple dislocations may be converted to complex ones with inappropriate reduction maneuvers. Reduction includes gentle traction and pressure to the base of the middle phalanx directed distally while trying to maintain contact between the base of the middle phalanx and the head of the proximal phalanx.
4. Injuries without dislocation or collateral ligament instability are treated with early mobilization. Buddy taping, compressive wrapping, and formal hand therapy are frequently used. Patients with instability with hyperextension only (i.e., volar plate insufficiency) are treated with an extension block splint at 20 degrees with active flexion-extension exercises in the splint for 4 weeks.
5. Open injuries require irrigation and débridement and may require pin stabilization before institution of early motion with protective splinting. Swelling and pain are common for 6 to 9 months with gradual improvement, but stiffness may be permanent.
6. The most common complications are stiffness and flexion contracture. These may respond to dynamic splinting in the first few months after injury. An indication for surgical release in the form of volar plate ("check rein" ligaments) or collateral ligament excision is the failure of a splinting program in a compliant patient without radiographic PIP arthrosis. "Pseudoboutonnière" deformity is a severe (>45 degree) flexion contracture of the PIP joint

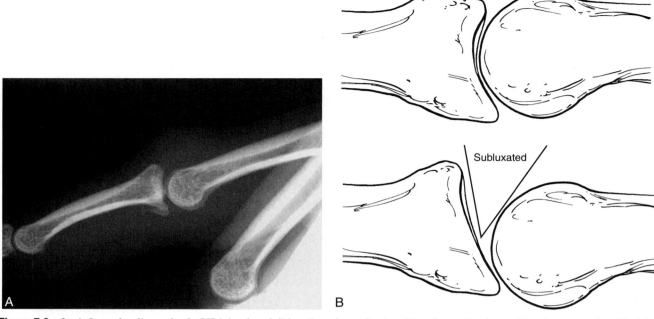

Figure 7-3 ◆ **A,** Lateral radiograph of a PIP joint dorsal dislocation after reduction. Note the small volar avulsion fracture and residual dorsal subluxation of the joint. **B,** Line drawing demonstrating subluxation of the joint and the dorsal "V" sign demonstrating residual incongruity of the joint. (**B** *from Blazar PE, Steinberg DR: Fractures of the proximal interphalangeal joint. J Acad Orthop Surg 8:383-390, 2000.*)

after a volar plate injury. Treatment includes surgical release of the PIP contracture. Hyperextension instability is unusual but may result in a swan-neck deformity. This can be treated with a volar plate reconstruction or a flexor digitorum superficialis tenodesis.

Volar Dislocation

Volar dislocations are less common. Both volar rotatory and pure volar patterns have been recognized.

1. In volar rotatory dislocations, one condyle of the proximal phalanx ruptures through the interval between the central slip and the lateral band (Fig. 7-4). These two components of the extensor mechanism form a noose around the condyle, making closed reduction impossible. One attempt at closed reduction is recommended with the wrist in mild extension, the metacarpophalangeal (MP) and PIP joints in 90 degrees of flexion to loosen the lateral band from the condyle. The reduction maneuver includes derotation and longitudinal traction in this position. If closed reduction is successful, the joint is immobilized in extension for 4 weeks. If it is unsuccessful, open reduction is required through a dorsal approach. The rent in the extensor is repaired. If the central slip is avulsed, repair is recommended. Motion is started at 4 weeks and progressed to passive and dynamic splints at 8 weeks.

2. Pure volar dislocations involve injury to a collateral ligament, the volar plate, and the central slip. These dislocations tend to be reduced easily but can demonstrate an extensor lag after reduction due to disruption of the central slip. K-wire fixation

across the PIP joint in full extension for 4 weeks with the DIP and MP joints left free for active mobilization is recommended.

FRACTURE-DISLOCATIONS

Three main patterns of injury are seen: volar lip, dorsal lip, and combined volar and dorsal lip (pilon-type injuries). The outcome of these injuries is most closely correlated with the restoration of articular congruity.

Volar Lip

1. Volar lip injuries may occur as part of a hyperextension mechanism (similar to dorsal dislocations) or with a longitudinal impaction of the extended or slightly flexed finger. The fracture patterns seen with these two mechanisms vary. Hyperextension injuries are avulsions with minimal comminution. In contrast, impaction injuries typically produce comminution of the articular surface. Impaction of the comminuted articular surface into the metaphysis is characteristic. Dorsal subluxation-dislocation is a concern because the primary anatomic structures resisting dorsal displacement (the volar plate and volar lip of the middle phalanx) are both detached from the body of the middle phalanx. In addition, if the volar fragment is large enough, the insertion of the collateral ligaments on the middle phalanx can be entirely on the fractured fragment, rendering the joint grossly unstable.

2. Stability depends on the percentage of the articular surface involved (Fig. 7-5). The treatment goal is congruent reduction and stability of the joint; anatomic restoration of the articular surface is

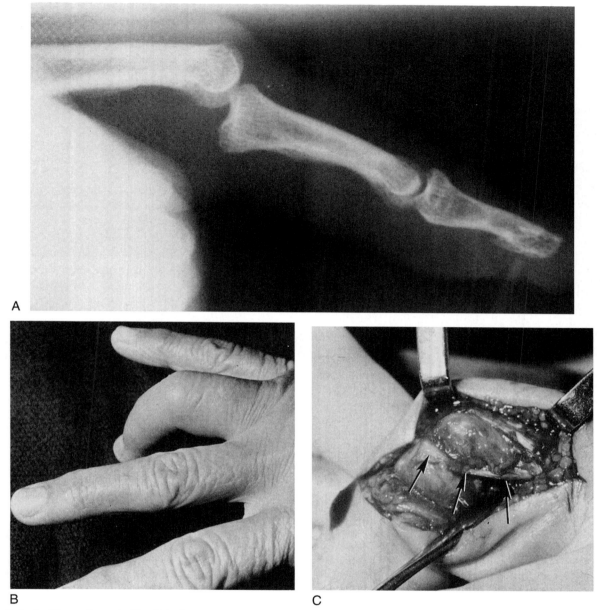

A

B   C

Figure 7-4 ⟡   The radiograph **(A),** clinical appearance **(B),** and operative pathology **(C)** of an irreducible volar dislocation. Note that the lateral band *(arrows)* has been split off the central slip and is interposed between the proximal phalangeal condyle and the displaced middle phalanx, impeding reduction. *(From Bowers WH: The anatomy of the interphalangeal joints. In The Hand and Upper Limb, vol 1. New York, Churchill Livingstone, 1987.)*

frequently technically challenging. If less than 30% of the joint surface is involved, the joint tends to be stable. Fracture of more than 50% of the articular surface leads to instability. Involvement of 30% to 50% of the articular surface leads to injuries that are potentially unstable. The assessment of stability is based on clinical assessment as well as radiographic parameters.

a. For stable injuries, buddy taping or extension block splinting with protected motion is recommended. At 6 weeks, passive motion may be added. All fractures must be clinically and radiographically re-examined within a week to check for signs of subluxation. If the joint remains stable, the outcome is dependent more on the time of immobilization than on reduction of the fragment or the presence of bone union. Slight PIP flexion contractures (<20 degrees) are common.

b. Potentially unstable injuries (30% to 50% of the articular surface involved) may be treated with static splinting, percutaneous pinning of the joint, extension block splinting, extension block K-wire, or a variety of other techniques.

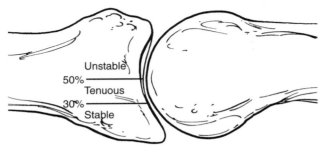

Figure 7-5 ◈ Classification of PIP fracture-dislocations. Stable (type I) injuries involve less than 30% of the articular surface and demonstrate no instability on stress testing. Tenuous (type II) injuries involve 30% to 50% of the articular surface, but reduction can be maintained with 30 degrees or less of joint flexion. All fracture-dislocations that have consumed 50% or more of the articular surface are unstable. Fractures with 30% to 50% joint surface involvement that will stay reduced only with more than 30 degrees of flexion are also classified as unstable. *(From Peimer CA: Surgery of the Hand and Upper Limb, vol 1. New York, McGraw-Hill, 1996.)*

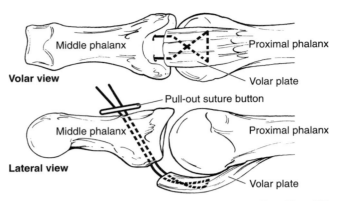

Figure 7-7 ◈ Volar plate arthroplasty technique. *(From Blazar PE, Steinberg DR: Fractures of the proximal interphalangeal joint. J Acad Orthop Surg 8:383-390, 2000.)*

Active flexion with an external block to extension is commonly chosen (Fig. 7-6). The digit is reassessed at 1 week, and the position is subsequently extended 10 degrees a week. The splint is removed after a week at full extension.

c. Injuries of more than 50% of the articular surface or clinically proven unstable are treated surgically. Restoration of the volar lip is necessary to prevent chronic subluxation. This may be done with traction applied through an external fixator, ORIF, volar plate arthroplasty, or "banjo" traction. ORIF, although theoretically attractive, must be approached with caution because radiographs may underestimate the comminution of the articular surface. The inability to proceed with early motion after attempted rigid internal fixation will invariably lead to a stiff PIP joint. Volar plate arthroplasty, a salvage option for comminuted fractures with an intact dorsal lip (Fig. 7-7), is performed through a volar approach, resurfacing the base of the middle phalanx with an advanced volar plate. Excision of 80% of the collateral ligaments is recommended to achieve reduction. The joint is held reduced with a K-wire or external fixator for a minimum of 2 to 3 weeks. This is followed by active and passive PIP motion with a dorsal blocking splint.

Dorsal Lip

These injuries are less common than volar lip injuries. The fracture fragment tends to be small and may include the insertion of the central slip. Dorsal lip fracture-dislocation occurs in the setting of an injury to one collateral ligament and can lead to varus-valgus instability. A PIP extensor lag is typically present if the fracture is displaced after the joint is reduced. ORIF should be considered for displacement of more than 1 mm.

Combined Volar and Dorsal Lip

1. Injuries that disrupt the volar and dorsal lips tend to occur with higher energy, axial-loading mechanisms. The articular surface is characteristically impacted and extensively comminuted. Because of the soft tissue and articular injuries, results of treatment are rarely completely satisfactory.

2. Treatment options include splinting, ORIF, traction, and external fixation. The last three options may allow early mobilization, although the extensive comminution rarely results in adequate stability for early motion after ORIF alone. Many authors prefer skeletal traction (Fig. 7-8) for 6 weeks with limited or no restoration of the articular surface in the most complex injuries. The patient is instructed to begin immediate mobilization of the PIP and DIP joints in traction. The base of the middle phalanx has shown some ability to remodel with time, and most patients achieve functional motion with some loss at both the PIP and DIP joints. These injuries have the highest risk for degenerative changes of any PIP injury. Restoration of articular congruence is the most important factor for a successful outcome.

CHRONIC DISLOCATIONS

Late presentation is not unusual. Patients usually have pain and swelling, and the digit is held in extension

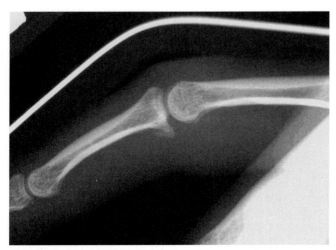

Figure 7-6 ◈ Residual PIP joint instability treated with extension block splinting. Note the congruent reduction of the joint.

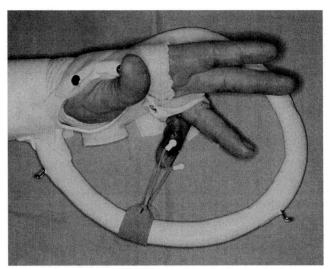

Figure 7-8 ◆ PIP pilon-type fracture-dislocation treated with traction and early motion.

with limited motion. If the articular surfaces are not destroyed, restoration of the joint is possible. An extensive release including the collateral ligaments is required to achieve reduction. Volar plate arthroplasty with or without dynamic external fixation is the procedure of choice for chronic dislocation with a salvageable joint, but it can be complicated by redislocation, angular deformity, and PIP and DIP joint stiffness.

Metacarpophalangeal Joint

ANATOMY

The articular surfaces of the MP joints are less congruent than those of the other digital joints. The metacarpal head is wider and the four metacarpal heads are slightly convergent volarly. The proximal phalanx articular surface is concave and is more congruent with the head in flexion than in extension. The supporting ligaments include the collateral ligaments, the accessory collateral ligaments, and the volar plate. The collateral ligaments arise from the radial and ulnar aspects of the head dorsal to the axis of rotation of the joint and insert on the volar half of the proximal phalanx. The accessory collateral ligaments arise from the metaphysis confluent with the proper collaterals and insert on the lateral aspect of the volar plate. The collateral ligaments are stretched as the joint is brought into flexion from their eccentric origin relative to the axis of motion and by the broader volar aspect of the head. This creates a "cam" effect, increasing lateral stability in flexion (see Fig. 1-6). The volar plate is firmly anchored to the base of the proximal phalanx and is the primary stabilizer against hyperextension. The volar plates of the ulnar four digits are interconnected through the deep transverse metacarpal ligament.

COLLATERAL LIGAMENT INJURIES

1. These are relatively uncommon injuries in the fingers. They occur more commonly on the radial side of the index finger and the ulnar side of the small finger. They may be associated with avulsion fragments that may be large distally and may go on to nonunion.
2. Stress testing of the ligament is performed in flexion because the collateral ligaments are taut in MP joint flexion.
   a. Injuries without instability are treated as simple sprains. Buddy taping for comfort and to protect against further injury is recommended for 3 weeks.
   b. Injuries with slight laxity on stress testing but with a solid endpoint represent partial ligament tears. These injuries are splinted for 3 weeks, and then intermittent active range of motion is started with buddy taping until range of motion and comfort improve. The position of splinting is midrange flexion, chosen as a compromise between removing tension from the ligament (with extension) and preventing extension contractures.
   c. Complete ligament ruptures present with instability and lack of an endpoint on stress testing. Patients with joint subluxation, rotational deformity (around the intact collateral), or associated sagittal band disruption are candidates for surgical repair. Displaced (>1 to 2 mm) avulsion fractures are also candidates for surgical repair. Patients presenting late (>3 to 6 weeks) may not be candidates for repair because of ligament scarring. Ligament reconstruction with a free palmaris longus tendon graft is the procedure of choice for symptomatic chronic instability.

DISLOCATIONS

Dorsal Dislocation

Dorsal MP joint dislocations are of two types, simple and complex. The most common digit involved is the index, and the mechanism is usually hyperextension. The ring and long fingers may dislocate along with the adjacent border digit but rarely in isolation.

1. Simple dislocations
   a. These injuries are reducible with manipulation and present with the more striking deformity, with the digit in almost 90 degrees of hyperextension. The base of the proximal phalanx is typically in contact with the dorsum of the metacarpal head.
   b. Simple dislocations must be reduced with caution. Longitudinal traction or hyperextension can convert a simple dislocation into a complex one. The preferred reduction maneuver is to push the proximal phalangeal base distally while flexing the joint and trying to maintain contact between the base of the phalanx and the metacarpal head.
   c. Simple dislocations are stable after reduction. The joint should remain reduced through a full range of active motion. Mobilization after 2 weeks in a splint at 60 degrees of MP joint flexion is recommended. Redislocation is a sign of

persistent subluxation or interposed osteochondral fragments. Surgical exploration is indicated in these cases.

2. Complex dislocations
   a. These injuries are not reducible because interposition of the volar plate blocks reduction. In the index finger, the lumbrical displaces radial to the metacarpal; the flexor tendons displace ulnar. These two structures are looped around the metacarpal neck. The small finger demonstrates a similar loop around the metacarpal neck with the flexor tendons radial and the abductor digiti minimi ulnar (Fig. 7-9).
   b. Complex dislocations show bayonet apposition of the joint surfaces. The metacarpal head is palpable in the palm, and there may be a characteristic dimple in the volar skin from attachments of the volar fascia to the transverse metacarpal ligament. The presence of dimpling or a sesamoid within the joint space is a pathognomonic sign of a complex dislocation.
   c. Complex dislocations are treated with operative reduction. Volar and dorsal approaches have both been recommended. The radial digital nerve to the index finger and the ulnar digital nerve of the small finger are displaced between the tethered skin and the metacarpal head. Extreme care must be taken to avoid injury to these structures because they are more superficial than expected from the volar approach. Longitudinal division of the volar plate allows relocation of the joint, although this is technically easier from the dorsal approach.
   d. After reduction, these injuries are inherently stable. Postoperative mobilization is started in about 1 week with an extension-blocking splint. Osteochondral injuries are more easily visualized and treated through the dorsal approach. Any tendency for resubluxation of the joint after attempted reduction suggests osteochondral fragments or interposed soft tissue between the articular surfaces.

Volar Dislocation

1. These injuries are much less common and are thought to occur from hyperflexion injuries. Digits may show malrotation and hyperextension.
2. Radiographs are often difficult to interpret; posteroanterior views may show overlap of the proximal phalanx on the metacarpal head. Lateral views are limited by overlap of adjacent digits, and careful scrutiny is required. Oblique views may reveal joint incongruity.
3. At least one collateral ligament and the volar plate are disrupted. Closed reduction may be successful, but the joint is usually unstable secondary to the associated soft tissue or bone disruption. Surgical repair of the affected collateral ligament is typically necessary to restore stability.

Chronic Dislocations

Open reduction is invariably necessary unless extensive articular destruction has occurred and requires extensive soft tissue release to achieve joint reduction.

Release of the dorsal capsule and collateral ligaments is required along with mobilization of the extensor tendon. After reduction, the joint may need to be percutaneously pinned for 3 to 4 weeks to avoid redislocation.

Multiple Dislocations

1. These injuries result from high-energy trauma and often present with massive hand swelling. Multiple MP dislocations are commonly simple dislocations and easily reducible.
2. One or more of the dislocations may be open and require irrigation and débridement and open reduction through the volar wound. If complex, all four MP joints can be reduced through two dorsal interspace incisions. Because of the high-energy nature of these injuries, there is a propensity for complications including compartment syndrome, intrinsic tightness, and loss of motion. After 48 to 72 hours of immobilization, patients begin aggressive mobilization, protecting against the terminal 20 degrees of extension for 4 weeks. At 4 weeks, protective splinting is discontinued and passive modalities into extension may be instituted.

Carpometacarpal Joint

ANATOMY

1. The bases of the index and long fingers are functionally fixed to the carpus by strong ligaments. The surface of the index metacarpal has articular facets for the trapezium, trapezoid, capitate, and third metacarpal. Strong dorsal and interosseous ligaments of the index and long fingers permit almost no motion at these articulations.
2. The ring and small metacarpal articular surfaces are more "saddle" shaped and articulate with the hamate. The surface of the hamate, which articulates with the small metacarpal, is more oblique to the long axis of the hand and has two facets. The ring carpometacarpal (CMC) joint typically has 10 degrees of motion in the sagittal plane, and the small CMC joint allows about 40 degrees of motion (flexion accompanied by supination).

DISLOCATIONS

1. Isolated CMC dislocations of the small finger are not uncommon and typically are caused by indirect trauma resulting in fracture-dislocations. A "reversed Bennett's" fracture pattern can occur with a volar-radial articular fragment left in situ and dorsal dislocation of the remainder of the metacarpal in continuity with the majority of the articular surface.
2. True lateral radiographs of the affected joints may be necessary to reveal the dislocation of the metacarpal base. Bora and Didizian describe a 30° pronated lateral view to assess the joint.
3. Fracture-dislocations usually occur with injury at multiple joints. The central three finger CMC dislocations are generally the result of high-energy trauma. These are frequently overlooked in the polytrauma patient in whom evaluation is delayed because of associated injuries.
4. Because of the high-energy nature of multiple injuries, there is a propensity for complications

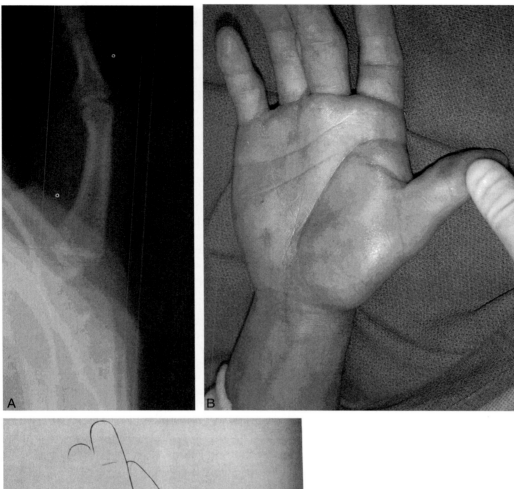

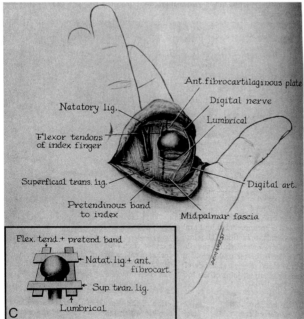

Figure 7-9 ◆ **A,** Lateral radiograph of a complex MP dislocation of the index finger. **B,** Note dimpling in skin over metacarpal head on the palm of the hand. **C,** Schematic of structures interfering with reduction of the metacarpal head. *(From Kaplan EB: Dorsal dislocation of the metacarpophalangeal joint of the index finger. J Bone Joint Surg Am 39:1081-1086, 1957.)*

including compartment syndrome, intrinsic tightness, and loss of motion.

MANAGEMENT

Small Finger CMC Dislocation

1. Fifth CMC fracture-dislocations are typically easily reduced closed but can be unstable after reduction. Percutaneous pinning is commonly used to maintain reduction.

2. Rarely, the fractured articular surface is in one or two fragments that can be treated by ORIF with rigid internal fixation. More commonly, the joint surface is comminuted. ORIF may be necessary for irreducible dislocations.

Multiple CMC Dislocations

1. Reduction is accomplished by traction and dorsal or volar pressure, depending on the direction of the dislocation, followed by percutaneous pinning, which is the treatment of choice. Pins are left in place for 4 to 6 weeks, followed by range-of-motion exercises.

2. Complex injuries or fracture-dislocations with large articular fragments can be treated by ORIF. This can be achieved through two incisions at the base of the index and ring fingers or one longer incision located centrally.

Thumb Joints

Interphalangeal Joint

ANATOMY

The head of the proximal phalanx is bicondylar, and the base of the middle phalanx is biconcave. This joint contour confers some stability, but the major stabilizers are ligamentous. The collateral ligaments and volar plate are analogous to the same structures in the finger interphalangeal (IP) joints (see Fig. 7-1).

COLLATERAL LIGAMENT INJURIES

1. In the thumb IP joint, collateral ligament injuries are much less common than at the MP joint level. Injuries without instability are splinted for comfort and treated with early mobilization. As for the MP joint, injuries to the ulnar side of the thumb are protected longer. Anatomic differences from the MP joint eliminate the potential for a Stener-type lesion, and therefore surgical repair is rarely required.

2. Injuries with instability to varus-valgus stress are immobilized for 10 to 14 days, and then protected mobilization is begun. Chronic instability may be seen in patients with rheumatoid arthritis or other inflammatory arthropathies. These patients may benefit from arthrodesis.

DISLOCATIONS

1. Closed dorsal dislocation of the thumb IP joint is an uncommon injury that is thought to occur from hyperextension. It may be simple or complex. Complex injuries are likely to have a rotational component and complete disruption of one collateral ligament. The volar plate or flexor pollicis longus may be interposed. Most reported complex cases are open volarly.

2. The majority of these dislocations are reducible with manipulation. Digital block anesthesia is used. After reduction, stability is assessed with active range of motion and stress testing of the collaterals. If stable, the joint is splinted for 10 days, and an extension block splint is subsequently used for 3 to 4 weeks. If the injury is open, surgical irrigation and débridement and reduction are necessary. For complex dislocations, the interposed soft tissue is removed and the volar plate is repaired.

Thumb Metacarpophalangeal Joint

ANATOMY

1. The base of the proximal phalanx is concave and shallow. The metacarpal head is more oval than circular when seen in cross section. There is relatively little bone stability.

2. The capsular soft tissues including the radial and ulnar collateral ligaments, the accessory collateral ligaments, and the volar plate primarily confer stability. The proper collateral ligaments originate from a fossa in the metacarpal neck dorsal to the axis of rotation and insert on the volar-lateral base of the proximal phalanx. The proper collaterals are the primary stabilizers against varus-valgus instability in flexion. The accessory collateral ligaments originate volar to the proper collateral and insert on the volar plate and sesamoid. The volar plate is a cartilaginous structure that incorporates the radial and ulnar sesamoids in its substance.

3. The thumb MP joint has the most widely varying range of motion in the body that has been ascribed to variations in the curvature of the metacarpal head in the volar-dorsal plane. The volar plate is the primary stabilizer against hyperextension. It is also an important secondary stabilizer against varus-valgus instability in extension. The accessory collaterals and the volar plate are the primary stabilizers against varus-valgus stress with the joint in extension. The proper collateral assumes that role with the joint in 30 degrees or more of flexion.

COLLATERAL LIGAMENT INJURIES

Ulnar Collateral Ligament

1. Ulnar collateral ligament injury of the thumb has come to be referred to as gamekeeper's thumb. The classic gamekeeper's thumb is a chronic attenuation of the ligament that was originally described from repetitive hyperextension against an adducted thumb.

2. Acute injuries (e.g., skier's thumb) are much more common in clinical practice. The injury occurs from forced hyperabduction-extension. Injuries are classified as complete (unstable joint) or incomplete. The majority of complete tears are at the distal attachment, although they can occur at any point.

3. Stener described the displacement of the proximal ligament superficial and proximal to the adductor aponeurosis with the distal attachment remaining deep to the aponeurosis (Fig. 7-10A). With a Stener lesion, the interposed tissue (adductor aponeurosis) forms a physical barrier that impedes healing of the injured ligament and leads to chronic instability.

4. Ligament insufficiency may occur with an avulsion fracture of the base of the proximal phalanx or the metacarpal head; however, fractures in this area may occur with or without ligament insufficiency.

Evaluation and Management

1. Distinction between complete and partial tears of the ulnar collateral ligament can be difficult.

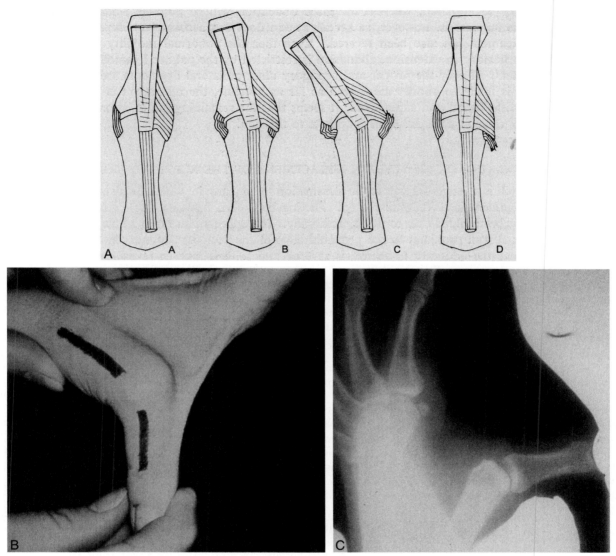

Figure 7-10 ◈ **A,** Schematic of a Stener lesion. *A,* The ulnar collateral ligament lies below the adductor aponeurosis. *B* and *C,* As the joint is forced into radial deviation, the collateral ligament becomes detached from the proximal phalanx. The adductor aponeurosis then covers the insertion of the collateral ligament. *D,* As the joint returns to normal alignment, the distal stump of the collateral ligament is forced proximally by the proximal edge of the aponeurosis, creating a Stener lesion and impairing the ability of the ligament to heal to its insertion point. **B** and **C,** Clinical photograph **(B)** and radiograph **(C)** of stress testing of the ulnar collateral ligament reveal instability due to complete rupture of the ligament. *(A from Stener B: Displacement of the ruptured ulnar collateral ligament of the metacarpophalangeal joint of the thumb. J Bone Joint Surg Br 44:869-879, 1962.)*

Because of the concern of displacing an avulsion fracture, radiographic evaluation before stressing the joint for stability is recommended. Injuries with nondisplaced avulsion fractures can also involve intrasubstance ligament tears.

2. The joint is stressed in full extension and at 30 degrees of flexion to isolate the ulnar collateral ligament. The injured side is compared with the uninjured side; 30 to 35 degrees of increased angulation in extension or 15 degrees in flexion is considered diagnostic of a complete rupture. Intra-articular local anesthetic or median and radial nerve blocks may be necessary for patients unable to tolerate the examination (Fig. 7-10*B* and *C*).

3. The reported incidence of Stener lesions and the ability to detect them on physical examination remain controversial. Stener reported a 64% incidence, but other studies have ranged widely with 14% to 83% of patients with this pathologic process. A painful, palpable mass on the ulnar aspect of the metacarpal head-neck junction in this setting is thought to be specific but of intermediate sensitivity for detecting Stener lesions. Stress radiography, arthrography, and magnetic resonance imaging (MRI) have been suggested to separate partial and complete ligament tears and to diagnose a Stener lesion, although none is routinely used by most hand surgeons.

Treatment

1. Partial tears are treated with immobilization in a thumb spica cast or splint for 4 to 6 weeks. Progressive mobilization is then begun with strengthening deferred until 8 weeks and restoration of full range of motion.
2. Complete tears are most commonly repaired surgically. Midsubstance tears and those with substantial ligament remnants are directly repaired with suture. The more common lesion (ligament detachment from the proximal phalanx) is repaired over a button with a pull-out suture or with a small suture anchor. Reattachment at a site as little as 2 mm volar, proximal, dorsal, or distal to the normal insertion alters MP joint motion in vitro. During surgery, volar plate and dorsal capsular injuries are also sought and may be repaired. If there is a fracture fragment sufficient in size for internal fixation, repair can be accomplished with K-wires, a tension band construct, or small screws. The presence of a nondisplaced avulsion fracture from the proximal phalanx does not preclude a concomitant ligament rupture. Unrepairable, smaller fragments are excised, and the ligament is repaired to the insertion site.
3. Postoperatively, the patient is immobilized for 4 to 5 weeks. Progressive mobilization and strengthening are then started.
4. A complete tear without a Stener lesion is controversial in its incidence, diagnosis, and treatment. Some authors recommend exploration of all complete injuries for repair and definitive diagnosis of the Stener lesion. Others use some of the diagnostic modalities mentioned before, and if a Stener lesion is not found, cast treatment is recommended.

Chronic Ulnar Collateral Ligament Instability

Patients with chronic instability typically present with pain or complaints of instability and weakness. Persistent pain, subluxation, and weakness are indications for surgical treatment. The static techniques employ a free tendon graft (commonly the palmaris longus) placed through drill holes to reconstruct the torn ligament. Dynamic techniques use a tendon transfer or tendon advancement. Both procedures have been shown to improve function but may lead to decreased motion of the MP joint. For MP joints with post-traumatic arthrosis, arthrodesis is the preferred procedure.

Radial Collateral Ligament

1. Varus instability is seen less commonly than ulnar-sided injuries are. There may be associated injuries to the abductor aponeurosis, the extensor hood, the EPB tendon, and the dorsal capsule. The abductor aponeurosis overlies the collateral ligament but is broader and prevents superficial displacement of the ligament as is seen on the ulnar side with Stener lesions.
2. Criteria for determining varus instability are usually analogous to those for determining injury to the ulnar side of the joint. There is a high degree of variation in the thumb MP joint, so comparison to

the opposite hand is mandatory. Volar and rotatory subluxation can occur with injury to one collateral ligament and the dorsal capsule. The rotation occurs about the intact ulnar collateral ligament with volar displacement of the proximal phalanx.

3. Treatment of incomplete tears is cast immobilization. Treatment of complete tears without joint subluxation is controversial. Radial collateral ligament instability in combination with joint subluxation is considered an indication for exploration and repair. Bone avulsions and insertional tears are repaired with suture anchors or over a button. Midsubstance tears are directly repaired. If there is volar subluxation of the joint, a repair of the dorsal capsule should be performed.
4. Chronic injuries (>8 weeks) may present with pain and a sense of instability with pinch. The instability tends to be rotational when it is present. Initial treatment includes splinting and anti-inflammatory medication. Reconstruction of the collateral ligament with free tendon graft or advancement of local tissue has been described for symptoms refractory to nonsurgical methods.

DISLOCATIONS

1. Most thumb MP joint dislocations are dorsal.
2. Most can be reduced in a closed fashion by flexion of the joint with downward pressure on the proximal phalanx to avoid soft tissue entrapment.
3. Irreducible dislocations can be due to entrapment of the flexor tendon, sesamoids, or volar plate. These require open reduction and pinning for 3 weeks.

Thumb Carpometacarpal Joint

ANATOMY

The thumb CMC joint has little intrinsic bone stability. The bases of the metacarpal and the trapezium have been described as two opposing saddle shapes. This allows circumduction and axial rotation. The stability of the joint is provided by the capsular ligaments. The restraints to dorsal trapezial-metacarpal dislocation include the dorsoradial ligament and the superficial and deep apical oblique (beak) ligaments. Attenuation or instability of the basilar joint has been implicated as a causative factor in thumb CMC arthritis.

DISLOCATIONS

1. Dislocations are the least common CMC injury pattern. The dorsal radial ligament on the trapezial-metacarpal joint is the primary soft tissue restraint. For this reason, most trapezial-metacarpal joint dislocations occur in a dorsal direction.
2. In general, these injuries are reducible in a closed manner. Resubluxation without internal fixation can occur.
3. Controversy exists whether closed management with or without percutaneous pinning is adequate treatment or whether ligament repair or reconstruction (tendon graft with use of half of the flexor carpi radialis) is required. Most authors favor early ligament repair or reconstruction because of concern for persistent instability.

FRACTURE-DISLOCATIONS (see Chapter 6)

Bennett's Fracture

1. Bennett's fracture represents fracture-dislocation of the thumb CMC joint with a fragment of variable size of the metacarpal base remaining attached to the beak ligament. Deforming forces include adductor pollicis and abductor pollicis longus. These two combine to supinate, adduct, and flex the metacarpal shaft.
2. Surgical treatment of these injuries is the norm in the form of percutaneous pinning or ORIF. Pin placement may be across the CMC joint, to the volar fragment or to the second metacarpal. Unlike in most articular fractures, the relationship between fracture congruence and subsequent degenerative change is unclear.

Rolando's Fracture

1. Rolando described T- or Y-shaped, three-part articular fractures of the base of the thumb metacarpal. The eponym is commonly used to describe comminuted fractures of the base of the thumb metacarpal.
2. The preferred management for the majority of these injuries is closed reduction and percutaneous pinning. ORIF may be performed, and external fixation is considered for comminuted fractures.

ATRAUMATIC INSTABILITY

1. Instability of the thumb CMC joint is a cause of radial-sided wrist pain. It typically occurs in women aged 25 to 40 years.
2. Symptoms may respond to medication and splinting, but surgical stabilization with half of the flexor carpi radialis tendon is indicated in patients with persistent symptoms.
3. The development of osteoarthritis in patients with joint laxity and subluxation has been suggested, but a definite association has not been demonstrated.

Wrist Joint

Carpal Instability

ANATOMY

Osteology

1. The wrist joint is composed of eight carpal bones (scaphoid, lunate, triquetrum, trapezium, trapezoid, capitate, hamate, pisiform), the distal ends of the radius and ulna, and the five metacarpals. The pisiform is considered a sesamoid bone within the flexor carpi ulnaris tendon. There are 13 intracarpal articulations, not including the CMC articulations and the distal radioulnar joint (DRUJ).
2. The carpal bones are often grouped into two rows, proximal (scaphoid, lunate, and triquetrum) and distal (hamate, capitate, trapezoid, and trapezium). The scaphoid is thought to "link" the two rows.
3. The distal radius articular surface is obliquely oriented volarly and ulnarly relative to the long axis of the radius. The articular surface of the distal radius is divided into the triangular scaphoid fossa and the quadrangular lunate fossa by the fibrocartilage interfossal ridge.

Soft Tissue

Wrist ligaments are described as extrinsic if they originate or insert on a non-carpal bone and intrinsic if they originate and insert on one or more of the eight carpal bones.

Extrinsic Ligaments

1. The supporting extrinsic ligaments are fibrous thickenings that reside within the capsule and contain collagen-filled bundles covered by a synovial lamina on the articular side. Some contain neurovascular structures that supply the carpal bones.
2. The extrinsic ligaments of the wrist, such as the radioscaphocapitate ligament and the long radiolunate ligament, have viscoelastic properties similar to other human ligaments, with loads to failure of approximately 100 to 200 N.
   a. The volar extrinsic ligaments are stronger than the dorsal ligaments (Fig. 7-11). They originate on the volar lip of the radius from the styloid

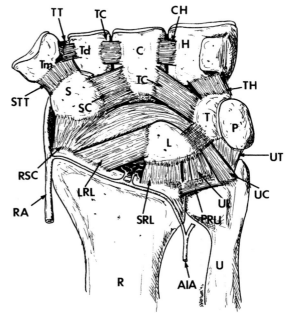

Figure 7-11 ◈ The palmar carpal ligaments from a palmar perspective. Note how the extrinsic ligaments tend to merge toward the midline from their more peripheral proximal attachments. Each set of adjacent carpal bones has an interosseous ligament connecting them, except the joint between the capitate and lunate. It is difficult to define planes separating the individual ligaments from the palmar perspective. Ligaments: RSC, radioscaphocapitate; LRL, long radiolunate; SRL, short radiolunate; UL, ulnolunate; UT, ulnotriquetral; UC, ulnocapitate; PRU, palmar radioulnar; STT, scaphotrapeziotrapezoid; SC, scaphocapitate; TC, triquetrocapitate; TH, triquetrohamate; TT, trapeziotrapezoid; TC, triquetrocapitate; CH, capitohamate. Bones: R, radius; U, ulna; S, scaphoid; L, lunate; T, triquetrum; P, pisiform; Tm, trapezium; Td, trapezoid; C, capitate; H, hamate. Note that the radial carpal arch (RCA), formed by branches from the radial (RA) and anterior interosseous (AIA) arteries, contributes to the vascular leash that penetrates the radiocarpal joint capsule between the LRL and SRL as the radioscapholunate "ligament." *(From Berger RA: The ligaments of the wrist: a current overview of anatomy with considerations of their potential functions. Hand Clin 13:63-82, 1997.)*

process to the volar radial aspect of the lunate fossa.

   i. These ligaments are best individually visualized arthroscopically.

   ii. From radial to ulnar, these ligaments include the radioscaphocapitate, long radiolunate, radioscapholunate, and short radiolunate.

   iii. The radioscapholunate ligament (ligament of Testut) is a neurovascular structure with no mechanical function; it is a remnant of the fetal mesenchymal division between the facets of the radius.

   iv. Viewed from the volar perspective, there is a central area over the distal lunate–midcarpal joint devoid of the stout ligaments of the remainder of the volar capsule known as the space of Poirier (see Fig. 7-11).

   v. Ulnarly, the ulnocapitate ligament forms the ulnar component of the arcuate complex at the distal aspect of the space of Poirier.

   vi. Three confluent ligaments form the ulnocarpal ligament complex: the ulnocapitate, ulnolunate, and ulnotriquetral ligaments. The ulnolunate and ulnotriquetral ligaments arise from the volar radioulnar ligament of the triangular fibrocartilage complex (TFCC) and insert into their respective carpal bones.

   vii. The ulnolunate ligament inserts on the ulnar portion of the volar aspect of the lunate, where it is confluent with the insertion of the short radiolunate ligament.

   viii. The ulnotriquetral ligament passes to the triquetrum and forms the distal portion of the extensor carpi ulnaris subsheath. The prestyloid recess lies within the ulnotriquetral ligament. The ulnotriquetral ligament also commonly has a small aperture that communicates between the radiocarpal and pisotriquetral joints and can be seen arthroscopically.

   ix. In contrast to the volar radial ligaments, the ulnar ligaments appear as a confluent capsule when viewed arthroscopically.

   x. The ulnocapitate ligament originates from the fovea of the ulnar head and the base of the ulnar styloid and lies just volar to the ulnolunate and ulnotriquetral ligaments to insert on the neck of the capitate.

  b. The dorsal extrinsic ligaments include the dorsal radiocarpal and dorsal intercarpal ligaments (Fig. 7-12).

   i. The dorsal radiocarpal ligament arises from the radius between Lister's tubercle and the sigmoid notch and inserts into the dorsal tubercle of the triquetrum.

   ii. The dorsal intercarpal ligament originates from the dorsum of the triquetrum and inserts on the dorsal aspects of the trapezoid and the waist of the scaphoid.

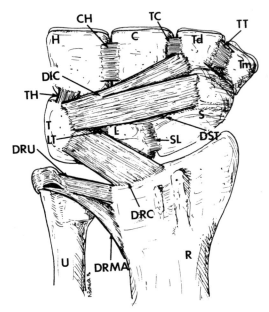

Figure 7-12 ◈ The dorsal carpal ligaments from a dorsal perspective. Ligaments: DRU, dorsal radioulnar; DRMA, dorsal radial metaphyseal arcuate; DRC, dorsal radiocarpal; DIC, dorsal intercarpal; DST, dorsal scaphotriquetral; SL, scapholunate; LT, lunotriquetral; TH, triquetrohamate; TT, trapeziotrapezoid; TC, trapeziocapitate; CH, capitohamate. Bones: R, radius; U, ulna; S, scaphoid; L, lunate; T, triquetrum; Tm, trapezium; Td, trapezoid; C, capitate; H, hamate. *(From Berger RA: The ligaments of the wrist: a current overview of anatomy with considerations of their potential functions. Hand Clin 13: 63-82, 1997.)*

Intrinsic Ligaments

1. The intrinsic ligaments are numerous, and every articulation within the proximal and distal carpal rows has an interosseous ligament or a pair of ligaments (volar and dorsal).

2. The intrinsic ligaments have been shown to have high loads to failure of approximately 300 N of longitudinal load.

3. The proximal row ligaments include the scapholunate interosseous ligament (SLIL) and lunotriquetral interosseous ligament (LTIL). They are U-shaped ligaments with three distinct anatomic regions, volar, central, and dorsal. The central region is composed of fibrocartilage.

  a. Mechanically, the strongest and anatomically thickest component of the SLIL is the dorsal region. The dorsal limb is the primary constraint for scapholunate translation; the volar component limits rotation.

  b. The LTIL ligament is similarly shaped, although the volar region is the thickest and resists lunotriquetral translation; the dorsal component resists lunotriquetral rotation.

4. Ligaments within the distal carpal row are found between the trapezium and trapezoid, trapezium and capitate, and capitate and hamate.

  a. These ligaments are short and stout, with dorsal and volar components. The combination of highly congruous articular surfaces and this stout ligament limits motion between the components of the distal carpal row and leads to a complex that functions mechanically as a single unit.

KINEMATICS

1. Kinematics is the study of the motion of objects without consideration of the forces acting on them.
2. The wrist is a unique human joint kinematically because the musculotendinous units that act on the carpus do not insert on or arise from any of the carpal bones (one exception: the flexor carpi ulnaris indirectly inserts onto the hamate by the pisohamate ligament). The implication of this anatomic observation is that the only constraints to normal (and abnormal) motion of the wrist are the bone and ligament restraints. As a result, motion of the proximal carpal row occurs only from pressure exerted by the distal row components or through tension from the ligamentous structures.
3. There are six articulations involved in wrist motion—radiocarpal, midcarpal, pisotriquetral, basilar joint, ulnar CMC, and DRUJ.
4. Global wrist motion (hand on forearm) is therefore the end product of the carpal bones moving on each other, influenced by their articulations, ligamentous attachments, and indirect actions of adjacent tendons.
5. Because of this complexity, the patterns of motion of the individual carpal bones are still being elucidated.
6. Whereas a great deal remains to be understood, several observations are central to our current understanding of carpal kinematics:
   a. Motions of the bones are similar to each other within a row more than between rows.
   b. There is relatively little motion between the carpal bones and the metacarpals, so the capitate, the hamate, and the distal carpal row move virtually as one unit with the index and long metacarpals.
   c. The proximal carpal row is much less constrained than the distal row, and thus the components of the proximal row exhibit greater three-dimensional motion.
   d. The center of rotation of the wrist joint lies in the head of the capitate.
   e. With radial deviation, the entire proximal row flexes. The scaphotrapeziotrapezoid (STT) joint demonstrates dorsal migration of the trapezium-trapezoid on the scaphoid. The distal row extends on the proximal row. The hamate disengages from the triquetrum.
   f. With ulnar deviation, the hamate engages the helicoid triquetrohamate joint. This has been described as the "high" position of the triquetrum because of the appearance of riding up the hamate on a posteroanterior view. The triquetrum extends, supinates, and translates radially and volarly. The remainder of the proximal row extends and translates volarly by its connections to the triquetrum. The distal row flexes slightly on the proximal row.
   g. With ulnar deviation, all three bones of the proximal carpal row extend; with radial deviation, they flex.

KINETICS

1. Kinetics is the study of the forces acting on an object and the changes in motion produced by those forces.
2. Longitudinal force transmission from the carpus to the forearm occurs primarily through the radius, which accepts 80% to 90% of the forces across the wrist. This force transmission is dependent on ulnar variance and the position of the wrist.
   a. Within the radius, the scaphoid fossa transmits a greater percentage of the load with a ratio of 1.1 to 1.7 relative to the lunate fossa.
3. Forearm pronation has been shown to increase the amount of force transmission across the ulna (up to 37%). This has been attributed to the relative increase in length of the ulna to the radius with pronation.
4. Ulnar deviation with the forearm in neutral rotation has been shown to increase the amount of force transmission across the ulna (up to 28%).
5. Alterations in carpal alignment (as seen in distal radius malunion, Kienböck's disease, or limited arthrodesis) have been shown to change the force transmission. Shortening of the radius by 2.5 mm shifts the loads toward the ulna (42%); lengthening of the radius by 2.5 mm diminishes the load to 4% (see Chapter 9).

CLASSIFICATIONS AND TERMS

1. *Carpal instability dissociative* is an instability pattern within the components of a row. Examples include tears of the scapholunate or lunotriquetral ligament leading to dorsal or volar intercalated segment instability patterns, respectively.
2. *Carpal instability nondissociative* is instability between rows in which the relationships within members of each row are maintained. Examples include ulnar translocation and midcarpal instability.
3. *Carpal instability combined* refers to patterns of instability in which two or more of the carpal instability dissociative or carpal instability nondissociative patterns are observed. The perilunate spectrum of injuries is an example.
4. *Static instability* is recognized on plain radiographs. *Dynamic instability* requires application of a stress for diagnosis. A classic example is scapholunate instability with normal alignment on standard radiographs (static) but an increased scapholunate interval on a clenched fist view (dynamic).
5. *Adaptive instability* occurs in response to a change in bone architecture. Dynamic and static instabilities have been described. An example of adaptive instability is the development of midcarpal instability in a patient with a distal radius fracture malunion.
6. An *intercalated segment* is the middle segment in a three-segment system under compression. In this type of mechanical system, the middle segment is

unstable unless it is connected to the proximal or distal segments. The proximal carpal row is an intercalated segment between the forearm and the distal carpal row–hand.

7. *Intercalated segment instability* refers to radiographic patterns of carpal instability (proximal row) that display a zigzag pattern of carpal alignment.

   a. One of the components of the proximal row will rotate with the lunate into abnormal flexion or extension, depending on the individual pathologic process.

   b. To simplify the understanding of this process, the following premises must be accepted:

      i. The scaphoid, if allowed, will have a tendency to flex.

      ii. The triquetrum, if allowed, will have a tendency to extend.

      iii. The lunate, if allowed, will have a tendency to remain neutral.

      iv. The flexion tendencies of the scaphoid and the extension tendencies of the triquetrum are equilibrated by their attachment to the lunate by the SLIL and LTIL ligaments, respectively.

   c. *Dorsal intercalated segment instability* (DISI) (Fig. 7-13)

      i. This pattern occurs when the scaphoid is dissociated from the lunate and triquetrum primarily because of disruption of the SLIL. The scaphoid is free to fall into a flexed position and the triquetrum is free to become extended, bringing the lunate into extension through the LTIL.

      ii. Because of the change in bone alignment, the scapholunate angle on the lateral radiograph is increased (normal, 30 to 60 degrees). In addition, the radiolunate angle is made more negative (normal, −15 to 15 degrees).

   d. *Volar intercalated segment instability* (VISI) (Fig. 7-13)

      i. This pattern occurs when the triquetrum is dissociated from the lunate and scaphoid because of disruption of the LTIL. The triquetrum is free to adopt an extended position and the scaphoid is free to flex, bringing the lunate into flexion through the SLIL.

      ii. Because of the change in bone alignment, the scapholunate angle on the lateral radiograph is decreased (normal, 30 to 60 degrees). In addition, the radiolunate angle is made more positive (normal, −15 to 15 degrees).

      iii. Incompetence of the dorsal radiocarpal ligament has been shown to be necessary but not sufficient to produce static VISI deformity.

      iv. To generate a VISI pattern in vitro, disruption of the LTIL and dorsal radiotriquetral ligaments is necessary.

SCAPHOLUNATE INSTABILITY

1. Scapholunate instability is primarily due to disruption of the SLIL. Most commonly, the ligament is disrupted at the point of attachment to the scaphoid.

2. Scapholunate instability can be dynamic or static. If it is static, widening at the scapholunate interval or a DISI pattern will be observed on plain radiographs. For the DISI pattern to develop, some of the supporting capsular ligaments in addition to the SLIL must be attenuated or injured.

Clinical Presentation

1. Patients present acutely with pain and some degree of swelling. With subacute or chronic presentation, patients may complain of pain or popping in the wrist particularly with loading. It is asymmetric with the other wrist.

2. Mechanism of injury involves wrist extension, ulnar deviation, and supination of the carpus on the radius.

3. Tenderness localized to the dorsal scapholunate interval is characteristic. The scaphoid shift test reproduces pain or a palpable clunk as the scaphoid proximal pole subluxates dorsally with respect to the radius (Fig. 7-14).

4. The diagnosis is frequently delayed (25%) because the patient and physician regard it as a sprained wrist.

5. Similar radiographic instability patterns can occur with inflammatory arthritis. Some patients may present without a clear traumatic event, suggesting chronic attenuation as a possible mechanism.

Imaging

1. In cases of static instability (DISI), radiographs show an increased scapholunate interval (Terry Thomas sign; normal, <3 mm), cortical ring sign (foreshortened view of volar flexed scaphoid), and extended lunate (trapezoidal in shape) on the posteroanterior view (Fig. 7-15). Lateral radiographs show a flexed scaphoid and extended lunate with an increase in the scapholunate angle.

2. These radiographic changes may not be present acutely and may develop with time as the asynchronous motion of the proximal row leads to attenuation of the capsular ligaments or articular changes resulting in static deformities.

3. Some authors recommend an anteroposterior view with the forearm in full supination to better evaluate scapholunate diastasis.

4. In cases of dynamic instability, stress radiographs (clenched fist posteroanterior view) are used to accentuate the scapholunate diastasis.

5. Fluoroscopy can help visualize dynamic instability by demonstrating displacement of the scaphoid out of the scaphoid fossa with motion.

6. Arthrography can demonstrate communication of contrast material between the midcarpal and radiocarpal joints in cases of SLIL disruption. The specificity of this test is relatively low, and this modality is no longer used routinely.

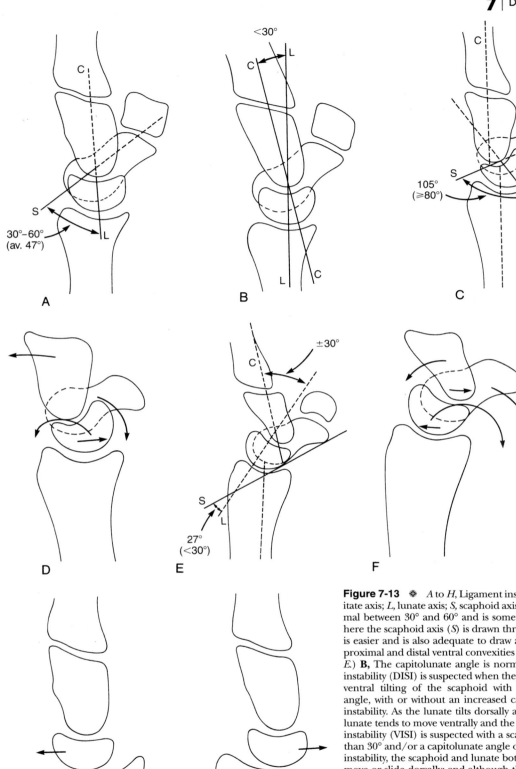

Figure 7-13 ◈ *A to H,* Ligament instability patterns of the wrist. *C,* capitate axis; *L,* lunate axis; *S,* scaphoid axis. **A,** The scapholunate angle is normal between 30° and 60° and is sometimes normal up to 80°. Although here the scaphoid axis (*S*) is drawn through the center of the scaphoid, it is easier and is also adequate to draw a scaphoid axis line tangent to the proximal and distal ventral convexities of the scaphoid. (See axis *S* in view *E.*) **B,** The capitolunate angle is normally less than 30°. **C,** Dorsiflexion instability (DISI) is suspected when there is dorsal tilting of the lunate and ventral tilting of the scaphoid with resultant increased scapholunate angle, with or without an increased capitolunate angle. **D,** Dorsiflexion instability. As the lunate tilts dorsally and the scaphoid tilts ventrally, the lunate tends to move ventrally and the capitate dorsally. **E,** Palmar flexion instability (VISI) is suspected with a scapholunate angle decreased to less than 30° and/or a capitolunate angle of 30° or more. **F,** In palmar flexion instability, the scaphoid and lunate both tilt ventrally. The lunate tends to move or slide dorsally; and although the distal pole of the capitate tends to tilt dorsally, the head (or proximal end) tends to move ventrally. **G,** With dorsal carpal subluxation, the center of the carpus is dorsal to the center of the midaxis of the radius. **H,** Palmar carpal subluxation is recognized when the central axis of the carpus and lunate is ventral to the midaxis of the radius. *(From Gilula LA, Weeks PM: Post-traumatic ligamentous instabilities of the wrist. Radiology 129:641-651, 1978.)*

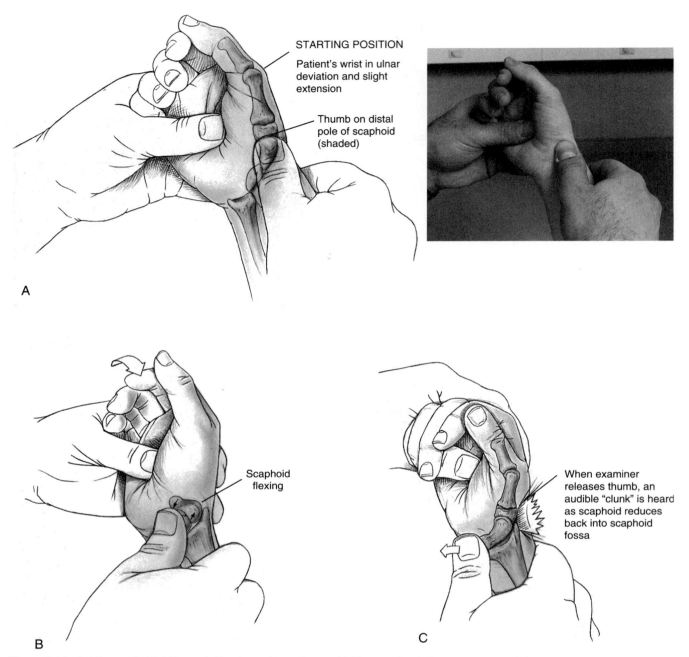

STARTING POSITION

Patient's wrist in ulnar deviation and slight extension

Thumb on distal pole of scaphoid (shaded)

A

Scaphoid flexing

B

When examiner releases thumb, an audible "clunk" is heard as scaphoid reduces back into scaphoid fossa

C

Figure 7-14 ❖ The scaphoid shift test. **A** *(drawing and inset photograph)*, The examiner's fingers are wrapped dorsally on the distal radius, and the examiner's thumb is placed on the distal pole of the scaphoid. **B,** With radial deviation, the scaphoid flexes to accommodate the decreased space between the trapezium, the trapezoid, and the distal radius. **C,** With lax periscaphoid ligaments, the proximal pole displaces dorsally out of the scaphoid fossa, over the dorsal rim. When the examiner releases the pressure, the scaphoid reduces back into the scaphoid fossa. *(From Torosian CM, et al: Physical examination of the wrist. In Lichtman DM, Alexander AH, eds: The Wrist and Its Disorders. Philadelphia, WB Saunders, 1997.)*

7. MRI has the advantage of being noninvasive and providing visualization of the intrinsic and extrinsic ligaments as well as other articular structures. Wrist MRI is highly technique and interpreter dependent, but some authors have reported accurate diagnosis of injuries to the scapholunate ligament.

8. Arthroscopy can be used as a diagnostic test for scapholunate instability because of the limitations of other imaging modalities. The "drive-thru" test (passing the arthroscope from the midcarpal joint to the radiocarpal joint through the scapholunate interval) is diagnostic. A classification of the spectrum of scapholunate ligament injuries seen arthroscopically has been proposed by Geissler, ranging from stretch injuries to partial tears to complete tears.

Treatment

1. Treatment depends on the time from injury and any secondary changes in the carpus.

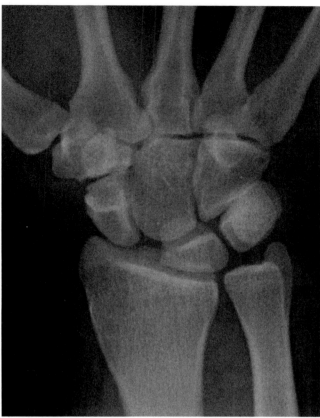

Figure 7-15 ❖ Posteroanterior wrist radiograph demonstrating widening of the scapholunate interval, foreshortening of the scaphoid, scaphoid cortical ring sign, and proximal migration of the capitate, all signs of scapholunate instability. The radiograph also demonstrates a radial styloid fracture.

2. Partial tears of the SLIL can be treated with a period of immobilization. If patients continue to be symptomatic, arthroscopic débridement of the partial tear can be helpful in decreasing symptoms.
3. Complete tears of the SLIL should be repaired surgically.

Acute Tears (<3-8 weeks)
1. The preferred method of treatment is a direct repair of the SLIL. The SLIL is repaired back to the scaphoid (more commonly) or lunate through drill holes or suture anchors.
2. Some advocate a dorsal capsulodesis (Blatt's procedure) in addition to the repair to impede flexion of the scaphoid (Fig. 7-16).
3. Closed reduction and closed reduction and pinning have been largely abandoned because of failure to maintain carpal alignment.

Subacute Tears (>8 weeks) in the Absence of Degenerative Changes
1. When SLIL tears go untreated, the torn ligament can become scarred and contracted, precluding the possibility of direct repair.
2. In some cases, the normal scapholunate relationship can be re-established. Eventually, the deformities

can become fixed, rendering the scapholunate diastasis and DISI pattern unreducible.
   a. Reducible injuries
      i. Because the ligament is not repairable, a reconstruction can be attempted.
      ii. Treatment options for reducible injuries include dorsal capsulodesis, free tendon grafts, and bone-ligament-bone composite grafts (from the capitohamate articulation, wrist retinaculum, or midfoot retinaculum). Scapholunate fusions have the highest rate of nonunion of any intercarpal arthrodesis.
   b. Unreducible injuries
      In these injuries, the normal intercarpal relationships cannot be re-established. Treatment options include limited carpal fusions, such as STT or scaphocapitate fusion. The complication rate after STT fusion has been noted to be as high as 52%. After STT fusions, motion averages about 60% and grip strength averages 74% of the contralateral wrist.

Chronic Tears with Degenerative Changes
1. Arthritic change after scapholunate injury is termed scapholunate advanced collapse (SLAC) wrist. This is the most commonly seen pattern of wrist arthritis, changes that develop as a result of alterations in the kinematics and contact areas of the carpus (as little as 5 degrees of malrotation of the scaphoid can decrease the radioscaphoid contact area by 45%).
2. Chronic instability leads to carpal collapse. Proximal migration of the head of the capitate between the scaphoid and lunate is observed. This leads to a decrease in the carpal height ratio. This ratio is defined as the distance from the base of the third metacarpal to the distal subchondral plate of the radius, divided by the length of the third metacarpal (Fig. 7-17). This carpal height ratio averages 0.54 in normal wrists.
3. The diagnosis, staging, and treatment of SLAC wrist are discussed in Chapter 9.

LUNOTRIQUETRAL INSTABILITY
1. In contrast to scapholunate instability, which is frequently a traumatic event, lunotriquetral (LT) instability is more likely to be seen as part of a degenerative process.
2. Isolated LT disruption has not been clearly associated with degenerative patterns analogous to a SLAC wrist either clinically or in the laboratory. Symptoms may be produced from dynamic instability noted in loaded positions, which may lead to synovitis or some cartilage deterioration.
3. Isolated LT ligament disruption in the laboratory does not produce a static radiographic instability. Division of the dorsal radiotriquetral and dorsal radiocarpal ligaments along with the LT ligament does produce a VISI radiographic pattern in vitro.
4. LT ligament lesions commonly present as ulnar-sided wrist pain. Symptoms occur with loading of the wrist, particularly with ulnar deviation or rotation of the wrist.

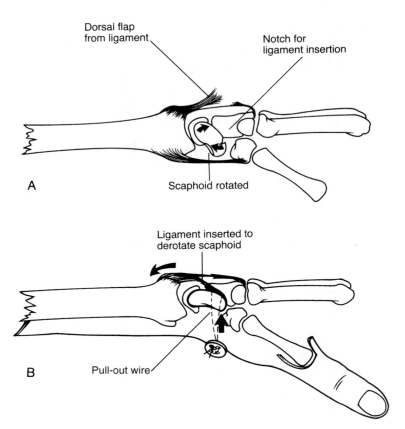

Figure 7-16 ❖ A graphic representation of the technique of dorsal capsulodesis. **A,** A proximally based ligamentous flap is developed from the dorsal wrist capsule. A notch for the ligament insertion is created in the dorsal cortex of the distal pole of the scaphoid, distal to the midaxis of rotation. **B,** The scaphoid has been derotated, and the ligament is inserted with a pull-out wire suture. *(From Blatt G, et al: Physical examination of the wrist. In Lichtman DM, Alexander AH, eds: The Wrist and Its Disorders. Philadelphia, WB Saunders, 1997.)*

5. Compression of the triquetrum against the lunate and LT ballottement or shear tests can reproduce symptoms.

Imaging
1. Radiographs may be normal initially or display a VISI deformity in cases of static instability.
2. Arthrography in combination with fluoroscopy has been used with moderate success.
3. MRI is widely used for TFCC disorders, but the resolution is generally not considered adequate for reliable evaluation of the LTIL in most centers.

Treatment
1. Initial management of LTIL disruption without static instability may include immobilization and anti-inflammatory agents.
2. In patients with ulnar positive variance, ulnar recession has been shown to tighten the extrinsic ligaments and can reduce instability and symptoms without associated carpal surgery.
3. LTIL repair through drill holes or with suture anchors can be performed in the minority of cases in which sufficient dorsal or volar LT ligament remains. The joint is typically pinned for 8 weeks in a cast, followed by 4 weeks of splint immobilization.
4. LTIL reconstruction is indicated when there is insufficient local tissue for a repair. Common techniques include a distally based strip of flexor carpi ulnaris or extensor carpi ulnaris tendon woven through drill holes in the lunate and triquetrum.

5. LT arthrodesis has been the most commonly reported reconstructive procedure for LT instability. Meta-analysis has revealed a nonunion rate of 26%. Persistent pain was reported in 46%. Range of motion averaged 84% of the opposite side, and strength averaged 74%.

MIDCARPAL INSTABILITY
1. Midcarpal instability is instability between proximal and distal rows (see carpal instability nondissociative).
2. It presents with a feeling of instability or mechanical symptoms. There may not be significant discomfort.
3. It can be post-traumatic in nature but can occur without a history of trauma in ligamentously lax individuals.
   a. It can also occur as an adaptive instability after a dorsally angulated malunion of the distal radius.
4. On physical examination, a palpable clunk can be elicited as the loaded wrist is taken from radial to ulnar deviation with the forearm in pronation. In addition, a palmar sag can be observed on the ulnar aspect of the wrist.
5. Plain radiographs are normal. Cineradiography can show a shift in the carpal relationship between both rows.
6. Treatment should be conservative initially with immobilization for 6 to 8 weeks.
7. If symptoms are persistent, surgical treatment in the form of partial intercarpal arthrodesis offers

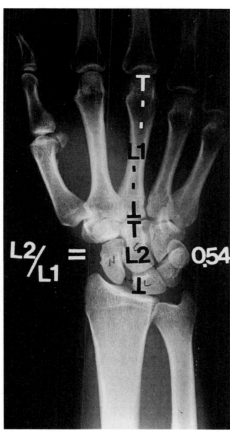

Figure 7-17 ❖ Use of the carpal height ratio allows one to evaluate carpal height (L2) compared with the third metacarpal length (L1). Normal ratio (L2/L1) is 0.54 ± 0.03. Abnormal ratios indicate shortening of the carpus, found in dislocations and fractures. *(From Markiewitz AD, et al: Carpal fractures and dislocations. In Lichtman DM, Alexander AH, eds: The Wrist and Its Disorders. Philadelphia, WB Saunders, 1997; modified from Youn Y, Flatt A: Kinematics of the wrist. Clin Orthop 149:21-32, 1980.)*

the most reliable results. Ligament reconstructions have yielded unreliable results. In patients with adaptive midcarpal instability, correction of the extra-articular disorder is necessary (e.g., osteotomy of a radius malunion).

ULNAR TRANSLOCATION

1. Ulnar translocation is a carpal nondissociative pattern of instability in which the entire carpus translates ulnarly on the distal radius, which occurs from disruption or attenuation of the volar capsular and radiocarpal ligaments.
2. It is a common pattern of deformity in rheumatoid arthritis and less commonly seen after trauma.
3. Ulnar translocation is recognized when less than 50% of the articular surface of the lunate articulates with the radius on a posteroanterior radiograph in the neutral position. Also seen is widening of the radial styloid to scaphoid distance.
4. Treatment depends on the cause and the presence of articular degeneration.
5. Radiolunate fusion in patients with rheumatoid arthritis offers reliable results.

6. In patients with ulnar translocation and DRUJ arthrosis, excision of the distal ulna can result in ulnar dislocation of the carpus from the distal radius.

SCAPHOID DISLOCATION

1. Scaphoid dislocation is an unusual radial sided carpal dislocation distinct from perilunate dislocations.
2. A spectrum of ligamentous injury exists, including injury to the radioscaphocapitate ligament, SLIL, long radiolunate ligament, and scaphotrapezial ligaments.
3. The mechanism of injury is unknown, but the majority in the literature result from high-energy trauma.
4. Treatment recommendations include closed reduction and percutaneous pinning or open reduction with repair of ligamentous structures and internal fixation.
5. Avascular necrosis has been reported as a complication.

AXIAL INSTABILITY

1. Axial instability is a rare, high-energy carpal injury usually secondary to a blast or crush injury.
2. The normal metacarpal arch is disrupted, and the digits may be rotationally displaced.
3. Disruption may occur in radial, ulnar, or both directions, depending on the direction of displacement of the CMC complex.
4. Treatment includes ORIF with careful attention to neurovascular injuries and the potential for compartment syndrome.

PERILUNATE INSTABILITY

1. These injuries are typically a result of high-energy trauma. Despite the severity of injury, the problem is often missed at presentation.
2. Mayfield described four stages of perilunate instability, starting at the scapholunate interval and rotating clockwise to the capitolunate, lunotriquetral, and radiolunate joints (Fig. 7-18A).
   a. An SLIL injury represents a Mayfield I injury.
   b. A dorsal perilunate dislocation is the equivalent of a Mayfield III injury.
   c. A perilunate injury with volar dislocation of the lunate from the lunate fossa into the carpal tunnel represents a Mayfield IV injury.
3. The injury can involve failure of the ligamentous structures and failure of bone structures (e.g., transscaphoid perilunate dislocation). In cases where the scaphoid is fractured, the SLIL is typically spared.
4. Diagnosis can be made on plain radiography. Disruption of Gilula's greater and lesser arcs on the posteroanterior view should raise the level of suspicion (Fig. 7-18C).
5. Given the significance of the injury, close attention should be paid to the potential for neurovascular injury, compartment syndrome, and acute carpal tunnel syndrome (particularly in Mayfield type IV injuries).
6. Treatment
   a. ORIF and ligament repair are recommended by volar, dorsal, or combined volar and dorsal approaches.

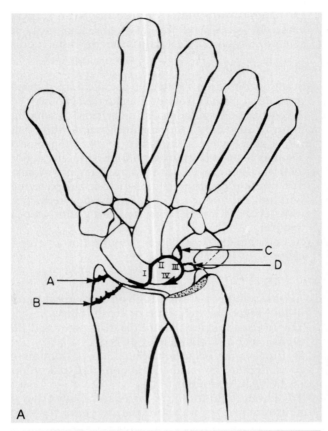

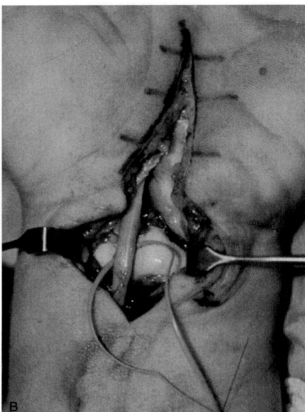

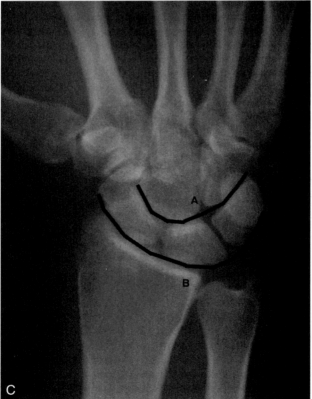

Figure 7-18 ◆ **A,** Mayfield stages of perilunar instability: Stage I: Scapholunate interosseous ligament disruption. Stage II: Capitolunate joint disruption. Stage III: Lunotriquetral ligament disruption. Stage IV: Radiolunate dislocation. A and B denote potential levels of radial styloid fractures. C denotes radiotriquetral ligament avulsion. D denotes ulnotriquetral ligament avulsion. **B,** Clinical photograph of a patient with a Mayfield IV injury. The volar approach reveals the median nerve (longitudinal structure identified with a vessel loop) after release of the carpal tunnel. The lunate can be seen extruded from the radiocarpal joint just below the median nerve. **C,** PA radiograph of a wrist depicting Gilula's arcs, demonstrating the articular contours of the proximal and distal carpal rows. Disruption of these arcs is indicative of perilunar instability. (*A from Mayfield JK, Johnson RP, Kilcoyne RK: Carpal dislocations: pathomechanics and progressive perilunar instability. J Hand Surg Am 5:226-241, 1980.*)

b. In cases in which the lunate dislocates from the lunate fossa of the radius and into the carpal tunnel, a volar approach is necessary for release of the carpal tunnel and reduction of the lunate (Fig. 7-18*B*).

7. Poor results can be correlated with persistent scapholunate diastasis.

8. Treatment of chronic or missed injuries can include reconstruction of the SLIL, proximal row carpectomy, wrist fusion, and carpal tunnel release.

9. Delay of surgical treatment (>6 weeks) may alter the biology of ligament healing and reduce the potential for healing of purely ligamentous variants compared with those involving bone injuries.

10. Persistent scapholunate diastasis is associated with poor outcomes.

SCAPHOCAPITATE SYNDROME

1. Scaphocapitate or naviculocapitate syndrome is the term applied to simultaneous fractures of the capitate and scaphoid.

2. The capitate head may be rotated 180 degrees.

3. Most scaphocapitate syndromes reported have been associated with perilunate dislocations. It is believed that scaphocapitate syndrome results from a spontaneously reduced transscaphoid, transcapitate perilunate fracture-dislocation.

4. Treatment includes ORIF of the scaphoid and capitate fractures from a posterior approach because of concern for avascular necrosis of the proximal fragments of both bones.

Distal Radioulnar Joint Instability

ANATOMY

1. Forearm rotation occurs through the radial-ulnar joints. At the DRUJ, the radius rotates about the fixed ulnar head. The joint is of limited congruity because the sigmoid notch (60 degrees) and ulnar head (105 degrees) have a different radius of curvature (Fig. 7-19).

2. Pronation of the forearm is accompanied by proximal migration of the distal radius relative to the ulna.

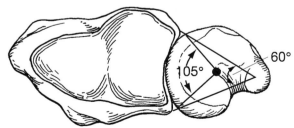

Figure 7-19 ◈ The radius of curvature of the seat of the ulna is 10 mm, with the arcs subtending an angle of 105 degrees. The radius of curvature of the sigmoid notch is approximately 15 mm, and the arcs subtend an angle of approximately 60 degrees. Thus, the distal radioulnar joint is not purely congruent. This anatomic feature allows the translational motion of the ulna within the sigmoid notch during prosupination. *(From Loftus JB, Palmer AK: Disorders of the DRUJ and TFCC. In Lichtman DM, Alexander AH, eds: The Wrist and Its Disorders. Philadelphia, WB Saunders, 1997.)*

Rotatory motions do not occur about a fixed point, so the DRUJ does not function as a simple hinge.

3. The ulnar head translates slightly dorsally in pronation with tightening of the volar radioulnar ligament. The bone curvature of the sigmoid notch provides some stability to the joint, but at extremes of pronation and supination, bone stability is lessened.

4. The DRUJ is supported by the TFCC, the ulnocarpal ligament complex, and the interosseous membrane of the forearm. The pronator quadratus muscle is also a dynamic stabilizer of the DRUJ.

TRAUMATIC INSTABILITY

1. Traumatic instability of the DRUJ is a common injury that occurs in association with forearm trauma.
   a. DRUJ instability is seen in association with extra-articular fractures (e.g., Galeazzi's fracture-dislocations), intra-articular fractures (e.g., distal radius fractures), or isolated disruptions of the bone and ligament supports (e.g., ulnar styloid fractures or TFCC disruptions).
   b. Injury mechanisms may be high or low energy and have been reported with repetitive events.
   c. A hyperpronation or supination mechanism is commonly identified.
   d. The ulnar attachment of the TFCC is the most common soft tissue disruption in cases of traumatic DRUJ instability.

2. The DRUJ must be examined in every forearm and wrist injury.
   a. Swelling and tenderness are commonly present over the joint, and symptoms are typically accentuated with rotation of the forearm.
   b. Increased translation of the DRUJ with anterior-posterior stress with the forearm in pronation, neutral, and supination may be present.
   c. Subacute or chronic instabilities may present with snapping with forearm rotation.

3. Routine wrist radiographs are frequently nondiagnostic or misleading.
   a. Dorsal or volar dislocation can be diagnosed on a lateral radiograph, but the radiograph must be a true lateral (established with overlap of the pisiform over the distal pole of the scaphoid).
   b. Small degrees of obliquity can lead to false-positive or false-negative results.
   c. Posteroanterior or oblique radiographs may show a widened distance between the ulnar head and the sigmoid notch in dorsal dislocations, while there may be narrowing of the distance in volar dislocations.
   d. Axial computed tomographic scanning of both wrists in pronation, supination, and neutral positions is commonly used.

Treatment

Treatment addresses any associated bone or soft tissue injury.

1. Isolated DRUJ dislocations typically reduce easily with closed manipulation in the acute period.

a. Dorsal dislocations (the majority) typically reduce with supination of the forearm, and volar dislocations reduce with pronation.

b. Irreducible dislocations require open reduction, extrication of interposed soft tissue, repair of ligaments and TFCC, and DRUJ pinning.

c. Instability of the DRUJ in association with displaced ulnar styloid fractures is likely to persist unless styloid ORIF is performed.

2. DRUJ instability due to extra-articular radius fracture (Galeazzi's fracture-dislocation) is treated with rigid internal fixation of the radius and DRUJ reduction.

a. Anatomic reduction of the distal radius fracture is mandatory because DRUJ instability can persist with very small degrees of radius malreduction.

b. The DRUJ must also be reduced. There is typically a dorsal dislocation of the DRUJ treated with closed manipulation into supination; however, interposed soft tissue (extensor carpi ulnaris tendon) may require open reduction.

c. If the DRUJ is stable after operative reduction of the fracture, closed treatment may be selected.

d. If the DRUJ is unstable, ORIF of the ulnar styloid fragment, repair of the TFCC, or closed pinning in a supinated position should be employed.

3. DRUJ instability due to articular fractures of the distal radius are treated by ORIF of the distal radius fracture and closed pinning of the DRUJ in a reduced position if the DRUJ is unstable after fracture fixation.

Chronic Instability

1. This is a more controversial and difficult problem to treat than traumatic instability.

2. There is a spectrum of injury and pathologic change that may include bone malalignment (at the radial shaft or metaphyseal level), nonunion of an ulnar styloid fragment, and soft tissue insufficiency.

3. Surgical solutions include osteotomy for the bone malalignment, repair of the TFCC or ulnar styloid, reconstruction of the ligamentous supports with a free tendon graft, and dynamic muscle transfer.

4. Salvage solutions for the DRUJ, such as distal ulna excision, Suave-Kapandji procedure, and distal ulnar prosthetic replacement, can be considered if the joint is irreparable or for failed prior surgery. Radioulnar fusion (one-bone forearm) is considered the ultimate salvage procedure for persistent DRUJ dysfunction (Fig. 7-20).

Triangular Fibrocartilage Complex Tears

Anatomy

1. The complex is composed of the triangular fibrocartilage, the volar and dorsal radioulnar ligaments, the subsheath of the extensor carpi ulnaris tendon, the ulnar collateral ligament, and the ulnolunate and ulnotriquetral ligaments (Fig. 7-21).

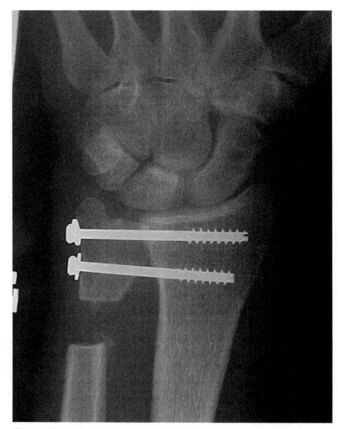

Figure 7-20 ◆ Patient treated with a Suave-Kapandji procedure for DRUJ arthrosis secondary to chronic instability from a radial shaft malunion. A segment of the distal ulnar shaft is removed to allow forearm rotation, and arthrodesis of the ulnar head to the sigmoid notch of the radius is performed with cannulated screws.

2. Blood supply originates from volar and dorsal branches of the anterior interosseous artery.

a. Vascularity is mostly peripheral, and the central 80% of the TFCC is avascular (Fig. 7-22).

b. For this reason, central tears are débrided and not repaired while peripheral tears are reparable.

3. The subsheath of the extensor carpi ulnaris tendon, which is confluent with fibers arising from the periosteum of the styloid, inserts on the ulnovolar triquetrum.

4. The volar and dorsal radioulnar ligaments are confluent with the triangular fibrocartilage.

a. The dorsal radioulnar ligament is the stouter of the two ligaments, and the volar radioulnar ligament is the origin for the ulnocarpal ligaments.

b. Both the dorsal and volar radioulnar ligaments arise from the respective rims of the sigmoid notch.

c. The radioulnar ligaments can be thought of as two separate laminae. The more proximal lamina inserts on the fovea adjacent to the styloid. The distal lamina inserts into the base of the styloid proper. The two sets of fibers are separated by the ligamentum subcruetum, primarily areolar tissue.

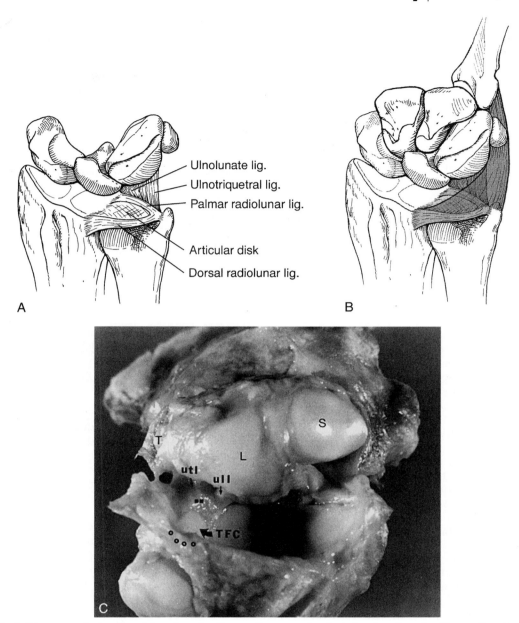

Figure 7-21 ❖ **A,** Diagrammatic drawing of the triangular fibrocartilage complex depicting the triangular fibrocartilage itself with its dorsal and palmar radioulnar ligaments. The ulnolunate and ulnotriquetral ligaments run from the fovea of the ulna to the carpus. **B,** Same view as in **A** with the addition of the meniscal reflection. **C,** Anatomic dissection of the triangular fibrocartilage complex. Of note is that the meniscus homologue, the ulnar collateral ligament, and the subsheath of the extensor carpi ulnaris tendon are not depicted in this anatomic dissection. TFC, articular disk of triangular fibrocartilage; open circles, dorsal radioulnar ligament; squares, palmar radioulnar ligament; utl, ulnotriquetral ligament; ull, ulnolunate ligament; T, triquetrum; L, lunate; S, scaphoid. *(From Loftus JB, Palmer AK: Disorders of the DRUJ and TFCC. In Lichtman DM, Alexander AH, eds: The Wrist and Its Disorders. Philadelphia, WB Saunders, 1997.)*

Labels in diagram A:
- Ulnolunate lig.
- Ulnotriquetral lig.
- Palmar radioulnar lig.
- Articular disk
- Dorsal radiolunar lig.

Biomechanics

1. The central component (triangular fibrocartilage) accommodates compressive stresses; the remainder of the complex acts to stabilize the DRUJ.
2. The TFCC increases the contact area between the distal radius and ulna and the carpal bones.
3. Removal of the TFCC decreases longitudinal stress on the ulna from 15% to 20% to about 5%.

Evaluation

HISTORY

1. Patients present with a history of ulnar-sided wrist pain, loss of strength, and painful forearm rotation.
2. It may be related to a forearm rotation injury or have an associated injury, such as a fracture of the distal radius.

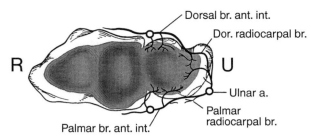

Figure 7-22 ❖ Diagrammatic drawing of the vascular supply to the triangular fibrocartilage through the following branches (labeled with abbreviated names): the dorsal and palmar radiocarpal branches of the ulnar artery, the palmar branch of the anterior interosseous artery, and the dorsal branch of the anterior interosseous artery. Note the avascularity of the central and radial aspects of the triangular fibrocartilage. R, radius; U, ulna. *(From Loftus JB, Palmer AK: Disorders of the DRUJ and TFCC. In Lichtman DM, Alexander AH, eds: The Wrist and Its Disorders. Philadelphia, WB Saunders, 1997.)*

❖ **Table 7-1**

CLASSIFICATION OF TFCC ABNORMALITIES

Class 1: Traumatic
A Central perforation
B Ulnar avulsion
    With distal ulnar fracture
    Without distal ulnar fracture
C Distal avulsion
D Radial avulsion
    With sigmoid notch fracture
    Without sigmoid notch fracture

Class 2: Degenerative (ulnocarpal abutment syndrome)
A TFCC wear
B TFCC wear
    Plus lunate and/or ulnar chondromalacia
C TFCC perforation
    Plus lunate and/or ulnar chondromalacia
D TFCC perforation
    Plus lunate and/or ulnar chondromalacia
    Plus lunotriquetral ligament perforation
E TFCC perforation
    Plus lunate and/or ulnar chondromalacia
    Plus lunotriquetral ligament perforation
    Plus ulnocarpal arthritis

From Loftus JB, Palmer AK: Disorders of the DRUJ and TFCC. In Lichtman DM, Alexander AH, eds: The Wrist and Its Disorders. Philadelphia, WB Saunders, 1997, p 393.

---

3. The patient may complain of mechanical symptoms such as locking and clicking.

PHYSICAL EXAMINATION

1. Tenderness is noted over the ulnar aspect of the wrist, particularly over the "fovea" of the distal ulna, which is the area that lies between the flexor carpi ulnaris and extensor carpi ulnaris.
2. Tenderness is elicited with TFCC "grind"—ulnar stress of the wrist with forearm rotation.
3. There may be instability with ballottement of the DRUJ.
4. Other possible causes of ulnar-sided wrist pain need to be ruled out: hamate hook fracture or nonunion, pisotriquetral joint degeneration, DRUJ arthrosis or instability, extensor carpi ulnaris tendinosis or instability, ulnocarpal abutment, and lunotriquetral instability, among others.

IMAGING STUDIES

1. Plain radiographs are typically normal. Radiography may help rule out other causes of ulnar wrist pain.
2. Arthrography, previously the "gold standard," has now been replaced with noninvasive modalities.
3. MRI is the new gold standard. Sensitivity and specificity are as high as 90% to 100% in some studies.
4. Arthroscopy is the most accurate diagnostic modality.

CLASSIFICATION (PALMER) AND TREATMENT (Table 7-1)

Type I: Traumatic

1. IA, central tear
   a. Treatment is initially conservative with immobilization for 6 to 8 weeks.
   b. If symptoms continue, arthroscopic débridement of the tear can yield 80% to 85% good results.
2. IB, peripheral tear from ulnar attachment
   a. MRI is the least sensitive in detecting these tears.
   b. The tear can be assessed at the time of arthroscopy with the "trampoline" sign—lack of triangular fibrocartilage tautness.

c. Half of these tears can be associated with extensor carpi ulnaris instability.
   d. Treatment is initially conservative with immobilization for 6 to 8 weeks.
   e. If symptoms continue, arthroscopic versus open repair of the tear can yield 85% to 90% good results.
3. IC, distal avulsion from insertions of ulnolunate and ulnotriquetral ligaments
   a. No data are available in the literature.
   b. Theoretically, it can be repaired because it is peripheral.
4. ID, peripheral tear from radial attachment
   a. This tear is most commonly associated with fractures of the distal radius.
   b. Open versus arthroscopic repair is technically demanding.

Type II: Degenerative

The ultimate goal of treatment is to decompress the ulnocarpal compartment, whether by TFCC débridement or by distal ulna recession, excision, or shortening.

The types represent a progression of degeneration at the ulnocarpal joint. All should have an attempt at conservative treatment with immobilization for 6 to 8 weeks. Treatment of degenerative tears in general has about 70% to 75% good results.

1. IIA, TFCC central wear or thinning
   a. Treat with arthroscopic synovectomy and ulnar shortening or wafer procedure (Feldon) (see Chapter 9).
2. IIB, TFCC central wear and lunate chondromalacia
   a. Treat with arthroscopic synovectomy and ulnar shortening or wafer procedure (Feldon).

b. Ulnocarpal impaction can be confused with Kienböck's disease on MRI.
  i. Increased signal intensity in Kienböck's disease is diffuse and should occupy more than 50% of the volume of the lunate.
  ii. In contrast, ulnocarpal impaction will reveal signal changes on the ulnar-proximal aspect of the lunate.
3. IIC, TFCC central wear and lunate chondromalacia
  a. Treat with arthroscopic TFCC débridement and ulnar shortening or wafer procedure (Feldon).
  b. The arthroscopic wafer procedure can be performed through the defect in the TFCC.
  c. Some authors recommend ulnar shortening in patients with central wears and ulnar neutral or positive variance.
4. IID, stage IIC and LTIL tear
  a. Treat with arthroscopic TFCC débridement and ulnar shortening.
  b. The ulnar shortening tends to tighten the ulnar extrinsic ligaments, stabilizing the lunotriquetral interval.
  c. If the lunotriquetral interval is unstable after the shortening, it should be pinned.
5. IIE, stage IID and ulnocarpal and DRUJ arthrosis
  a. Treat with distal ulna resection (Bowers) or Suave-Kapandji procedure.

Ulnar Styloid Impaction Syndrome
1. The ulnar styloid impaction syndrome is seen in patients with long ulnar styloids. The tip of the styloid will abut on the triquetrum with ulnar deviation of the wrist.
2. Ulnar styloid process index = (ulnar styloid length - ulnar variance)/ulnar head width.
  a. Ulnar styloid process index above 0.22 is elevated.
3. All should have an attempt at conservative treatment with immobilization and activity modification.
4. Styloidectomy is successful in refractory cases.

Wrist Arthroscopy

1. Arthroscopy is gaining a prominent role in the diagnosis and treatment of wrist and hand problems.
2. Its uses include débridement or repair of TFCC tears; débridement of partial intercarpal ligament tears; visualization during fixation of distal radius and scaphoid fractures; débridement of articular defects; excision of ganglion cysts; removal of the radial styloid, distal ulna, and proximal pole of the scaphoid; synovectomy; lavage of septic joints; and contracture releases.

Equipment

1. The extremity is typically placed under 10 to 15 pounds of distraction force. A distraction tower is commercially available for this purpose.
2. The arthroscopes are typically between 2 and 3 mm in diameter, and usually a 30-degree angled lens is used.
3. The procedure is typically performed under gravity inflow, but low-pressure pumps are also available for this purpose.
4. Small shavers, graspers, and thermal ablation probes are also available for use in small joint arthroscopy.

Portals (Fig. 7-23)

1. Portal nomenclature typically refers to the extensor compartment used (e.g., the 4-5 portal is between the fourth and fifth dorsal extensor compartments) and whether the portal is placed radial (R) or ulnar (U) to the compartment (e.g., the 6-R portal is just radial to the sixth dorsal compartment).
2. There are a total of five radiocarpal portals that can be used as visualization and work portals (1-2, 3-4, 4-5, 6-R, and 6-U). The 1-2 and 3-4 portals are

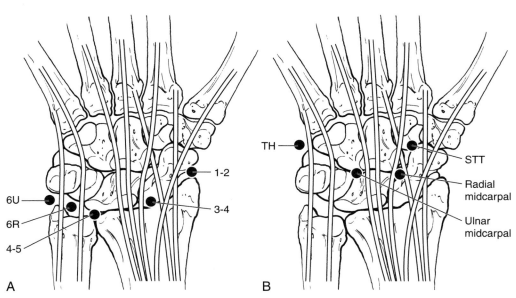

Figure 7-23 ◈ Commonly used portals in wrist arthroscopy. STT, scaphotrapeziotrapezoid; TH, triquetrohamate. *(From Gupta R, Bozentka D, Osterman AL: Wrist arthroscopy: principles and clinical applications. J Acad Orthop Surg 9:200-209, 2001.)*

primarily visualization portals, the 4-5 is a work portal, and the 6-R and 6-U are outflow portals, but all can be used interchangeably.

3. There are a total of four midcarpal portals (STT, radial midcarpal, ulnar midcarpal, and triquetrohamate). The radial and ulnar midcarpal portals are located at the junction of the capitate head, scaphoid, and lunate.
4. There are two radioulnar portals.
5. Nerve injuries during arthroscopy include
   a. Dorsal cutaneous branch of the ulnar nerve at the time of 6-U portal placement.
   b. Superficial radial and lateral antebrachial cutaneous nerves at the time of 1-2 portal placement.

Bibliography

Abrams RA, Petersen M, Botte MJ: Arthroscopic portals of the wrist: an anatomic study. J Hand Surg Am 19:940-944, 1994.

Berger RA: The ligaments of the wrist: a current overview of anatomy with considerations of their potential functions. Hand Clin 13:63-82, 1997.

Bilos ZJ, Vender MI, Bonavolenta M, Knutson K: Fracture subluxation of proximal interphalangeal joint treated by palmar plate advancement. J Hand Surg Am 19:186-196, 1994.

Blazar PE, Steinberg DR: Fractures of the proximal interphalangeal joint. J Acad Orthop Surg 8:383-390, 2000.

Bora FW, Didizian NH: The treatment of injuries to the carpometacarpal joint of the little finger. J Bone Joint Surg Am 56:1459-1463, 1974.

Bowers WH, Wolf JW Jr, Nehil JL, et al: The proximal interphalangeal joint volar plate. I. An anatomical and biomechanical study. J Hand Surg Am 5:79-88, 1980.

Bowers WH, Wolf JW Jr, Nehil JL, et al: The proximal interphalangeal joint volar plate. II. A clinical study of hyperextension injury. J Hand Surg Am 6:77-81, 1981.

Bowers WH: Distal radioulnar joint arthroplasty: the hemiresection-interposition technique. J Hand Surg Am 10:169-178, 1985.

Breen TF, Gelberman RH, Jupiter JB: Intra-articular fractures of the basilar joint of the thumb. Hand Clin 4:491-501, 1988.

Dinowitz M, Trumble T, Hanel D, et al: Failure of cast immobilization for thumb ulnar collateral ligament avulsion fractures. J Hand Surg Am 22:1057-1063, 1997.

Eaton RG, Malerich MM: Volar plate arthroplasty of the proximal interphalangeal joint. A review of ten years' experience. J Hand Surg Am 5:260-268, 1980.

Feldon P, Terrono AL, Belsky MR: Wafer distal ulna resection for triangular fibrocartilage tears and/or ulna impaction syndrome. J Hand Surg Am 17:731-737, 1992.

Geissler WB, Freeland AE: Arthroscopically assisted reduction of intraarticular distal radial fractures. Clin Orthop 327:125-134, 1996.

Geissler WB, Freeland AE, Weiss APC, Chow JCY: Techniques of wrist arthroscopy. J Bone Joint Surg Am 81:1184-1197, 1999.

Gelberman RH, Cooney WP III, Szabo RM: Carpal instability. J Bone Joint Surg Am 82:578-594, 2000.

Herzberg G, Comtet JJ, Linscheid RL, et al: Perilunate dislocations and fracture-dislocations: a multicenter study. J Hand Surg Am 18:768-779, 1993.

Kaplan EB: Dorsal dislocation of the metacarpophalangeal joint of the index finger. J Bone Joint Surg Am 39:1081-1086, 1957.

Kiefhaber TR, Stern PJ: Fracture dislocations of the PIP joint. J Hand Surg Am 23:368-380, 1998.

Kihara H, Short WH, Werner FW, et al: The stabilizing mechanism of the distal radioulnar joint during pronation and supination. J Hand Surg Am 20:930-936, 1995.

Lavernia CJ, Cohen MS, Taleisnik J: Treatment of scapholunate dissociation by ligamentous repair and capsulodesis. J Hand Surg Am 17:354-359, 1992.

Lawlis JF, Gunther SF: Carpometacarpal dislocations. J Bone Joint Surg Am 73:52-59, 1991.

Linscheid RL, Dobyns JH, Beabout JW, et al: Traumatic instability of the wrist: diagnosis, classification and pathomechanics. J Bone Joint Surg Am 54:1612-1632, 1972.

Mayfield JK, Johnson RP, Kilcoyne RK: Carpal dislocations: pathomechanics and progressive perilunar instability. J Hand Surg Am 5:226-241, 1980.

McElfresh WC, Dobyns JH, O'Brien ET: Management of fracture-dislocation of the proximal interphalangeal joints by extension-block splinting. J Bone Joint Surg Am 54:1705-1711, 1972.

Morgan JP, Gordon DA, Klug MS, et al: Dynamic digital traction for unstable comminuted intra-articular fractures—dislocations of the PIP joint. J Hand Surg Am 20:565-573, 1995.

Palmer AK: Triangular fibrocartilage complex lesions: a classification. J Hand Surg Am 14:594-606, 1989.

Stener B: Displacement of the ruptured ulnar collateral ligament of the metacarpophalangeal joint of the thumb. A clinical and anatomical study. J Bone Joint Surg Br 44:869-879, 1962.

Trousdale RT, Amadio PC, Cooney WP, Morrey BF: Radio-ulnar dissociation. J Bone Joint Surg Am 74:1486-1497, 1992.

Watson HK, Ballet FL: The SLAC wrist: scapholunate advanced collapse pattern of degenerative arthritis. J Hand Surg Am 9:358-365, 1984.

Watson HK, Ryu J, Akelman E: Limited triscaphoid intercarpal arthrodesis for rotatory subluxation of the scaphoid. J Bone Joint Surg Am 68:345-349, 1986.

Watson HK, Ashmead D IV, Makhlouf MV: Examination of the scaphoid. J Hand Surg Am 13:657-660, 1988.

Weiland AJ, Berner SH, Hotchkiss RN, et al: Repair of acute ulnar collateral ligament injuries of the thumb metacarpophalangeal joint with an intraosseous suture anchor. J Hand Surg Am 22:585-591, 1997.

8

✧ Mark A. Katz, MD   ✧ L. Scott Levin, MD
✧ Richard D. Goldner, MD   ✧ James R. Urbaniak, MD

MICROVASCULAR HAND SURGERY

Replantation

Introduction

GENERAL PRINCIPLES

1. Progress in the field of microsurgery has led to the high viability rates of greater than 80% for amputated parts.
2. The patient's perspective, measured outcomes, predicted morbidity, and cost containment along with other significant factors are critical to the decision-making process.
3. Survival of an amputated limb does not equate with function. Anticipated function of the replanted part should be equal to or better than function with the alternative choice of revision amputation with or without use of a prosthesis, although cosmesis should not be ignored.

REPLANTATION VERSUS REVASCULARIZATION

1. Distinction is essential for discussing methods and results of reattachment of amputated parts.
2. Replantation involves the reattachment of a part that has been completely amputated with no tissue connection to the patient.
3. Revascularization is the repair of an incompletely amputated part that has some intact soft tissue (skin, nerve, or tendon) and no perfusion because of arterial injury.

Care of the Amputated Part

ISCHEMIA TIME

1. Warm ischemia. Warm ischemia becomes most critical in proximal amputations involving skeletal muscle. Replantation is generally not recommended if warm ischemia time is longer than 6 hours for amputations proximal to the carpus and 12 hours for digital amputations.
2. Cool ischemia. Proper cooling and care of amputated parts protects against ischemic injury and prolongs allowable ischemia time. Cooling (4°C to 10°C) of amputated parts may prolong the ischemia time to 10 to 12 hours for levels proximal to the carpus and to 24 hours or more for digits.

HANDLING OF THE AMPUTATED PART

1. Digits should be wrapped in gauze moistened with lactated Ringer's or saline solution and then placed in a sterile specimen container or plastic bag. The digit can also be placed in a specimen container filled with either solution if gauze is not available. The container or bag is then placed on ice.
2. For proximal amputations, the part can be wrapped in gauze or sterile towels moistened with lactated Ringer's or saline solution and placed in a plastic bag, which is then placed on ice.
3. The amputated part should never be placed directly on ice, nor should dry ice ever be used; this can result in frostbite or permanent tissue damage.

Factors Influencing Replantation: Indications and Contraindications

LOCATION AND LEVEL OF INJURY

1. Anatomic location and level of injury remain the most important criteria for replantation.
2. In general, good candidates for replantation are those with the following amputations.

Thumb

Replantation of the thumb should be considered in most cases because of its functional importance of opposition and pinch. Good results have been shown, and replantation should be considered even in an avulsion injury, which may require shortening of the thumb, metacarpophalangeal arthrodesis, or neurovascular grafting. Successful thumb replantation is often functionally and cosmetically superior to reconstructive alternatives. Replanted thumbs with good sensibility tend to perform better with tasks requiring fine dexterity.

Single Digit Distal to the Flexor Digitorum Superficialis Insertion

Although replantation of a single digit may be controversial, amputated digits replanted distal to the flexor digitorum superficialis (FDS) insertion often function well. The proximal interphalangeal (PIP) joint and metacarpophalangeal joint typically regain some motion, and sensibility of the digit is generally good. In addition, the cosmetic results are satisfying. Replantation of single digits proximal to the FDS insertion is seldom indicated. Hand function is usually not improved, particularly regarding the border digits. Limited PIP joint motion (mean, 35 degrees) is expected. The index finger is usually bypassed to the long finger and may interfere with function in a manual laborer. Loss of motion of the small finger may result in decreased grip strength.

Multiple Digits

Multiple digits are always given consideration for replantation because hand function is greatly affected. These attempts may be limited to replantation of the least damaged digit or digits to the most functional or least damaged position on the hand. At times, these measures are necessary to provide the basic function of pinch. With respect to function, the order of importance from greatest to least is as follows: thumb, long, ring, small, and index fingers.

Partial Hand Through the Palm, Wrist, or Forearm

The significance of complete loss of hand function for amputations at the level of the palm, wrist, or distal forearm warrants an attempt at replantation whenever possible. The functional results of replantation at these levels are generally better than those achieved with a prosthesis. Extrinsic motor function is typically sufficient for grasping and releasing items. In contrast, intrinsic function is often poor. Sensibility is poor but usually adequate.

Sharply Amputated or Moderately Avulsed Elbow and Above-Elbow Levels

Amputations through the proximal third of the forearm, elbow, or humerus require cautious consideration. In some individuals, useful hand function can be obtained. In others, survival of the amputated part may allow the conversion of an above-elbow amputation to a more functional below-elbow amputation with the use of a prosthesis. Careful selection of patients is recommended. Sharply amputated or moderately avulsed limbs are best for consideration. The morbidity associated with more proximal levels of replantation is generally higher, and the results are less predictable. Muscle necrosis and subsequent infection can severely complicate replantation at these anatomic levels and can be life threatening in cases in which myoglobinuria leads to renal failure.

Almost Any Part in a Child

An attempt at replantation in healthy children should always be considered in nearly all amputated parts. Children usually have greater potential for functional recovery compared with adults. Epiphyseal growth can continue, and nerve recovery is good, particularly in children younger than 9 years. Bone shortening should be kept to a minimum (less than 5 mm). Interphalangeal joint involvement may require joint arthrodesis with an effort to maintain the physes of the distal articular segment.

Distal Fingertip

Replantation of distal fingertip injuries remains controversial. Advantages include maintenance of digital length, sensibility, soft tissue coverage, preservation of the nail plate, and cosmesis. Disadvantages include associated cost and morbidity (e.g., long hospitalization stay, blood transfusions). Replantation for amputations distal to the distal interphalangeal (DIP) joint is technically difficult because of the small vessel diameter and vessel branching. Although the arterial diameter may be large enough to obtain a patent anastomosis, the venous diameter is often too small for repair. Distal digital replantation is indicated for amputations of the dominant thumb tip and with factors affecting the patient (e.g., musician's fingertip). Three zones are described distal to the FDS insertion on the basis of vascular and flexor tendon anatomy:

1. Zone I: amputations distal to the nail base. The digital arteries on both the ulnar and radial sides form an arch and branch into smaller arteries.
2. Zone II: amputations between the DIP joint (interphalangeal joint of the thumb) and the nail base.
3. Zone III: amputations proximal to the DIP joint to the FDS insertion.

TYPE AND MECHANISM OF INJURY

1. Mechanism of injury significantly influences the decision to perform replantation or revascularization of amputated parts. Patients sustaining a sharp or guillotine amputation are ideal candidates for replantation. Severe crush, mangling, or avulsion injuries are not suitable for replantation or revascularization, although these injuries are not absolute contraindications. Segmental or multilevel injuries are also poor candidates for replantation. Major contamination of an amputated part may jeopardize viability. These injuries are susceptible to serious infection and possible systemic sequelae.
2. With avulsion or crush injuries, the degree of arterial injury can be difficult to establish, and careful inspection of the adjacent tissues along with meticulous débridement is critical. The red-line sign and ribbon sign are caused by traction injuries to the neurovascular bundle (Fig. 8-1). Traction on the digital artery tears branches along the course of the vessel, producing hemorrhage and a characteristic red line or streak along the lateral border of the digit. The ribbon sign describes a twisted, tortuous, or coiled artery resulting from the traction force followed by the elastic recoil of the artery. The vessel adventitia becomes distorted, and the media layer separates from the intima. Presence of either sign typically contraindicates replantation. In select cases, the zone of injury may be bypassed with the use of interpositional vein grafts connecting two healthy vessel ends.

Ring Avulsion Injuries

Significant digital vascular damage can occur in ring avulsion injuries despite a relatively benign appearance of injury to the skin. Therefore, careful assessment of digital perfusion is warranted in these types of injuries, which may require 3 to 5 days of observation. The evaluation and management of ring avulsion injuries can be separated into three classes as described by Urbaniak:

1. Class I: circulation adequate. Standard bone and soft tissue treatment is sufficient.
2. Class II: circulation inadequate. Vessel repair preserves viability, permitting immediate or delayed

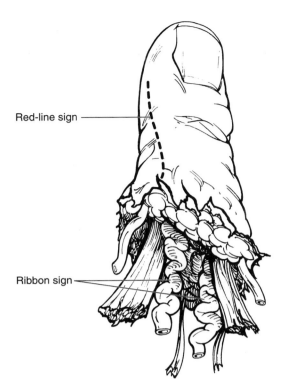

Red-line sign

Ribbon sign

Figure 8-1 ◆ The red-line and ribbon signs. (©1998 American Academy of Orthopaedic Surgeons. Reprinted from the Journal of the American Academy of Orthopaedic Surgeons, Volume 6[2], pp 100-105, with permission.)

repair of other tissues. The incomplete ring degloving or amputation injuries with vascular compromise can be successfully revascularized in most cases, achieving good sensibility and useful motion.

IIa: bone, tendons, nerves, and veins intact.

IIb: bone, tendon, or nerve injury.

IIc: venous compromise only.

3. Class III: complete degloving or complete amputation. Complete degloving injuries of the ring finger have the worst prognosis and are often best managed by surgical amputation of the digit. Although a complete amputation can be reattached successfully, the functional outcome is limited; in degloving injuries, the potential for functional use exists, but tissue revascularization can be difficult or impossible. The degloved finger with intact tendons allowing full flexion and extension is doomed without satisfactory skin coverage. Tubed pedicle coverage results in poor appearance, inadequate sensibility, and possible loss of motion due to joint stiffness. Some studies have reported successful replantation of class III avulsion injuries (69% to 85%), resulting in a useful digit with 90 degrees or more of PIP joint motion.

AGE OF THE PATIENT

Children

Unlike in adults, replantation of nearly all amputated parts is considered in healthy children. However, success of viability can be lower owing to the increased technical difficulty of repairing smaller vessels and a higher proportion of crush and avulsion injuries in the young

compared with adults. In addition, the more aggressive approach toward attempting replantation in children may correlate with lower survival rates of amputated parts. Vasospasm associated with pain and anxiety in the pediatric population can further compromise perfusion and thus viability.

Adults

The aging patient can negatively affect potential outcomes of replantation, although age is not necessarily a barrier. Elderly patients may have preexisting medical conditions that may compromise replantation surgery, diminish functional outcome, or increase the risk of surgical morbidity. For example, severe arteriosclerosis complicates vascular repair, or significant cardiovascular disease increases the risks of surgery related to prolonged anesthesia and significant blood loss. These patients may not tolerate the lengthy period of rehabilitation and the possible need for future operations.

ASSOCIATED INJURIES AND MEDICAL CONDITIONS

Polytrauma

Serious or life-threatening systemic injuries in the polytrauma patient must take priority over replantation surgery. During the initial examination, the patient needs a thorough multisystem evaluation, and focus on the site of amputation is discouraged. In addition, complete assessment of the patient may reveal the presence of a serious proximal injury that may preclude distal reattachment. For example, brachial plexus avulsion should be regarded as a contraindication in upper extremity replantations.

Past Medical History

Preexisting conditions, such as prior trauma to or severe osteoarthritis of the involved amputated part, cardiac disease, diabetes, peripheral vascular disease, hypercoagulopathy, mental illnesses, bleeding gastrointestinal ulcers, and other serious medical conditions, may adversely affect the viability and functional results of replantation or increase risks to the patient. In particular, the risks of surgery unique to replantation are prolonged anesthesia, hemorrhage, transfusion of blood products, compartment syndrome, infection, and metabolic disturbances (related to major limb amputations involving muscle) including acidosis, hyperkalemia, and myoglobinuria. Replantation in patients with a history of severe psychiatric disease is contraindicated.

SOCIAL FACTORS

Occupation

Special consideration may be given to patients on the basis of their profession. For example, a musician may be a candidate for replantation of a single digit, whereas the same procedure in a laborer may be of limited value and interfere with the patient's ability to work. The lengthy period of rehabilitation required after replantation surgery results in significant time away from work, substantial loss of wages, and potential risk to job security.

Social Habits

The patient's ability to comply with postoperative management and instructions is critical for successful viability and function of the replanted part. A discussion with the patient about any history of substance abuse, smoking, and caffeine consumption is imperative before surgery. The patient must be willing to avoid these habits and understand the negative effects on outcome. In addition, the patient must be motivated to endure the extensive therapy after replantation.

Patient's Beliefs

For some individuals, cosmesis can be an important consideration and at times can be the primary reason for replantation despite a potentially poor functional result. Loss of a body part in some ethnic groups can be associated with severe social humiliation. These beliefs may be the overwhelming influence in the decision to proceed with restoration of body image while ignoring any functional improvement.

Operative Sequence and Techniques

DIGITAL AND DISTAL HAND REPLANTATION

Sequence

For digital and hand replantation, the operative sequence of repair after identification of structures and débridement of necrotic tissue is as follows (BEFANV mnemonic):
1. **B**one shortening and fixation.
2. **E**xtensor tendon repair.
3. **F**lexor tendon repair.
4. **A**rtery anastomosis.
5. **N**erve repair.
6. **V**ein anastomosis.
7. In multiple digital amputations, following this sequence, repair of the same anatomic structures in each digit ("structure by structure") improves overall efficiency compared with completion of all aspects in one digit before the next digit is addressed ("digit by digit").

Technique

Identification of Structures and Débridement

Careful isolation and tagging of the neurovascular structures are important steps before any débridement. Failure to label vessels and nerves, particularly in multiple amputations, makes for a difficult time in attempting to identify these structures in a bloody field and can lead to extreme frustration at the later stages of replantation. Slightly dorsal midlateral incisions on each side of the digit are used to create dorsal and volar flaps for isolation of digital arteries, nerves, and dorsal veins. Subsequently, the distal and proximal wounds are débrided to decrease risks of infection. For transmetacarpal levels, débridement should include the distal interosseous and lumbrical muscles, which allows the distal intrinsic tendon position and scarring to be controlled by splinting. Importantly, careful identification and ligation of multiple superficial and deep arteries are necessary to help prevent later hematoma formation at the replantation site.

Bone Shortening and Fixation

Bone shortening and fixation are critical aspects of replantation. Bone shortening of 0.5 to 1 cm may be necessary to allow primary anastomosis of vessels without tension and primary closure of the skin. However, vein grafts should be used when indicated to avoid excessive tension on an anastomosis. Shortening of more than 1 cm can interrupt the balance between the extensor mechanism and flexors with loss of mechanical advantage. In thumb amputations, the majority of bone shortening should be done on the amputated part. Maintaining maximal stump length facilitates thumb reconstruction in case the replantation surgery fails.

Bone stabilization can be accomplished with different methods of fixation:
1. Longitudinal or crossed Kirschner wires (K-wires). Fixation by K-wires is commonly used for digital replantation. The advantages of K-wire fixation are quick fixation, less skeletal exposure and stripping, fixation in the presence of deficient bone stock, correction of rotational deformities, and ease of reshortening of bone if indicated for neurovascular repair or soft tissue coverage. Problems associated with K-wires include lack of rigidity, difficulty with accurate bone apposition, and transfixation of soft tissues. Reported rates of nonunion are as high as 21% when crossed K-wires are used.
2. Intraosseous wiring. Intraosseous wiring (90-90 wiring) decreases the chance of angulation and nonunion compared with K-wires. Intraosseous wiring is recommended for replantations at the metaphyseal level to permit early motion. However, precise technique and additional bone exposure are required.
3. Intramedullary fixation.
4. Miniplates and screws. Plates and screws offer improved stabilization and early joint mobilization, but their application may be time consuming and requires further soft tissue stripping and damage, particularly to the dorsal veins.

Extensor Tendon Repair

After bone stabilization, the extensor tendon is repaired by standard tendon repair techniques. For amputations involving the proximal phalangeal region, repair of the lateral bands is critical in the hope of re-establishing distal joint extension. In severe avulsion or crush injuries, direct repair may be impossible in the presence of significant extensor tendon damage or loss. An arthrodesis of the interphalangeal joints or an extensor tendon grafting as a secondary procedure may be required.

Flexor Tendon Repair

Primary flexor tendon repair should be performed if at all possible. Secondary surgery for flexor tendons in these patients usually requires two-stage flexor tendon grafting procedures with the use of a silicone rod, which can be safely performed 3 months after replantation. In the presence of an avulsion or crush injury, liberal or extensive dissection is not recommended to retrieve and repair avulsed tendons primarily. For amputations involving the proximal portion of the digit, placement of sutures in each free flexor tendon end without tying the repair until the neurovascular structures are repaired on the flexor surface can expedite and facilitate the microvascular surgery. The exposure for the artery and nerve repairs in this zone is greatly improved because the digit can be placed in full extension. When multiple tendon repairs are necessary in the palm or wrist, placement of all the sutures in the proximal and distal tendon ends is generally done before any knot tying; the tendon ends are then appropriately matched and tied.

Arterial Repair

In a digit, at least one artery and two veins (or two arteries and three veins when possible) should be repaired. Repair of only one digital artery can help conserve time; however, even in multiple digit amputations, repair of both arteries can increase the survival rate. In a partial wrist or hand amputation, all restorable arteries should be repaired. The redundant vascular supply of the hand may provide perfusion of multiple digits with each arterial repair within the hand. However, this abundant collateral circulation can result in hematoma at the site of replantation if care is not taken to identify and repair or ligate multiple deep and superficial arteries. Arterial repair should only proceed once good pulsating blood flow is achieved from the proximal artery. In the absence of good proximal blood flow, methods to induce flow include the following:

1. Relief of vascular compression or tension.
2. Resection of proximal vessel to healthy vessel walls.
3. Warming of the environment and patient.
4. Ensuring adequate hydration of the patient.
5. Elevation of the patient's blood pressure (without vasopressors).
6. Warm irrigation of proximal vessel.
7. External or intraluminal flushing with papaverine, chlorpromazine (Thorazine), or lidocaine (Xylocaine) solutions.
8. Avoidance of metabolic causes (per discussion with the anesthesiologist) for vasospasm (e.g., acidosis).
9. Time (waiting!).

Arterial repair also requires identification of normal intima under the highest possible magnification, which may require resection of damaged vessels, particularly in avulsion or crush injuries. If healthy intima is not identifiable or large gaps between vessels exist, interpositional vein grafts or vessel shifts of uninjured arteries may be necessary. The shifting principle is typically used when one of the distal vessels of a digit is not salvageable. Previously, in avulsed thumb amputations, the index finger radial digital artery was often shifted to replace a severely damaged princeps pollicis artery. This method has been abandoned, however, because of scar contracture of the first web space, frequent small size of the index radial digital artery, and concomitant injury to the index radial artery and princeps pollicis artery. Our recommendation is the use of an interposition vein graft sewn end to side to the radial artery in the anatomic snuffbox in an avulsed thumb replantation because it is easier, quicker, and more reliable.

Vessels should never be repaired under tension. Vessels repaired with excessive tension on the anastomosis have a high incidence of aneurysm and thrombosis. Both arteries and veins have been used for interpositional grafting, but vein grafts have the highest patency rate and are the most readily available. When an interpositional graft is necessary, there has been some concern that two anastomoses may be more susceptible to thrombosis than a single anastomosis, as in direct vessel repair. However, if a direct repair is done under tension, interpositional vein grafting is unequivocally superior, and its advantages far outweigh the potential disadvantages in these difficult situations.

Nerve Repair

Direct nerve repairs are generally possible, particularly after bone shortening. Careful fascicular bundle alignment is better ensured with the use of the microscope. However, even with the use of high-power magnification, the extent of nerve injury can be difficult to determine, particularly in severe avulsion or traction-type mechanisms. In most cases of digital replantation surgery, primary nerve repair should be done.

Primary nerve grafting can be done when a direct end-to-end repair is not possible. The medial antebrachial cutaneous nerve is an ideal choice as the donor nerve graft for digital nerve grafting. The medial antebrachial cutaneous nerve is localized two fingerbreadths anterior and distal to the medial epicondyle of the elbow and is found superficial to the forearm muscle fascia. The terminal posterior interosseous nerve to the dorsal wrist is also an alternative. In the presence of multiple finger amputations, digital nerve grafts can be harvested from the discarded parts. In digital replantation, no statistical difference in nerve recovery is noted between primary and secondary repairs.

Vein Repair

Two veins should be repaired for each arterial anastomosis. Again, venous repair should not be done under tension. To alleviate tension on repairs or to increase the number of available veins for anastomosis, a method of mobilization or harvesting (ligation and mobilization of branches, creating additional veins for outflow) of veins from the dorsal venous system of the amputated part can be employed. If direct repair without tension is not achievable, vein grafting is recommended. Dorsal veins require skin coverage to prevent desiccation of the vessels. Split-thickness, full-thickness, or local rotational skin flaps can be used for coverage. However, if a venous deficit coincides with skin loss, a venous flap may afford both venous repair and skin coverage. This composite flap can be based on a proximal venous pedicle from an adjacent digit, or it can be harvested as a free tissue transfer from the volar wrist or dorsal hand. In situations of an arterial repair requiring both an interposition vein graft and skin coverage, the venous flap may be reversed for digital artery reconstruction. Unfortunately, these methods are not completely reliable.

Skin Coverage

The skin wounds may be loosely approximated, ensuring no tension on the skin or compression of the digital vessels. Frequently, the midlateral incisions may be left open to heal secondarily, which avoids undue constriction of the digital vessels. Skin coverage or digital neurovascular coverage can also be accomplished with local rotation of skin flaps, split-thickness skin, or full-thickness skin grafts.

DISTAL DIGITAL REPLANTATION

Amputations at the DIP joint, base of the nail plate, or more distally can be successfully replanted, but adequate venous drainage to prevent venous congestion must be possible for survival of the amputated part. Typically, dorsal veins and digital arteries are difficult to find in the amputated parts at these levels. About 1 cm of dorsal skin on the amputated tip proximal to the base of the nail plate is necessary to locate dorsal veins. Adequate venous drainage can be achieved by several techniques, as follows:

1. Repair of volar veins (although less than ideal, these vessels are smaller in diameter, are more difficult to repair, and have thinner vessel walls).
2. Creation of an arteriovenous shunt after one digital arterial repair by anastomosis of the other distal digital artery of the amputated part with arterial backflow to a proximal vein. A technique involving a single arteriovenous anastomosis of the proximal artery with a volar vein from the distal part has been described, but an external bleeding technique for postoperative care must be done.
3. Removal of the nail plate and rubbing of the nail plate with a cotton applicator every 1 to 2 hours to invoke bleeding and continued venous oozing by placement of a heparin-soaked pledget to the raw nail matrix.
4. A paraungual stab incision of the skin or fish mouth incision of the fingertip followed by continuous heparinized saline drip to the site to maintain external bleeding for 5 to 7 days and by systemic heparinization (substantial blood loss often occurs in most patients [88%], requiring blood transfusions).
5. Use of medical-grade leeches or chemical leech implantation.
6. Periodic digital massage of the replanted digital tip (usually unsuccessful if necessary beyond 48 hours).

Nail regeneration depends on the level of the distal injury. Replantations distal to the lunula generally result in nearly normal nail growth, but more proximal injuries, particularly at the level of the germinal matrix, tend to cause problems with nail regeneration.

MAJOR LIMB REPLANTATION

Replantation of amputated parts at the level of or proximal to the wrist requires techniques and principles similar to those of digital replantation, but some modifications are necessary.

Sequence

Major limb amputations must be approached by a sequence of repair different from that of digital amputations because ischemia time is more critical. The sequence is typically as follows:

1. Extensive débridement and fasciotomies.
2. Arterial shunting (not anastomosis).
3. Skeletal shortening and fixation.
4. Arterial anastomosis.
5. Venous anastomosis.
6. Nerve repair.
7. Muscle repair.
8. Soft tissue coverage.

Technique

Débridement and Fasciotomies

Extensive soft tissue and muscle débridement of the detached limb is essential to prevent myonecrosis and subsequent infection, which is a significant problem in major limb replantation. Fasciotomies are routinely performed of the forearm, hypothenar, thenar, and interosseous compartments to avoid the development of a postoperative compartment syndrome. The two most common causes of failure of major limb replantation are myonecrosis with subsequent infection and inadequate compartmental decompression.

Arterial Shunting

Duration of ischemia of the amputated part becomes a critical factor because the proximal injuries involve more skeletal muscle mass. Despite proper cooling of the detached limb, major limbs are in great jeopardy at 10 to 12 hours of ischemia. Therefore, rapid revascularization is the goal to prevent or to diminish muscle necrosis for amputations proximal to the metacarpal level. A synthetic shunt is usually inserted to provide arterial inflow from the proximal vessel to the amputated part. Arterial shunting before bone fixation allows reperfusion of muscle as quickly as possible, particularly for limbs approaching 4 to 6 hours of ischemia time. Some authors believe that perfusion of the amputated part before replantation helps dilute the accumulated toxic metabolites and lactic acid. Perfusion of the amputated limb with lactated Ringer's solution containing sodium bicarbonate by gravity drip can be done initially.

Bone Fixation

After the initial débridement with the synthetic shunt in place, rapid bone stabilization is necessary. Bone shortening is often necessary, which enables adequate débridement as well as better soft tissue approximation for repair. The bone is typically stabilized with plate and screw fixation of the long bones and crossed Steinmann pin fixation at the joint levels. Adequate bone shortening must be carefully planned on the basis of the type and level of injury. At the forearm level, up to 4 cm of bone shortening may be necessary; the humerus can be shortened up to 8 cm to permit soft tissue closure.

Vascular Repairs

Arterial repairs should always be done before venous anastomoses. This sequence of vascular repair allows a physiologic washout of lactic acid and other noxious breakdown products of anaerobic metabolism before venous repair. If venous anastomoses are completed first, rapid systemic influx of these catabolites can be harmful to the patient, causing myoglobinuria with subsequent renal failure, systemic acidosis, and hypercalcemia. Intravenous sodium bicarbonate given before completion of the venous repairs may be beneficial. The disadvantage of initial arterial repair is an increase in blood loss, which may require blood transfusions. Judicious, intermittent use of a tourniquet can help lessen blood loss because great care must be taken to maintain the patient's blood volume and pressure. In general, more venous repairs, including both the deep and superficial, help reduce the massive swelling of the limb and reduce the fluid and protein losses from the limb in the postoperative period. If a vein graft is required in regions of soft tissue loss, placement of the graft in nonanatomic positions out of the zone of injury can provide adequate vessel soft tissue coverage. Heparin is not used postoperatively for forearm or transhumeral replantations because lacerated muscle may bleed excessively in anticoagulated patients.

Nerve Repairs
Peripheral nerve repairs should be executed meticulously because these repairs have a major influence on the ultimate functional outcome. Proper anatomic identification and isolation of each involved nerve are initially done without excision of nerve length during the débridement. At the time of neurorrhaphy, the damaged nerve ends are resected to a length that allows repair without tension. An epineural neurorrhaphy is preferred; a group fascicular repair has not been shown to improve the quality of nerve repair.

Muscle and Tendon Repair
Repair of these remaining structures follows an order from deep to superficial. In general, muscle bellies are repaired with a large whipstitch, cylindrical tendons are repaired by crisscross or side-locking stitches, and flat tendons are approximated with multiple horizontal mattress stitches.

Soft Tissue Coverage
Complete closure of the wound should be avoided at the initial procedure. Exposed neurovascular structures may be covered safely by partial closure or with skin grafts. Coverage or closure of other areas of soft tissue injury may be delayed, particularly if further débridement is required within 48 to 72 hours. If there is no evidence of sepsis, definitive closure is carried out in the first postoperative week. A distant or local pedicle skin flap may be necessary to obtain coverage over bone or neurovascular structures.

Postoperative Management

ROUTINE PRECAUTIONS

Protective dressings and splints are carefully applied to avoid undue compression. The extremity is elevated to the level of the heart with adjustments in elevation based on the arterial and venous status of the replanted part. If arterial inflow is diminished, the hand is lowered; if venous outflow is compromised, the hand may need further elevation. The patients are kept at bed rest for 2 to 3 days in a quiet, warm room. Peripheral circulation is also enhanced by adequate hydration of the patient. Elimination of nicotine and caffeine products is important. Antibiotics are administered for 5 to 7 days. Anticoagulation of some type is typically used, although it is controversial and depends on the surgeon's preferences. Some surgeons use none. Various anticoagulants, and vasodilators, used alone or in combination, are aspirin, heparin, low-molecular-weight dextran (a plasma expander), dipyridamole (Persantine), and chlorpromazine. Several factors that influence the use of anticoagulation are the degree of crush or avulsion, the appearance of the vessels before and after anastomosis,

and the use of vein grafts. In guillotine or sharp amputations that allow technically easier vessel anastomoses and brisk blood flow, heparin is generally not indicated. In contrast, heparin is used for 5 to 7 days after surgery for crush or avulsion injuries. Periodic inspection of dressings is important in anticoagulated patients because excessive bleeding into the dressings may cause constriction by a "blood cast." Again, heparin is not used in amputations proximal to the wrist level.

EVALUATION

Replanted parts are typically evaluated hourly for assessment of color, pulp turgor, capillary refill, and warmth. Quantitative skin temperature measurements by use of surface temperature probes on the replanted part are the most reliable and noninvasive means of monitoring perfusion. Poor perfusion is indicated if the temperature of the replanted part drops below 30°C or by more than 2°C in 1 hour. The compromised circulation warrants assessment of the possible causes and often requires re-exploration of the vessel anastomoses.

USE OF LEECHES

Medical-grade leeches are readily available and may be placed on the surface of failing replanted parts when venous congestion occurs. The leeches become engorged in 15 to 30 minutes and subsequently detach from the digit or part. While attached, the leech secretes a local anticoagulant, hirudin, that allows bleeding from the incision for 8 to 12 hours, preventing congestion of the replanted part. Once bleeding stops, a leech is again applied. This leech treatment may be required for 5 to 7 days until venous outflow is established. Leeches will not attach to or remain on avascular tissue and may infect patients with a gram-negative anaerobic rod, *Aeromonas hydrophila*. This gram-negative rod has been identified from wound smears of patients treated with leeches. The bacteria are endosymbiotic within the leech by inhibiting growth of other bacteria and by producing essential digestive enzymes to break down red cells and hemoglobin. These enzymes include amylase, lipase, and proteolytic hemolysin. Early surgical débridement is required in the presence of infection after the use of leeches followed by antibiotic treatment (aminoglycosides, tetracycline, chloramphenicol, trimethoprim-sulfamethoxazole, third-generation cephalosporins, or aztreonam).

Results of Replantation

Critical comparison of revision amputation with replantation is difficult because the complexity of injury varies widely. Functional results, no matter the treatment, will reflect the severity of injury to multiple digits and other anatomic structures of the hand. Some patients may have concomitant injuries to other digits not requiring replantation, thereby confounding the comparison of results of functional outcome of these cases.

THUMB REPLANTATION

In most reports, thumb replantation success rates are approximately 75% to 85% for sharp amputations.

This success rate is lower for avulsion injuries, averaging approximately 50%. Protective sensation is generally regained, and an average two-point discrimination of 9 to 11 mm is achieved. Thumb total active motion averages about 60 to 70 degrees. Hypersensitivity, difficulty grasping small objects, cold intolerance, and pain are the most frequent complaints.

DIGITAL REPLANTATION

As in thumb replantation, finger replantation success rates are approximately 75% to 85% for sharp amputations. Survival after revascularization of ischemic digits is about 90%. The anatomic level of injury appears to have the greatest effect on functional outcome. For digits replanted distal to the insertion of the FDS, the average PIP joint motion was 82 degrees; digits replanted for amputations proximal to the FDS insertion had an average range of PIP joint motion of only 35 degrees. Mean two-point discrimination after amputation is about 8 mm for sharp amputations compared with an average of 15 mm for fingers sustaining a crush or avulsion injury. Factors influencing return of sensibility after replantation include age of the patient (better in children; in children younger than 9 years, about 70% of replanted parts can achieve two-point discrimination of less than 5 mm), level of injury (better in distal replantations), mechanism of injury, digital blood flow, cold intolerance, and sensory re-education postoperatively. Recovery of sensibility in the replanted digit is comparable to that achieved by simple nerve repair and techniques of nerve grafting. Tobacco smoking results in poor survivorship of digits.

MAJOR LIMB REPLANTATION

The overall survival rate of major limb replantations and revascularizations is about 70%.

Hand and Distal Forearm

Young patients with complete, sharply amputated limbs at the wrist level with minimal soft tissue injury and those with incomplete injuries or uninjured peripheral nerves have the best functional results. Diffuse crush, multiple-level, and avulsion injuries and high-level peripheral nerve injury have poorer results with less return of function. Intrinsic motor function is uniformly absent or poor in all patients with these proximal injuries. Loss of intrinsic function commonly results in most digital total active motion occurring across the interphalangeal joints with proportionally less motion at the metacarpophalangeal joint. Most patients will have absent or weak pinch and grasp strength despite good to fair digital total active motion. Cold intolerance occurs commonly. Two-point discrimination is generally poor, but protective and normal ranges can be obtained, particularly for incomplete injuries.

Elbow Region

1. Proximal forearm: an overall survival rate of 65% has been reported of 20 cases reviewed in the literature. Most failures resulted from vascular thrombosis.
2. Transarticular level: a limited number of cases have been reported in detail with a survival rate of 70% to 85%. Functional results were good to fair in all surviving limbs. Multiple secondary procedures (average of two procedures) were nearly always required to maximize functional outcome.

Transhumeral

Limb survival is about 50%. Failure is usually due to sepsis or arterial thrombosis. Intraoperative or postoperative death is not uncommon. It is suggested that transhumeral replantation may be of value for recovery of elbow function in most patients. This recovery may allow conversion of an above-elbow amputation to a functional below-elbow level.

Free Tissue Transfer (see Chapter 3 for pedicle flaps)

Introduction

DEFINITION

1. Free tissue transplantation describes the transfer of autologous tissue from one location in the body to another site by use of techniques of microvascular surgery for small vessel anastomoses.
2. Free flap types include isolated tissue transfer, composite tissue transfer, and functioning free muscle transfer. Structural tissue transfers, such as vascularized bone grafts or toe transplantations for hand reconstruction, are also included in this category.

GENERAL PRINCIPLES

1. Free tissue transfer is generally considered for any tissue deficit that is not amenable to skin grafting, adjacent tissue rearrangement, regional tissue transfer, or local pedicle flaps.
2. Free tissue transfer not only provides coverage and reconstitution of the soft tissue envelope but can facilitate function. For the hand, early mobilization can be achieved after injury, which decreases limb edema and stiffness.
3. Free flaps allow the possibility of composite tissue reconstruction in one stage by transfer of various combinations of skin, muscle, tendon, bone, and nerve at once.
4. A thorough understanding of the rationale, timing, and type or selection of tissue transplantation is critical for successful reconstruction.

Soft Tissue Reconstruction Ladder

ALGORITHM

1. The reconstruction ladder is applicable to acute or chronic soft tissue injury with or without fractures, limb-sparing tumor resections, and chronic conditions such as osteomyelitis and fracture nonunions.
2. Limb reconstruction may require simultaneous use of techniques from different levels of the reconstruction ladder for different problems.
3. Adequate débridement is the first major step of the reconstruction ladder. All nonviable tissue should be removed because the border of débridement should include healthy tissue. Nerves are the only structures in which débridement is more conservative.

4. Free tissue transfer represents the most complex rung on the reconstruction ladder.

"RUNGS" OF THE RECONSTRUCTION LADDER (see Chapter 3)

1. Primary wound closure. After adequate débridement, primary wound closure may be possible in cases of minor trauma, such as minor hand injuries. However, primary closure is not always possible or desirable (e.g., open fractures). This is particularly true of lower extremity injuries because the degree of contamination and associated soft tissue loss may be significant. Serial débridements may allow delayed primary closure.

2. Delayed primary closure. Delayed primary closure is usually done on return to the operating room at 24 to 48 hours after an initial débridement.

3. Healing by secondary intention. A wound may be left open to heal by granulation, epithelialization, and wound contraction. This technique can be applied to small wounds or skin graft donor areas or in abrasions over muscle compartments, which have small areas that can rapidly epithelialize.

4. Skin grafting. Skin grafts may be full thickness or split thickness, either meshed or unmeshed. Skin grafting will successfully close many wounds in the extremities. Indications are for wounds beyond primary or delayed primary closure. The wound bed must have good vascularity with smooth, pink granulation tissue. Also, skin grafts will take to fat, muscle fascia, paratenon, and intact periosteum. The wound beds must be cleaned before grafting to avoid infection and subsequent loss of the graft. Immobilization is critical for successful graft healing.

5. Local or distant flaps. More complex wounds with exposed neurovascular structures, bone devoid of periosteum, insufficient vascularity, or poor soft tissue beds require the importation of well-vascularized tissue to achieve wound closure. Rotation flaps, in isolation or in combination with muscle, fascia, or cutaneous tissue, can provide vascularized tissue for obliteration of dead space and wound closure without tension. However, these options may be limited because of wound location or regional donor site deficiencies.

6. Free tissue transfer. The highest rung of the reconstruction ladder may be used in combination with lower rungs of the ladder, such as skin closure, skin grafting, or rotational flaps.

Indications for Free Tissue Transfer

Trauma, tumor, and infection are the indications for free tissue transfer in the upper and lower extremities. In addition, reconstruction of brachial plexus injury is described.

UPPER EXTREMITY

Trauma
Mutilating Trauma
Patients who sustain mutilating trauma to the upper extremity often have the greatest need for free tissue transfer. Severe trauma to the hand requires resurfacing with free cutaneous, muscle, or fascial flaps. In cases of severe trauma, free tissue transfer is preferable to use of island pedicle flaps because further compromise to the upper extremity occurs (e.g., ipsilateral radial forearm island pedicle flap for dorsal hand coverage sacrifices the radial artery).

Fracture Nonunion
Recalcitrant nonunion of upper extremity long bone fractures for which standard methods of fixation and bone grafting have failed can be reconstructed by free vascularized bone grafting. Advantages of vascularized bone grafting include faster hypertrophy and remodeling than with nonvascularized structural grafts.

Thumb or Digit Reconstruction

1. Digit or partial digit transfers offer replacement of all or partial loss of a thumb or finger from prior injury. Reconstruction may include skin, nail, nerve, bone, joint, and tendon. Microvascular toe to hand transfer offers superior results for reconstruction of thumbs or fingers compared with other reconstruction techniques. In a single composite tissue transfer, a digit transfer can provide an appearance of a thumb or finger and allow the functional necessities of stability, sensibility, and mobility. Donor sites include the great toe, second toe, two toes in combination, and fingers.

2. Thumb reconstruction by great-toe transplantation is considered if at least one third of the proximal portion of the thumb metacarpal bone is present. Second-toe to thumb transplantation is indicated when a large discrepancy in size exists between the thumb and great toe, when loss of the great toe is not acceptable, or when the amputation level is proximal to the proximal third of the first metacarpal and considerable length is necessary. Harvesting of the first metatarsophalangeal joint should be avoided. Second-toe or multiple-toe transfers are indicated in a hand with all fingers lost and no opposable post for the thumb. Second toes are not cosmetic and should be used only if the great toe is too short. Patients with congenital deformities, such as constriction band syndrome (in which proximal structures are relatively normal), can benefit from these transfers (see Chapter 12).

3. Another reconstructive option for thumb loss is the wraparound procedure. This procedure involves harvest of the soft tissue of the great or second toe, leaving the toe osseous structures intact. The bone structure of the thumb is reconstituted by bone graft, followed by coverage with the free soft tissue transfer from the foot. Microvascular great-toe transfer, second-toe transfer, and wraparound procedure have in common the vascular pedicle anatomy, which is the first dorsal metatarsal artery of the dorsalis pedis artery. In 78% of cases, the first dorsal metatarsal artery runs superficial to the first dorsal interosseous muscle. Wraparound toe transfer is cosmetically better than free toe transfer. Some graft bone resorption should be anticipated; 30% to 50% of pinch strength is regained, and return of two-point discrimination of about 15 mm

is expected. Great-toe transfer is preferred when motion, length, and stability are needed, for example, in amputations in which the metacarpophalangeal joint is missing.

4. Partial toe transfer of the second toe can be used for finger amputations at the level of the DIP joint. The distal aspect of the second toe can provide pulp, nail plate, sensibility, and osseous length. Pulp flaps can also be harvested as partial distal toe transfers for distal volar thumb and finger resurfacing. Major indications for pulp transfer are as follows:
   a. Acute loss from trauma.
   b. Unstable skin or failure of previous pulp reconstruction with skin grafting or local flap.
   c. Distal fingertip post-traumatic insensibility with pulp atrophy and distal neuroma with no possibility of nerve repair.

5. Vascularized joint transfers from the foot have been described. These transfers are indicated in active young patients in whom articular injury (especially of the thumb) is functionally limiting and joint arthroplasty is not desirable because of age.

Tumor

Limb-sparing compartment resections of tumor are best treated with free tissue transfer, including free cutaneous, muscle, or bone flaps in isolation or in combination.

Infection

Soft tissue sepsis can usually be managed with local débridement, unless massive tissue necrosis is present and requires coverage of vital structures, bones, or joints. Complicated osteomyelitis with or without fracture nonunion may necessitate resection of large intercalary bone segments. In these cases, composite tissue transfer, such as an osteoseptocutaneous fibula flap, can offer an excellent means of reconstructing the arm or forearm.

Brachial Plexus Injury

Different procedures using microsurgical techniques have been described for brachial plexus reconstruction. Techniques include conventional and vascularized (e.g., ulnar nerve) nerve grafting, neurotization, nerve crossing procedures, and free muscle transfer (e.g., free gracilis) in combination with neurotization of the muscle flap. A combined technique of double free muscle and multiple nerve transfers has been described.

LOWER EXTREMITY

Trauma

Severe, open fractures (Gustilo grade IIIB or IIIC open injuries) typically involve simultaneous management of fractures and associated soft tissue injury. Expeditious soft tissue reconstruction with the use of free tissue transfer allows optimal soft tissue repair and bone fixation and helps facilitate bone vascularity; it facilitates additional reconstruction, such as bone grafting, and avoids the adverse sequelae of failed fixation, sepsis, and ultimately amputation. Nerve injuries do not preclude salvage of a severely damaged limb, but the potential for return of sensibility becomes a critical factor. Therefore, complex lower limb injuries with nerve damage (particularly proximal injuries) are frequently considered for amputation because the return to a functional status is usually more rapid with an appropriate prosthesis. Advanced age should not be a contraindication to microvascular limb salvage. Delayed post-traumatic reconstruction may be accomplished with free vascularized bone grafting, as in cases of chronic fracture nonunion.

Tumor

Free tissue transfer is indicated after tumor resection for coverage of large soft tissue defects, neurovascular structures, bone devoid of periosteum, and allografts or tumor prostheses when local tissue is insufficient. Free muscle flaps may be used for coverage and can be innervated to assist in foot and ankle function. Wounds that follow irradiation therapy for sarcomas have a high incidence of wound complications after primary closure. These wounds have poor vascularity and are susceptible to breakdown. Patients may also require secondary limb reconstruction either in the early postoperative period or several months or years after tumor resection.

Infection

Osteomyelitis

Extensive débridement after sequestrectomy can create a large dead space requiring free tissue transfer for coverage. Free muscle flaps provide coverage for the bone and soft tissue, obliterate dead space, improve vascularity, and enhance leukocyte function at the site. Advances in reconstruction and fixation by use of vascularized bone grafts or bone lengthening techniques have allowed successful treatment of patients with osteomyelitis and large (>6 cm) segmental bone defects. In addition, failed arthrodesis due to sepsis can be successfully treated with vascularized bone grafting to achieve joint fusion.

Infected Implants

1. Total joint arthroplasty. Compromised wound healing increases the risk of infection for patients with total joint arthroplasty. Diseases such as rheumatoid arthritis, peripheral vascular disease, chronic renal failure, and diabetes can compromise wound healing. Other risk factors contributing to poor wound healing include irradiation, corticosteroids, immunosuppressive therapy, multiple previous surgeries, and malnutrition. An exposed total joint prosthesis requires immediate intervention with flap coverage, which can prevent osteomyelitis, adequately cover the defect, and provide a healthy, vascularized tissue bed for later revision total joint arthroplasty. A local rotational gastrocnemius muscle flap can be used for coverage of smaller wounds on the proximal third of the leg, and a soleus muscle flap can be used for the middle third of the leg. However, local rotational muscle flaps will not reliably cover defects larger than 25 cm² or those on the distal third of the leg, ankle, or foot. Free muscle flaps are the preferred choice for treatment of these distal defects.

2. Internal fixation. Compromised wound healing or infection after open reduction and internal fixation of fractures can lead to hardware exposure. Factors contributing to wound complications include

significant tissue edema, fracture blistering, wide zones of injury, and poor tissue handling. Treatment of exposed hardware typically requires local muscle or free tissue coverage. The medial pretibial surface of the distal leg is affected more often than the lateral malleolus region. Indications for wound coverage of the leg are as discussed for total joint arthroplasty.

Nonhealing Wounds

Wound healing problems are common in patients with diabetes and peripheral vascular disease. Management of these patients requires close collaboration between the orthopedic surgeon, the vascular surgeon, and the microsurgical team for optimal assessment and treatment of the vascular problems and for appropriate and timely planning of wound care. In this population of patients, morbidity is lower with free cutaneous flaps than with free muscle flaps, but diabetic patients generally have a higher incidence of repeated surgeries. Mortality, however, has not been found to be higher in this group of patients who undergo microsurgical reconstruction alone or in combination with vascular reconstruction. In general, defects of the foot can be appropriately reconstructed once the extremity has been revascularized and is well perfused. Free flap coverage is indicated for patients who have an intact vascular supply without apparent compromise but have large, colonized wounds involving major soft tissue, tendon, or bone. Free tissue transfer ideally allows the following:

1. Resurfacing of any size defect.
2. Aggressive débridement by resection of unhealthy, bacterial colonized tissue.
3. Replacement of the defect with healthy, atraumatic tissue.
4. Revascularization of the defect.

Diabetic patients and patients with peripheral vascular disease require a high degree of observation to avoid problems with wound healing at the donor and recipient sites. Most important, the results of lower extremity salvage in these patients must be critically reviewed with respect to ambulatory function. Salvage of a nonfunctional limb in such patients is of limited value to the patient and the overall management. In addition, heroic limb salvage is contraindicated for patients who are significantly compromised medically (e.g., severe cardiovascular disease) and have a high risk of mortality. A high degree of success can be achieved only when patients are carefully selected.

Free Tissue Selection and Timing of Transfer

TYPES OF FREE TISSUES

Isolated Tissue

Muscle, skin, fascia, bone, and nerve are examples of an isolated tissue type for transplantation.

Classification of Muscle Flaps

Muscle types are classified on the basis of five patterns of muscle circulation. A muscle used for free tissue transfer must be able to survive on one dominant vascular pedicle that can support the entire muscle mass. Classification is as follows:

1. Type 1: one vascular pedicle (extensor digitorum brevis, tensor fascia lata).
2. Type 2: one dominant pedicle and minor pedicles (abductor hallucis longus, gracilis).
3. Type 3: two dominant pedicles (rectus abdominis, serratus anterior).
4. Type 4: segmental vascular pedicles.
5. Type 5: one dominant and secondary pedicles (latissimus dorsi, pectoralis major, pectoralis minor).

Composite Tissue

Composite flaps are a combination of tissue types and provide more than one function. Toe transplantation, which includes vascular, neural, tendinous, osseous, and nail components as a composite, is the best example of composite tissue transfer. Other examples are myocutaneous, fasciocutaneous, osteocutaneous, and innervated myocutaneous flaps (e.g., functioning free muscle transfer).

SELECTION OF FREE FLAP

Donor site morbidity, recipient site requirements (i.e., size, anatomic location, structural loss, dead space, presence of infection or colonization), vascular pedicle length, and anticipated aesthetic results are important factors for appropriate free flap selection. Free tissue flaps are not always selected to cover soft tissue defects or to replace missing tissue. Some instances require augmentation of an existing soft tissue envelope insufficient in texture or quality.

Recipient Site

The type of tissue deficiency and surfacing requirements typically determine selection of the type of free flap, in isolation or as a composite flap. For example, a myocutaneous latissimus dorsi flap is not a good choice for the dorsum of the foot or for resurfacing the dorsal hand for secondary tendon reconstruction because of its bulkiness and lack of donor tissue matching the dorsum of the foot or hand. An isolated cutaneous flap, such as a radial forearm or lateral arm flap, would be considered a better selection. A lateral arm flap, however, would not afford enough tissue bulk to fill dead space created by aggressive débridement and sequestrectomy for osteomyelitis. In addition, muscle flaps are more effective than cutaneous flaps for the treatment of osteomyelitis.

Use of Skin Paddle

Incorporation of a skin paddle as a composite tissue transfer can serve multiple purposes. A skin paddle can provide necessary soft tissue contouring and aesthetics, or it can solely function as a monitor for flap perfusion during the postoperative period.

Vascular Pedicle and Recipient Vessels

The vessel anastomosis should be done in a "safe zone" where the recipient vessels have not been previously damaged. The concept of "zone of injury" refers to the inflammatory response within the soft tissue of the traumatized limb that extends beyond the grossly evident wound. Perivascular changes of blood vessels within the zone of injury can result in increased friability of vessels and increased perivascular scar tissue, which ultimately contribute to a higher failure rate of free tissue transfer, especially for the lower limb.

A higher rate of microvascular thrombosis is believed to occur. The zone of injury can be avoided with extensive proximal dissection of the recipient vascular pedicle or with use of interpositional vein grafts. The condition of the recipient pedicle with regard to vessel wall pliability and quality of blood flow is more important than the distance of the recipient vessels from the wound. Angiography is frequently used to evaluate the vasculature of the recipient site, although there is some debate about its necessity. Meticulous use of the Doppler probe for clinical evaluation can obviate the need for routine recipient site angiography.

Intercalary Bone Defects

Vascularized bone flap selection should be based on the cross section of the bone defect, the available vascular supply, and the possible need for simultaneous soft tissue reconstruction.

TIMING OF FREE TISSUE TRANSFER

General Principles

Two key factors are considered in determining wound coverage with a free flap transfer: (1) the presence of exposed vital structures and (2) the risk of infection. Vital structures include vessels, nerves, joint surfaces, tendons, and bone denuded of periosteum. These tissues will necrose rapidly if they are inadequately covered and may lose function with prolonged exposure. The risk of infection increases with increased exposure time and in the presence of tissue necrosis.

Trauma

Important factors related to an extremity injury that influence the timing of definitive wound management include the general condition of the patient, bacterial status of the wound, type of fracture, types of tissues injured, and exposed structures. In severe extremity trauma with associated soft tissue defects and exposure of underlying structures, acute coverage of the wound by 5 to 7 days is generally accepted as having a good prognosis. Early aggressive wound débridement with soft tissue coverage by a free flap within 5 days has been shown to reduce the risks of postoperative infection, flap failure, nonunion, and chronic osteomyelitis. Some authors emphasize the importance of radical débridement in cases of high-energy trauma and recommend free flap coverage at the time of the initial débridement to within the first 72 hours after injury. Others recommend that free tissue transfer be done between 7 and 14 days after injury and several débridements. This algorithm favors continued assessment and evaluation of the zone of injury, which is often not apparent on presentation. Consideration should be given to an arteriogram in the severely injured limb with suspected major vascular injury or a large zone of injury that may compromise potential sites of microvascular anastomosis.

Tumor

1. Irradiated wounds are associated with a high incidence of wound complications after tumor resection and attempted primary closure of surgical incisions because of poor vascularity and tissue quality. Free tissue transfer for coverage of these wounds affords improved local vascularity and results in more rapid wound healing. For this reason, some surgeons implement immediate free tissue transfer after tumor resection in these cases; results show decreased hospital stay, decreased costs, decreased morbidity, and increased rate of limb salvage with high satisfaction of the patient. When patients receive adjuvant therapy consisting of chemotherapy or radiotherapy, the appropriate window for the timing of surgery, inclusive of tumor resection and free tissue transfer, is determined by a multidisciplinary evaluation involving the oncologist, radiation therapist, oncologic surgeon, and microsurgical team.

2. Secondary limb reconstruction with free tissue transplantation can be divided into two subsets: (1) acute reconstruction for wound complications in the early postoperative period after tumor resection and (2) late (several months or years) reconstruction for chronic unstable soft tissue, wound dehiscence, failed or infected prosthesis, or limb growth complications. Patients who experience acute complications after surgery, such as skin flap necrosis, may require débridement and free flap coverage within the first or second week from surgery. Serial débridements and continual wound inspection allow demarcation of questionable areas before free tissue transplantation. Patients who later present with impending exposure of an allograft or prosthesis should have immediate débridement and tissue coverage to avoid infection of the implant or allograft.

Specific Free Flaps

See Table 8-1 (see Chapter 3 for pedicle flaps).

Postoperative Care and Monitoring

GENERAL PRINCIPLES

Patients require adequate hydration, proper maintenance of body temperature, and maintenance of hematocrit. Routine heparinization and anticoagulation are not used. Monitoring of free flaps is essential. Flaps are typically monitored for a minimum of 5 days by use of clinical acumen and adjunctive devices such as a laser Doppler probe. The immediate 24 to 48 hours after surgery are the most critical, but occasional late free flap failure warrants continued monitoring for 5 days. Extremities are elevated at all times to avoid venous congestion. Patients with lower extremity flaps do not bear weight for a minimum of 3 weeks, and timing of allowed weight bearing is determined on the basis of flap selection (i.e., muscle or skin) and assessment of flap healing and maturation. Foot and ankle sites are most susceptible to increased venous pressure and ensuing edema of the flap, which can result in free flap dehiscence.

FREE FLAP MONITORING

Many different devices and techniques have been used with varying levels of success. Flap monitoring is ideally harmless to the patient, objective, applicable

◈ **Table 8-1**

TYPES OF FLAPS

Tissue Types	Flap	Vascular Anatomy	Notes
Fascial and fasciocutaneous flaps	Radial forearm	Pedicle: radial artery	Radial artery is sacrificed Complications are most commonly due to skin graft problems at the donor site Can be innervated by the medial and lateral antebrachial cutaneous nerves
	Posterior interosseous	Pedicle: posterior interosseous artery (septocutaneous perforators between extensor carpi ulnaris and extensor digiti minimi) Anastomoses between posterior and anterior interosseous arteries at the level of distal radioulnar joint maintain viability	Useful for defects on dorsum of hand Advantage over radial forearm flap is that a large artery is not sacrificed Elevation of flap limited by posterior interosseous nerve branch to extensor carpi ulnaris
	Lateral arm	Pedicle: posterior radial collateral artery (pedicle length is 7-8 cm)	Can be used for coverage after severe thumb web space contracture release Harvest leads to numbness in the posterolateral elbow due to transection of posterior cutaneous nerve of forearm Can be innervated by the posterior cutaneous nerve of the forearm
	Ulnar artery	Pedicle: ulnodorsal artery (arises 2.5 cm proximal to pisiform) (pedicle length can be up to 20 cm)	Cause of paresthesias in the hand after flap elevation due to transient ischemia of ulnar nerve during flap elevation
	Brachioradialis	Pedicle: anterior recurrent radial artery	Can be innervated by the radial nerve
	Temporoparietal fascial	Pedicle: superficial temporal artery	
	Scapular	Pedicle: circumflex scapular artery	
	Groin	Pedicle: superficial circumflex artery	Superficial circumflex artery runs 1 inch below inguinal ligament Numbness in the thigh after groin flap related to meralgia paresthetica (lateral femoral cutaneous nerve)
	Anterolateral thigh	Pedicle: lateral femoral circumflex artery (descending branch between rectus femoris and vastus lateralis)	Can be innervated by the medial and lateral cutaneous nerves of the thigh
	Lateral thigh	Pedicle: profunda femoris artery (third perforator)	Can be innervated by the medial and lateral cutaneous nerves of the thigh
	Dorsalis pedis	Pedicle: anterior tibial–dorsalis pedis artery	
Muscle and myocutaneous flaps	Latissimus dorsi	Pedicle: thoracodorsal artery (pedicle length can be up to 11.2 cm)	Release of tendon insertion has the greatest effect on the axis of rotation of a pedicled latissimus flap Can be innervated by the thoracodorsal nerve Can be used as a functional muscle transfer
	Vastus lateralis	Pedicle: lateral circumflex artery (proximal); profunda femoris artery (distal)	
	Serratus anterior	Pedicle: thoracodorsal artery	No scapular winging occurs if only lower slips of the muscle are harvested Can be used as a functioning muscle transfer Can be innervated by the long thoracic nerve
	Rectus abdominis	Pedicle: inferior epigastric artery	
	Tensor fascia lata	Pedicle: lateral circumflex artery (proximal); profunda femoris artery (distal)	
	Gracilis	Pedicle: medial femoral circumflex artery	Can be used as a functional muscle transfer

continued

◆ Table 8-1—cont'd

TYPES OF FLAPS—cont'd

Tissue Types	Flap	Vascular Anatomy	Notes
Osseous and osteocutaneous flaps	Fibula and osteocutaneous fibula	Pedicle: peroneal artery	Can be transferred as an osteocutaneous flap by including fasciocutaneous perforators in the mid to distal third of the fibula The vascularized fibular graft remodels and hypertrophies more quickly than nonvascularized grafts do
	Iliac crest and osteocutaneous iliac crest	Pedicle: superficial circumflex artery	Can be harvested as an osteocutaneous flap with iliac crest bone
Composite tissue flaps	Great toe, second toe	Pedicle: first dorsal metatarsal artery	In 78% of cases, the first dorsal metatarsal artery runs superficial to the first dorsal interosseous muscle
	Toe wraparound	Pedicle: first dorsal metatarsal artery	

to all flap types, and cost-effective. Monitors must be capable of prolonged continuous use and must respond rapidly to changes in perfusion. Methods of monitoring include clinical evaluation, direct vessel monitoring, tissue circulation monitoring, and metabolic parameters.

Clinical Evaluation

This method remains the "gold standard." Clinical assessment includes observation of skin color, temperature, capillary refill, and bleeding characteristics. Experienced personnel are necessary, and unfortunately, clinical examination is limited to the surfaces of skin flaps and muscle flaps. Initial detrimental changes are often subtle and may not be clinically apparent before irreversible tissue damage has occurred.

Direct Vessel Monitoring

Direct monitoring of the vessels can be done by electromagnetic flowmeters, ultrasonic Doppler probe, and thermocouples.

1. Electromagnetic flowmeter. Readings are based on the measured electrical potential induced by blood flow.
2. Ultrasonic Doppler probe. Reflected sound waves from columns of moving blood cells are measured.
3. Thermocouples. Two microthermocouples are used to measure the difference in temperature between preceding and succeeding sites relative to the anastomosis on the vascular pedicle.

Circulation Monitoring

Tissue circulation can be monitored by temperature probes, photoplethysmography, laser Doppler examination, and pulse oximetry.

1. Temperature probes. Changes in temperature measurements can indicate changes in cutaneous blood flow.
2. Photoplethysmography. Readings indicate changes in the amount of light reflected as based on changes in local cutaneous blood volume.
3. Laser Doppler examination. Measurements are based on the frequency changes of light reflected from moving red blood cells.

4. Pulse oximetry. Blood flow is indirectly measured by continuous monitoring of both oxygen saturation and pulsatility.

Metabolic Parameters

Transcutaneous oxygen monitoring and invasive PO_2 measurements assess tissue perfusion. The level of tissue oxygen tension measured has been shown to reflect the quality of capillary flow.

Management of Flap Failure

ACUTE COMPLICATIONS

The initial 48 hours are the most critical because most complications occur during this time. Complications include arterial insufficiency, venous insufficiency, hematoma, hemorrhage, and excessive flap edema. These complications can occur alone or in any combination.

Arterial Insufficiency

This problem manifests as decreased capillary refill, pallor, reduced temperature, and absence of bleeding after pinprick. Arterial spasm, thrombosis, poor vessel quality (e.g., plaque, small vessel disease), torsion or kinking of the pedicle, pressure on the flap, technical error of the anastomosis, and flap tissue harvested too large for its blood supply are possible causes of arterial insufficiency.

Prompt surgical intervention is required to restore blood flow. Adjuvant pharmacologic agents used for flap salvage include vasodilators, calcium channel blockers, and anticoagulants.

Venous Compromise

Obstructed venous outflow can be manifested as flap cyanosis, rapid capillary refill, normal or elevated temperature, and presence of dark blood after pinprick. Thrombosis, torsion or kinking of the pedicle, flap edema, hematoma, and excessively tight closure of tissue over the pedicle are possible causes of venous compromise. Because microcirculatory disruption can occur rapidly, early recognition of venous compromise is critical. Leeches can be used in the presence of venous congestion despite a patent venous anastomosis with insufficient outflow. Hematoma can be drained at the bedside by the removal of limited sutures to decrease pressure.

LATE FLAP FAILURES

Cause of Failure
Technical or physiologic factors can result in flap failure. Technical errors, the most frequent cause of failure, may include an error in flap harvest, pedicle compromise during harvest, improper microsurgical technique, poor insetting of the flap with resultant increased tissue tension or edema, or pedicle avulsion from postoperative extremity motion (rare, but it occurs).

Options for Failure
Options for management include a second free flap transfer, delayed débridement (Crane principle) and skin grafting, and amputation.
1. Second free flap. When a second free tissue transfer is considered, physiologic conditions and technical errors that lead to flap failure must be recognized before proceeding. Additional studies, such as arteriography or blood coagulation profiles, may be considered.
2. Delayed débridement. On the basis of the Crane principle, the unsalvageable free flap can be left in place as a biologic dressing or eschar over the wound. If no infection is present, the eschar can be left over the wound bed in the hope of some healing with sufficient granulation tissue. Ultimately, the eschar could be removed, and with an appropriate granulation bed, the wound can be skin grafted, obviating the need for a second free flap for wound closure. If sufficient healing of the underlying tissue is absent, a second flap must be considered. However, as a word of caution, the failed flap can become a source of infection, which can further compromise local tissues.
3. Amputation. When flaps fail in severely compromised extremities, consideration should be given to amputation. Treatment decisions must account for the additional morbidity of a second free tissue transfer and the expected outcome for the salvaged extremity to determine whether reconstruction or amputation is more favorable.

Bibliography

REPLANTATION

Akyurek M, Safak T, Kecik A: Fingertip replantation at or distal to the nail base: use of the technique of artery-only anastomosis. Ann Plast Surg, 46(6):605-612, 2001.

al-Shammari S, Gupta A: Revascularization of the digits and palm. Hand Clin, 17:411-417, 2001.

Arakaki A, Tsai TM: Thumb replantation: Survival factors and reexploration in 122 cases. J Hand Surg, 18B:152-156, 1993.

Backman C, Nystrom A, Backman C, et al: Arterial spasticity and cold intolerance in relation to time after digital replantation. J Hand Surg, 18B:551-555, 1993.

Boulas JH: Amputations of the fingers and hand: Indications for replantation. J Am Ac Orthop Surg, 6:100-105, 1998.

Bowen CVA, Beveridge J, Milliken RG, et al: Rotating shaft avulsion amputations of the thumb. J Hand Surg, 16A:117-121, 1991.

Brown ML, Wood MB: Techniques of bone fixation in replantation surgery. Microsurg, 11:255-260, 1990.

Fukui A, Maeda M, Inada Y, et al: Arteriovenous shunt in digit replantation. J Hand Surg, 15A:160-165, 1990.

Glickman L, Mackinnon S: Sensory recovery following digital replantation. Microsurg, 11:236-242, 1990.

Goldner RD: Postoperative Management. Hand Clin, 1:205-215, 1985.

Goldner RD, Howson MP, Nunley JA, et al: One hundred eleven thumb amputations: replantation versus revision. Microsurg, 11:243-250, 1990.

Goldner RD, Nunley JA: Replantation proximal to the wrist. Hand Clin, 8:413-425, 1992.

Goldner RD, Stevanovic MV, Nunley JA, et al: Digital replantation at the level of the distal interphalangeal joint and the distal phalanx. J Hand Surg, 14A:214-220, 1989.

Hovius SE, van Adrichem LN, Mulder HD, et al: Comparison of laser Doppler flowmetry and thermometry in the postoperative monitoring of replantations. J Hand Surg, 20A:88-93, 1995.

Janezic TF, Arnez ZM, Solinc M, et al: Functional results of 46 thumb replantations and revascularisations. Microsurg, 17:264-267, 1996.

Jupiter JB, Pess GM, Bour CJ: Results of flexor tendon tenolysis after replantation in the hand. J Hand Surg, 14A: 35-44, 1989.

Kim WK, Lim JH, Han SK: Fingertip replantations: clinical evaluation of 135 digits. Plast Reconstr Surg, 98:470-476, 1996.

Koshima I, Soeda S, Moriguchi T, et al: The use of arteriovenous anastomosis for replantation of the distal phalanx of the fingers. Plast Reconstr Surg, 89:710-714, 1992.

Lowen RM, Rodgers CM, Ketch LL, et al: Aeromonas hydrophilia infection complicating digital replantation and revascularization. J Hand Surg, 14A:714-718, 1989.

Meyer VE: Hand amputations proximal but close to the wrist joint: prime candidates for reattachment (long-term functional results). J Hand Surg, 10A:989-991, 1985.

Patradul A, Ngarmukos C, Parkpian V: Distal digital replantations and revascularizations. 237 digits in 192 patients. J Hand Surg, 23B:578-582, 1998.

Povlsen B, Nylander G, Nylander E: Cold-induced vasospasm after digital replantation does not improve with time. A 12 year prospective study. J Hand Surg, 20B:237-239, 1995.

Russell RC, O'Brien BM, Morrison WA, et al: The late functional results of upper limb revascularization and replantation. J Hand Surg, 9A:623-633, 1984.

Saies AD, Urbaniak, JR, Nunley JA, et al: Results after replantation and revascularization in the upper extremity in children. J Bone Joint Surg, 76A:1766-1776, 1994.

Soucacos PN: Indications and selection for digital amputation and replantation. J Hand Surg, 26B(6):572-581, 2001.

Sud V, Freeland AE: Skeletal fixation in digital replantation. Microsurg, 22:165-171, 2002.

Taras JS, Nunley JA, Urbaniak JR, et al: Replantation in children. Microsurg, 12:216-220, 1991.

Urbaniak JR, Evans JP, Bright DS: Microvascular management of ring avulsion injuries. J Hand Surg, 6A:25-30, 1981.

Urbaniak JR, Roth JH, Nunley JA, et al: The results of replantation after amputation of a single finger. J Bone Joint Surg, 67A:611-619, 1985.

Wang H: Secondary surgery after digit replantation: its incidence and sequence. Microsurg, 22:57-61, 2002.

Wei FC, el-Gammal TA: Toe-to-hand transfer. Current concepts, techniques, and research. Clin Plast Surg, 23:103-116, 1996.

Weil DJ, Wood VE, Frykman GK: A new class of ring avulsion injuries. J Hand Surg, 14A:662-664, 1989.

Whitney TM, Lineaweaver WC, Buncke HJ, et al: Clinical results of bony fixation methods in digital replantation, J Hand Surg, 15A:328-334, 1990.

Wood MB, Cooney WP: Above-elbow limb replantation: functional results. J Hand Surg, 11A:682-687, 1986.

FREE TISSUE TRANSFER

Armenta E, Fisher J: Vascular pedicle of the tensor fascia lata myocutaneous flap. Ann Plast Surg, 6:112-116, 1981.

Arnez ZM: Immediate reconstruction of the lower extremity: an update. Clin Plast Surg, 18:449-457, 1991.

Bartlett SP, May JW, Yaremchuk MJ: The latissimus dorsi muscle: a fresh cadaver study of the primary neurovascular pedicle. Plast Reconstr Surg, 67:631-636, 1981.

Barwick WJ, Goodkind DJ, Serafin D: The free scapular flap. Plast Reconstr Surg, 69:779-787, 1982.

Brown DM, Upton J, Khouri RK: Free flap coverage of the hand. Clin Plast Surg, 24:57-62, 1997.

Chen S, Tsai YC, Wei FC, et al: Emergency free flaps to the type IIIC tibial fracture. Ann Plast Surg, 25:223-229, 1990.

Chuang DC, Jeng SF, Chen HT, et al: Experience of 73 free groin flaps. J Plast Surg Br, 45:81-85, 1992.

Chung KC, Wei FC: An Outcome Study of Thumb Reconstruction Using Microvascular Toe Transfer. J Hand Surg 25A:651-658, 2000.

Costa H, Soutar DS: The distally-based island posterior interosseous flap. J Plast Surg Br, 41:221-227, 1988.

el-Gammal TA, Wei FC: Microvascular reconstruction of the distal digits by partial toe transfer. Clin Plast Surg 24:49-55, 1997.

Giordano PA, Abbes M, Pequignot JP: Gracilis blood supply: anatomical and clinical reevaluation. J Plast Surg Br, 43:266-272, 1990.

Godina M: Early microsurgical reconstruction of complex trauma of the extremities. Plast Reconstr Surg, 78:285-292, 1986.

Govila A, Sharma D: The Radial Forearm Flap for Reconstruction of the Upper Extremity. Plast Reconstr Surg, 920-927, 1990.

Han CS, Wood MB, Bishop AT, Cooney WP: Vascularized Bone Transfer. J Bone Joint Surg, 74A:1441-1449, 1992.

Hausman M: Microvascular applications in limb-sparing tumor surgery. Orthopaed Clin N Am, 20:427-437, 1989.

Hirase Y, Kojima T: Use of double-layered free temporal fascia flap for upper extremity coverage. J Hand Surg, 19A:864-870, 1994.

Isenberg JS, Sherman R: Zone of injury: a valid concept in microvascular reconstruction of the traumatized lower limb. Ann Plast Surg, 36:270-272, 1996.

Katsaros J, Schusterman M, Beppu M, et al: The lateral upper arm flap: anatomy and clinical applications. Ann Plast Surg, 12:489-500, 1984.

Lassen M, Krag C, Nielsen IM: The latissimus dorsi flap: an overview. J Plast Reconstr Surg Scand, 19:41-51, 1985.

Levin L: Debridement. Tech Orthop, 10:104-108, 1995.

Levin L: Microsurgical autologous tissue transplantation. Tech Orthop, 10:134-145, 1995.

Levin LS: The reconstructive ladder: an orthoplastic approach. Orthopaed Clin N Am, 24:393-409, 1993.

Lister G, Scheker L: Emergency free flaps to the upper extremity. J Hand Surg, 13A:22-28, 1988.

Lister GD, Kalisman M, Tsai TM: Reconstruction of the Hand with Free Microneurovascular Toe-to-Hand Transfer: Experience with 54 Toe Transfers. Plast Reconstr Surg, 71:372-384, 1983.

Man D, Acland RD: The microarterial anatomy of the dorsalis pedis flap and its clinical applications. Plast Reconstr Surg, 65:419-423, 1980.

Manktelow RT, Zuker RM, McKee NH: Functioning free muscle transplantation. J Hand Surg, 9A:32-39, 1984.

Mathes SJ, Alpert BS, Chang N: Use of the muscle flap in chronic osteomyelitis: experimental and clinical correlation. Plast Reconstr Surg, 69:815-829, 1982.

Mathes SJ, Nahai F: Classification of the vascular anatomy of muscles: experimental and clinical correlation. Plast Reconstr Surg, 67:177-187, 1981.

McCabe SJ, Breidenbach WC: The role of emergency free flaps for hand trauma. Hand Clin, 15:275-288, 1999.

Muhlbauer W, Herndl E, Stock W: The forearm flap. Plast Reconstr Surg, 70:33-44, 1982.

Park S, Han SH, Lee TJ: Algorithm for recipient vessel selection in free tissue transfer to the lower extremity. Plast Reconstr Surg, 103:1937-1948, 1999.

Scheker LR, Kleinert HE, Hanel DP: Lateral arm composite tissue transfer to ipsilateral hand defects. J Hand Surg, 12A:665-672, 1987.

Song R, Gao Y, Song Y, et al: The forearm flap. Clin Plast Surg, 9:21-26, 1982.

Urbaniak JR, Koman LA, Goldner RD, et al: The vascularized cutaneous scapular flap. Plastic Recon Surg, 69:772-778, 1982.

Wheatley MJ, Meltzer TR: The management of unsalvageable free flaps. J Reconstr Microsurg, 12:227-229, 1996.

Yaremchuk MJ, Brumback RJ, Manson PN, et al: Acute and definitive management of traumatic osteocutaneous defects of the lower extremity. Plast Reconstr Surg, 80:1-14, 1987.

Yousif NJ, Warren R, Matloub HS, et al: The lateral arm fascial free flap: its anatomy and use in reconstruction. Plast Reconstr Surg, 86:1138-1145, 1990.

❖ Sanjiv Naidu, MD, PhD   ❖ John D. Temple, MD

ARTHRITIS

Osteoarthritis

Introduction

1. Osteoarthritis (OA) is a degenerative condition involving hyaline cartilage in diarthrodial joints, distinct from inflammatory arthropathies and post-traumatic arthrosis. The most common type is idiopathic. Osteoarthritic articular cartilage has decreased tensile stiffness.
2. Prevalence increases with age; men are more commonly affected than are women until menopause. After the age of 65 years, it is estimated that 99% of women and 78% of men will have radiographic evidence of OA in the hand. Patterns vary by race (e.g., OA in the carpometacarpal [CMC] joint of the thumb is more common in whites).
   a. Joints most commonly affected in decreasing order are distal interphalangeal (DIP) joint, CMC joint of the thumb, proximal interphalangeal (PIP) joint, and metacarpophalangeal (MP) joint.
   b. OA in one or more joints in a row is a predictor of subsequent OA in all other joints in a row.
3. Radiographic appearance of OA is characterized by osteophytes, sclerosis, asymmetric joint narrowing, and subchondral cysts.

Osteoarthritis in the Carpometacarpal Joint of the Thumb (Fig. 9-1)

1. The CMC joint of the thumb is the joint that most often requires surgical treatment for OA in the upper extremity. Several anatomic factors predispose the joint to OA.
   a. It resembles two saddles with perpendicular opposing surfaces resulting in a semiconstrained and incongruous joint. This construct allows a wide range of motion in several planes (flexion-extension, abduction-adduction, and rotation to allow thumb opposition).
   b. The critical stabilizer is the palmar (beak) ligament. Incompetence of this ligament results in pathologic laxity and increased shear forces between the two joint surfaces. Other stabilizing ligaments of the CMC joint are the intermetacarpal, ulnar collateral, posterior oblique, and dorsoradial ligaments.

2. Patients present with pain at the base of the thumb with movement, particularly with actions that generate stress across the joint (e.g., pinch). Pain and grinding of the joint occur in compression. Aching may be localized to the thenar or abductor muscle group; pressure over the dorsal, volar, or radial CMC capsule reproduces symptoms.
3. It should be differentiated from first dorsal compartment (de Quervain's) tenosynovitis, MP arthrosis, and intercarpal or radiocarpal arthrosis.

RADIOGRAPHIC STAGING

Radiographic staging as described by Eaton and Littler is as follows:
1. Stage 1: articular contours normal; joint space may be widened and possible mild subluxation.
2. Stage 2: slight narrowing of the joint space; articular contours remain normal. Mild subchondral sclerosis at the joint level and osteophytes < 2 mm.
3. Stage 3: CMC joint narrowing with sclerotic or cystic changes in subchondral bone and osteophytes > 2 mm in diameter; scaphotrapezial joint intact.
4. Stage 4: pantrapezial arthrosis; both the CMC and scaphotrapezial joints are affected with severe articular degeneration.

TREATMENT

Treatment of all stages is initially conservative; splints, nonsteroidal anti-inflammatory drugs (NSAIDs), and corticosteroid injections are appropriate. Surgical treatment is indicated for severe pain and disability independent of radiographic findings. Surgical treatment typically results in improvement of grip and pinch strength.
1. Stage 1: CMC synovectomy and débridement (arthroscopic); metacarpal osteotomy; ligament reconstruction with flexor carpi radialis tendon in cases of joint laxity.
2. Stage 2: arthroscopic débridement and tendon transposition; partial trapeziectomy with tendon interposition; metacarpal osteotomy; prosthetic arthroplasty (Fig. 9-2); complete trapeziectomy and ligament reconstruction and tendon interposition (LRTI); trapeziometacarpal arthrodesis (optimal position for CMC fusion: 30 to 40 degrees of palmar abduction, 35 degrees of radial abduction, 15 degrees of pronation). Arthrodesis is reserved

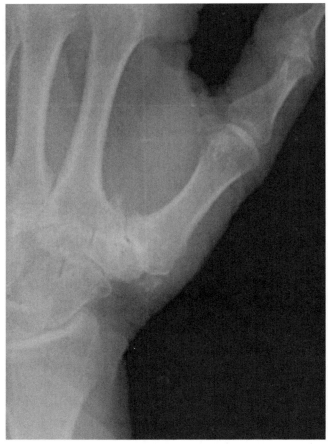

Figure 9-1 ◆ Osteoarthrosis of the CMC joint of the thumb. Note the destruction of the articular surface and osteophyte formation.

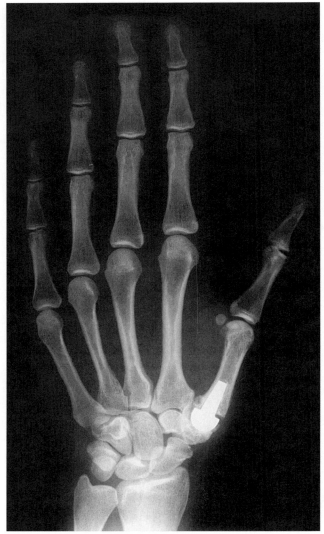

Figure 9-2 ◆ Osteoarthrosis of the CMC joint of the thumb treated with metallic prosthetic arthroplasty.

for the young laborer. Limitations of fusion include inability to lay the hand flat with the thumb in the plane of the hand (Table 9-1).

3. Stage 3: partial trapeziectomy with tendon interposition; prosthetic arthroplasty; complete trapeziectomy and LRTI; trapeziometacarpal arthrodesis.
4. Stage 4: complete trapeziectomy and LRTI; after trapeziectomy and LRTI, the amount of subsidence of the thumb metacarpal directly correlates with lateral pinch stress.

SILICONE IMPLANT ARTHROPLASTY

Silicone implant arthroplasty is contraindicated in the population of active patients with OA. Recurrent pain, instability, and localized synovitis develop after a period of pain relief (after silicone trapezial arthroplasty) as a result of silicone synovitis. Dislocation is the most common reason for reoperation in patients treated with silicone implants for CMC arthrosis. The biologic response to silicone particles starts with adsorption of protein molecules onto the surface of the particles, which are hydrophobic. This protein adsorption then leads to an inflammatory response to the silicone particles. The treatment of choice for failed implants is implant excision and conversion to soft tissue arthroplasty.

Thumb Metacarpophalangeal Joint Deformity in Carpometacarpal Joint Arthrosis

If hyperextension deformity is present, the MP joint must be surgically addressed to diminish stress across the CMC joint.

1. MP hyperextension of less than 10 degrees: pin the joint in flexion.
2. MP hyperextension of 10 to 20 degrees: volar plate advancement and pinning of MP joint.
3. MP hyperextension of more than 25 degrees: consider arthrodesis, especially if radiographic OA in the MP joint is visible. The optimal position for MP joint fusion is 15 degrees of flexion and 10 degrees of pronation. Other options include extensor pollicis brevis transfer and sesamoid fusion.

✦ Table 9-1	
OPTIMAL POSITION FOR ARTHRODESIS	
DIP	10-20 degrees of flexion
PIP	30-45 degrees of flexion, cascading from the index to the small fingers in 5-degree increments
Thumb MP	15 degrees of flexion
	10 degrees of pronation
Thumb CMC	30-40 degrees of palmar abduction
	35 degrees of radial abduction
	15 degrees of pronation
Wrist	10 degrees of extension
	Neutral deviation (one side should be in neutral extension in bilateral cases)

Osteoarthritis in the Distal Interphalangeal Joints

1. OA in the DIP joint is characterized by enlargement of the joint (Heberden's nodes). Patients complain of pain and deformity.
2. Nodular involvement and bone spurs lead to formation of mucous cysts that are often associated with an osteophyte. The cysts may lead to draining sinus tracks or septic arthritis. Nail plate involvement may occur with loss of normal gloss, splitting, and deformity (see Chapter 10).

TREATMENT

1. Mucous cysts: aspiration, or open excision of the mucous cyst and débridement of the distal and middle phalangeal osteophytes.
2. DIP joint arthrosis: arthrodesis of the DIP joint in 10 to 20 degrees of flexion. Poor bone stock is the major reason for DIP joint nonunion after attempted arthrodesis. Herbert screw fixation has the highest union rate in DIP fusions (Fig. 9-3).
3. Arthroplasty is rarely performed at the DIP joint. The literature supports similar function and pain relief with arthroplasty and arthrodesis.

Osteoarthritis in the Proximal Interphalangeal Joints (Fig. 9-4)

1. Complaints are similar to those of OA in the DIP joints, although the PIP joint is less often involved. Enlargement is characterized by Bouchard's nodes.
2. Joint contractures may develop with fibrosis of the collateral ligaments.

TREATMENT

1. Mucous cysts: less common than in the DIP joint; treatment options are similar.
2. When contracture is predominant and joint involvement is minimal, collateral ligament excision, volar plate release, and osteophyte excision can be helpful.
3. Arthroplasty: consideration must be given to joint replacement with Swanson implants before arthrodesis, especially in the long and ring fingers. There should be intact bone stock without any angulation or rotational deformity. In the border digits (index and small fingers), consideration must be given to

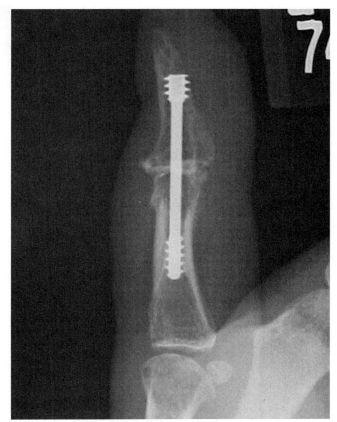

Figure 9-3 ✦ Arthrodesis of the interphalangeal joint of the thumb with a compression (Herbert) screw.

arthrodesis before arthroplasty. If the bone stock is inadequate, the implant is more likely to fail.
4. Arthrodesis: highest rate of fusion is in patients with OA treated with screw fixation (Herbert or cannulated screw system). The position for arthrodesis is 30 to 45 degrees of flexion, cascading from the index to the small fingers in 5-degree increments.

Osteoarthritis in the Scaphotrapezial-Trapezoidal Joint

1. The scaphotrapezial-trapezoidal (STT) joint is the second most common site of OA in the wrist.
2. It may be post-traumatic in origin. Although a specific ligament injury is unknown, rotatory subluxation of the scaphoid may contribute to altered mechanics of the STT joint. Palmar flexion of the scaphoid progresses until the articular contact surfaces of the trapezium and trapezoid are increasingly dorsal on the distal scaphoid. Shear forces develop across the STT joint, resulting in STT arthrosis.
3. It can be associated with the SLAC wrist in 15% of cases.

TREATMENT

1. If OA is isolated to the STT joint without involvement of the thumb CMC joint, STT arthrodesis is an option. Consider arthroscopy of the CMC joint

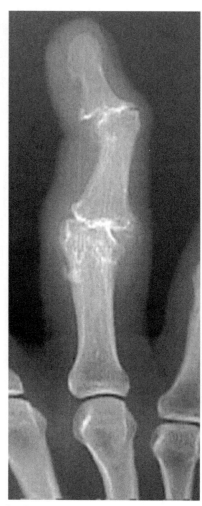

Figure 9-4 ◆ Osteoarthrosis of the DIP and PIP joints of the long finger. Note the destruction of the articular surface and osteophyte formation.

to confirm absence of CMC arthrosis before proceeding with STT fusion.
2. If pantrapezial arthrosis is present, the surgical treatment of choice is trapeziectomy and LRTI.

Osteoarthritis in the Pisotriquetral Joint

1. Patients present with pain in the base of the hypothenar eminence.
2. It may be post-traumatic in origin.
3. Symptoms are elicited with loading of the pisotriquetral joint. Oblique radiographs of the wrist in 30 degrees of pronation reveal the arthritic joint.
4. Treatment is conservative with splinting and corticosteroid injections. The pisiform can be excised in refractory cases.

Erosive Osteoarthritis

1. Erosive OA is a form of advanced OA characterized by intermittent inflammatory episodes that destroy articular cartilage and adjacent bone. Synovial change resembles that of rheumatoid arthritis; however,

there are no systemic effects. Hands, feet, and spine are most commonly affected.
2. It is most common in women (10:1 ratio) and affects primarily DIP joints. Patients are generally asymptomatic.
3. Radiographs reveal joint destruction with osteophytes and erosions.

TREATMENT

1. Erosive OA is a self-limited disease.
2. The patient is observed if symptoms are tolerable. Many go on to ankylosis if left untreated.
3. Arthrodesis can correct the deformity.

Pulmonary Hypertrophic Osteoarthropathy

1. This condition is associated with digital clubbing, abnormal deposition of periosteal bone, arthralgias, and synovitis.
2. Patients complain of burning pain with morning joint stiffness.
3. On radiography, periosteal thickening is observed and periosteal elevation appears as a continuous, sclerotic line of new bone.
4. Pulmonary hypertrophic osteoarthropathy is typically seen in patients with a pulmonary neoplasm. Hypertrophic osteoarthropathy occurs in 5% to 10% of patients with thoracic malignant neoplasms. Bronchogenic carcinoma is the most common, followed by non–small cell lung cancers. It is occasionally seen with other lung diseases and in familial cases.

Post-traumatic Arthrosis

Thumb and Digits

The same principles as for OA apply to post-traumatic arthrosis of the thumb and digits.

Wrist

SCAPHOLUNATE ADVANCED COLLAPSE

Scapholunate advanced collapse (SLAC) is the most common pattern of wrist OA (Fig. 9-5).
1. Injury to the scapholunate interosseous ligament and extrinsic ligament complex attenuation lead to rotatory subluxation of the scaphoid. The scaphoid falls into palmar flexion. As a result, the radioscaphoid joint becomes incongruous, normal radioscaphoid mechanics are altered, contact forces are increased, and arthrosis develops. As the scaphoid flexes and the scapholunate diastasis increases, the capitate migrates proximally. The altered intercarpal mechanics lead to arthrosis at the capitolunate joint. As the collapse progresses, pancarpal arthrosis develops. The radiolunate joint is typically spared because of its spheroid shape. Advanced disease is associated with loss of carpal height and progressive ulnar displacement of the lunate, causing ulnocarpal impingement in some patients.
2. Patients complain of decreased grip and pinch strength and stiffness with extension and radial deviation. Physical examination demonstrates

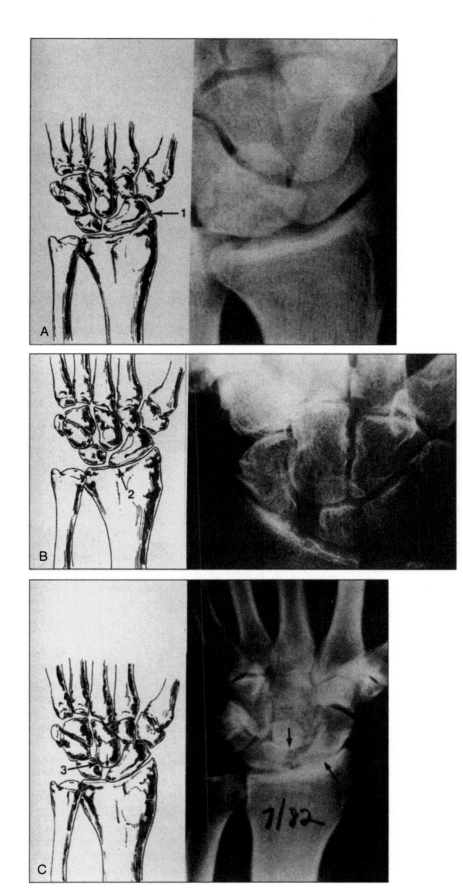

Figure 9-5 ❖ SLAC wrist. The progression of scapholunate advanced collapse follows a predictable pattern. **A,** Early degenerative process is visualized at the tip of the radial styloid and distal scaphoid. **B,** Eventually, the entire radioscaphoid joint is involved in the degenerative process. **C,** The capitolunate joint becomes involved with the degenerative process, which leads to proximal migration of the capitate. At this point, the radiolunate joint is still preserved. (*From Watson HK, Ballet FL: The SLAC wrist: scapholunate advanced collapse pattern of degenerative arthritis. J Hand Surg [Am] 9:358-365, 1984.*)

localized tenderness at the radial scaphoid articulation (at the base of the thumb in STT arthrosis). Wrist motion is decreased, especially extension and radial deviation. Carpal tunnel syndrome, de Quervain's tenosynovitis, or volar ganglion cyst may be present in up to a third of patients.

3. Watson recognized a pattern of progression of arthritic changes and eventual carpal collapse:
   a. Stage I: arthrosis localized to the radial side of the scaphoid and the radial styloid region of the distal radius with sharpening of the radial styloid.
   b. Stage II: arthrosis extending to the entire radioscaphoid joint with progressive radioscaphoid changes.
   c. Stage III: arthrosis progressing to the capitolunate joint due to proximal migration of the capitate.

Treatment by Stage

Patients with asymptomatic SLAC wrists do not need surgical treatment.

1. Stage I
   a. If the scapholunate relationship is reducible: radial styloidectomy plus scapholunate reduction and stabilization (dorsal capsulodesis, scapholunate ligament reconstruction) (see Chapter 7).
   b. If the scapholunate relationship is not reducible: radial styloidectomy plus scaphoid stabilization (STT fusion, scaphocapitate fusion).
2. Stage II: radioscaphoid joint must be eliminated because of arthrosis. Options include proximal row carpectomy versus scaphoid excision and four-corner (lunate-capitate-hamate-triquetrum) fusion (SLAC procedure). Other options include radioscaphoid fusion, radioscapholunate fusion, and total wrist arthrodesis. If there are capitate head degenerative changes, proximal row carpectomy should be avoided. Both proximal row carpectomy and SLAC procedures lead to reduction of wrist motion (about 50% to 60% of normal) and decrease in grip strength (about 50% to 60% of normal). Some believe that the SLAC procedure results in better grip strength. The volar radiocarpal ligaments must be preserved during a proximal row carpectomy to prevent instability.
3. Stage III: options include the SLAC procedure and total wrist arthrodesis. There is no role for proximal row carpectomy here because of the capitate head degenerative changes. With total wrist arthrodesis, the nonunion rate is 10 times greater if an AO fusion plate is not used. A spanning AO plate must be used to maximize fusion rates. Caveat about AO technique: extending the plates to the distal third of the metacarpal increases extensor tendon irritation. Scapholunate fusions have the lowest healing rates of all intercarpal arthrodeses. The optimum position for wrist fusion is 10 degrees of extension and neutral deviation. In cases requiring bilateral fusions, one side should be fused in neutral to allow personal hygiene.

SCAPHOID NONUNION ADVANCED COLLAPSE

Scaphoid nonunion advanced collapse is a less common form of post-traumatic wrist arthrosis.

1. Natural history and staging are similar to those of the SLAC wrist. Scaphoid nonunion or malunion may occur. Changes in carpal mechanics lead to carpal collapse. Incongruity of the radioscaphoid joint results in degenerative changes. Loss of scaphoid stabilization of the carpal rows leads to proximal migration of the capitate and arthrosis between the capitate head and the scapholunate complex.
2. Pattern of progression
   a. Stage I: arthrosis localized to the distal scaphoid and radial styloid.
   b. Stage II: above plus scaphocapitate arthrosis (in contrast to stage II SLAC, the proximal scaphoid and corresponding radial articular surface are spared).
   c. Stage III: periscaphoid arthrosis involving radiostyloid, distal scaphoid, scaphocapitate, and capitolunate (proximal lunate and capitate may be preserved, depending on nonunion site).

Treatment by Stage

1. Stage I: radial styloidectomy and fixation of scaphoid nonunion with bone graft.
2. Stage II: proximal row carpectomy, SLAC procedure, wrist arthrodesis.
3. Stage III: SLAC procedure and wrist arthrodesis.

ULNOCARPAL IMPINGEMENT

Ulnocarpal impingement is a degenerative condition associated with a discrepancy in the relative length of the distal articular surfaces of the radius and ulna (positive ulnar variance). Increased forces across the ulnocarpal articulation lead to wearing of the triangular fibrocartilage complex, chondromalacia of the ulnar head and proximal ulnar aspect of the lunate, and disruption of the lunotriquetral ligament.

1. Load sharing across the wrist varies with ulnar variance:
   Neutral = 80% radius, 20% ulna
   + 1 mm = 30% ulna
   + 2 mm = 40% ulna
   − 1 mm = 10% ulna
   − 2 mm = 5% ulna
2. Post-traumatic causes include fractures of the distal radius with shortening, Galeazzi or Essex-Lopresti fractures, and epiphyseal injuries. It may occur with advanced stages of SLAC wrist as the lunate migrates ulnarly.
3. Congenital causes include dyschondroplasia, such as Madelung's disease, and naturally occurring positive ulnar variance.
4. Patients complain of pain at the dorsal aspect of the wrist at the distal radioulnar joint (DRUJ) and an intermittent clicking sensation. Extremes of forearm rotation and ulnar deviation exacerbate symptoms. Physical findings include pain with axial loading of the ulnar side of the wrist and a positive result of the ballottement test (dorsal and palmar displacement of the distal ulna with the wrist in

ulnar deviation increases symptoms). Arthrography reveals triangular fibrocartilage complex tear and lunotriquetral ligament tear. Magnetic resonance imaging shows changes primarily on the ulnar border of the lunate, unlike avascular necrosis of the lunate, which shows radial-sided or diffuse changes.

Treatment

1. Open excision of distal ulnar head (wafer resection [Feldon]).
2. Wrist arthroscopy and arthroscopic wafer resection.
3. Ulna shortening osteotomy.
4. Ulnocarpal impingement after distal radius fracture malunion is best treated by corrective osteotomy of the distal radius.
5. Ulnocarpal impingement after wrist arthrodesis is best treated by triquetral excision; avoid wafer resection, distal ulna hemiresection, and Darrach procedures.

DISTAL RADIOULNAR JOINT ARTHROSIS (Fig. 9-6)

DRUJ arthrosis must be differentiated from instability, subluxation, and ulnocarpal impaction. Diagnosis is difficult secondary to numerous joints within the small area.

Patients complain of pain at the dorsum of the wrist with limitation of forearm rotation. Snapping and crepitation are often present. Pain is increased with proximal rotation of the forearm and compression of the ulna against the radius. Confirmation of DRUJ involvement is improvement in rotation and grip strength with injection of local anesthetic into the DRUJ.

Treatment

1. Darrach resection and distal ulna stabilization (extensor carpi ulnaris suspensionplasty). The most common complication of the Darrach procedure is distal ulnar stump instability.
2. Distal ulna hemiresection and tendon interposition (Bowers). An advantage of this procedure is the preservation of the TFCC insertion.

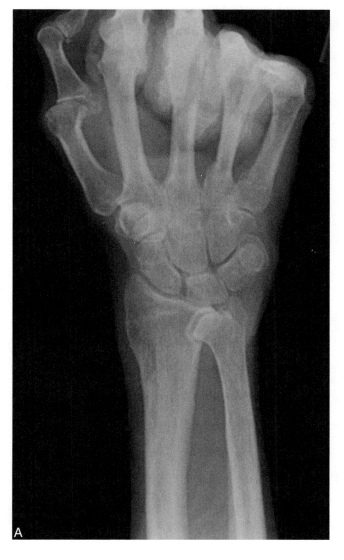

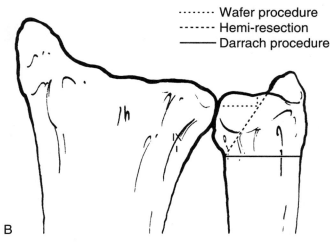

•••••••• Wafer procedure
------- Hemi-resection
—— Darrach procedure

Figure 9-6 ◆ **A,** Primary osteoarthrosis of the distal radioulnar joint. **B,** Surgical margins of distal ulna excision.

3. Metallic prosthetic replacement of the ulnar head (silicone implants are no longer in use).

Rheumatoid Arthritis

Introduction (Fig. 9-7)

1. Rheumatoid arthritis (RA) is a systemic autoimmune disorder resulting in erosive synovitis in peripheral joints, particularly the hands and wrist. Injury to synovial microvascular endothelial cells triggers an inflammatory reaction, causing influx of polymorphonuclear leukocytes, monocytes, and macrophages. Inflammatory mediators produced by these cells stimulate osteoclasts, which are responsible for the subchondral osteopenia.
2. The cause is thought to be a combination of genetic and environmental factors.
3. Extra-articular manifestations include vasculitis, pericarditis, pulmonary nodules, episcleritis, and subcutaneous nodules. Of these extra-articular processes, subcutaneous nodules are the most common and are seen in 25% of patients with RA.
4. Subcutaneous nodules are usually found over the olecranon, ulnar border of the forearm, and interphalangeal (IP) joints dorsally and less common volarly (Fig. 9-7A). These may cause pain and ulcerations, and they can be unsightly. The condition known as rheumatoid nodulosis is characterized by multiple subcutaneous nodules generally on the hands, intermittent polyarthralgias, absent or minimal joint involvement, subchondral cysts, and positive rheumatoid factor. Treatments include corticosteroids and surgical excision, although the recurrence rate is high. Hematoma formation after nodule excision is a common complication.
5. Epidemiology: women are affected more commonly than are men (2.5:1). Prevalence increases with age. RA has been associated with HLA-DR4/DR1.

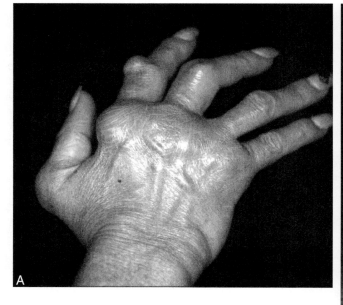

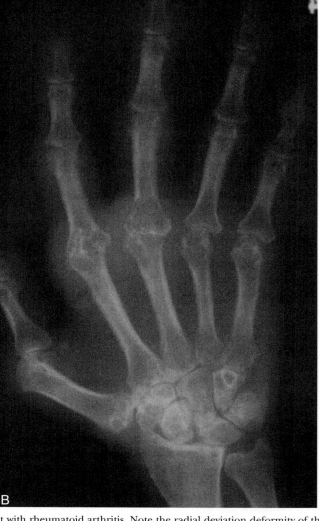

Figure 9-7 ◆ Clinical photograph **(A)** and radiograph **(B)** of a patient with rheumatoid arthritis. Note the radial deviation deformity of the wrist and ulnar deviation of the digits. Soft tissue swelling is noted over the articulations. Note the rheumatoid nodule over the PIP joint of the index finger.

6. Medical treatment: NSAIDs (prostaglandin inhibition), methotrexate, sulfasalazine, gold, penicillamine. New directed therapies (e.g., anti–tumor necrosis factor antibodies) are resulting in significant improvement of symptoms.
7. Surgical treatment: the three primary goals are pain relief, restoration of function, and cosmetic improvement of the hand.
   a. In patients with multiple joint involvement, proximal joints are addressed before distal ones.
   b. Lower extremity procedures should be performed before upper extremity surgery.
   c. Stabilizing procedures (arthrodesis) should be staged with mobilizing ones (arthroplasty) and not performed simultaneously.

Extensor Tendon Involvement

Potential causes include tendon erosion over bone prominences, infiltration of synovial tissue into the tendon proper, and ischemia.

TENOSYNOVITIS

1. Presentation is typically as a painless dorsal wrist mass distal to the extensor retinaculum.
2. It should initially be treated medically or conservatively with splinting and corticosteroid injections.
3. If symptoms persist more than 4 to 6 months despite medical management, tenosynovectomy is indicated to prevent tendon rupture.

TENDON RUPTURE

1. Patients present with sudden loss of finger extension. There is no tenodesis effect, and patients are unable to maintain the fingers in extension if they are passively placed in that position. In addition, the tendon defect may be palpable.
2. Extensor digiti minimi, extensor digitorum communis to the ring and small fingers, and extensor pollicis longus are most commonly affected, in order of decreasing incidence.
3. Caput ulnae syndrome. Synovitis in the DRUJ leads to capsular and ligamentous stretching and bone and cartilage damage. As the extensor carpi ulnaris subsheath stretches, the extensor carpi ulnaris will subluxate into volar and ulnar position. This leads to supination of the carpus away from the ulnar head, further stretching dorsal restraints. This developing instability allows the radius, carpus, and hand to subluxate in a palmar direction with respect to the ulna. The prominent ulnar head places pressure on the overlying extensor compartments, in which pressure is already elevated by synovitis. This increased pressure may result in ischemic necrosis and lead to rupture of the extensor tendons (Vaughn-Jackson syndrome). Alternatively, the tendon can also rupture through attrition over the prominent bone. Vaughn-Jackson syndrome is the most common tendon rupture in patients with RA.

Treatment

1. If the problem is recognized before the DRUJ subluxates, synovectomy can slow the disease process.

2. Extensor carpi radialis longus to extensor carpi ulnaris transfer corrects wrist radial deviation and supination deformities.
3. If rupture occurs, treatment should address the prominent distal ulna (shaving dorsal prominence, hemiresection, resection [Darrach], or Suave-Kapandji procedure), tenosynovectomy, and extensor indicis proprius transfer to extensor digiti minimi. This transfer provides better function than does extensor digiti minimi to extensor digitorum communis ring piggyback tenorrhaphy. In patients with RA, the Darrach procedure may potentiate ulnar translocation of the carpus.
4. In cases with multiple tendon ruptures, consider flexor digitorum superficialis (FDS) transfer or bridge graft with free palmaris longus tendon autograft.
5. In cases with multiple tendon ruptures and dislocated MP joints, MP arthroplasties should be performed before proceeding with tendon transfers and bridge grafts.

Differential Diagnoses

Differential diagnoses for loss of finger extension include the following:
1. Ulnar subluxation of the extensor tendons over the MP joints due to attritional lengthening of the radial sagittal band. This is differentiated from rupture by the ability to maintain the fingers in extension if they are passively placed in that position. The treatment of choice is sagittal band reconstruction, extensor realignment, and MP joint synovectomy.
2. Posterior interosseous nerve palsy. Posterior interosseous nerve compression is common in patients with RA because of synovitis in the elbow joint. It is differentiated from rupture by an intact tenodesis effect and from tendon subluxation by the inability to maintain the fingers in extension if they are passively placed in that position.
3. MP joint subluxation-dislocation. This problem can be diagnosed radiographically.

Flexor Tendon Involvement

1. The flexor tendon is usually involved by tendon attrition over a bone prominence or direct invasion by rheumatoid synovium.
2. Patients may complain of weak grip, morning stiffness, nerve compression symptoms, and finger locking or triggering.

WRIST TENOSYNOVITIS

1. Symptoms of median nerve compression can develop because of tenosynovial proliferation of the flexor tendons in the carpal tunnel. Bone spicules may be present within the canal.
2. Nerve conduction studies may be misleading.
3. The treatment of choice is carpal tunnel release and flexor tenosynovectomy. Wide exposure for the tenosynovectomy and to address occult tendon ruptures is recommended.

PALMAR TENOSYNOVITIS

1. The palm is the most common location of flexor tenosynovitis.
2. This results in pain, triggering, and tendon rupture, with passive finger flexion that is greater than active flexion.
3. Tenosynovectomy with resection of one of the FDS slips provides the best result by lowering reoperation rates; clinical recurrence rate is about 30%, and reoperation rate is 15%.
4. The A1 pulley should be preserved to avoid increasing the lever arm of the tendon and thus potentiating the flexion deformities at the MP joints.

DIGITAL TENOSYNOVITIS

1. The bulk of the tenosynovial mass is unable to smoothly pass through the annular pulleys.
2. Triggering results with the digit usually locked in flexion. However, with a profundus tendon nodule distally at the A2 pulley, the finger will be locked in extension.
3. In distal stenosing tenosynovitis, perform a tenosynovectomy and consider release of up to 50% of A2 and A4 if needed.

RUPTURE

Flexor tendon rupture may occur in the carpal canal, palm, or digits.

Carpal Region

The carpal region is the most common site of tendon ruptures. Ruptures in the distal palm and tendon sheath are much less common.

1. Flexor pollicis longus rupture (Mannerfelt-Norman syndrome) is the most common attritional flexor tendon rupture in RA.
   a. The most common location for rupture is at the scaphoid because of a spur at the level of the STT joint.
   b. If the IP joint of the thumb is in good condition, consider FDS transfer or free interposition tendon graft in addition to spur excision. Otherwise, consider IP arthrodesis.
   c. If untreated, the bone spur will lead to tendon ruptures of the flexor digitorum profundus (FDP) tendons in a radial to ulnar progression.
2. FDP rupture within the carpal canal may be masked by an intact superficialis.
   a. If an adjacent FDP tendon in the palm is available, side-to-side tenorrhaphy is indicated. Otherwise, free interposition tendon graft to an adjacent FDP is performed.
   b. If DIP joints are severely affected, DIP arthrodesis is the procedure of choice.
3. FDS rupture is usually without functional significance.

Palm Region

FDP ruptures are treated with side-to-side tenorrhaphy with or without a graft. FDS rupture is also of little functional significance.

Digital Sheath

FDP ruptures are treated with DIP arthrodesis and digital tenosynovectomy to preserve FDS function.

Staged tendon reconstructions are not indicated. FDS ruptures should be observed.

Wrist Joint (Fig. 9-7*B*)

1. Wrist synovitis begins on the ulnar aspect of the wrist with the DRUJ and radiocarpal joint first affected; the midcarpal joints are usually spared. Erosive changes are seen at the prestyloid recess of the ulnar styloid, the sigmoid notch of the radius, the insertion of the radioscapholunate ligament, and the scaphoid waist. Along with loss of ligamentous stability, these changes result in carpal supination, palmar dislocation, radial deviation, and ulnar translocation. These changes also produce relative ulnar head prominence and facilitate the progression of deformities distally (MP ulnar drift).
2. Scapholunate ligament disruption will result in rotatory subluxation of the scaphoid and characteristic SLAC-type changes with carpal collapse.

TREATMENT

1. Consider synovectomy of radiocarpal joint and DRUJ for pain relief if medical treatment fails after a trial of 6 months in the absence of any advanced radiographic changes.
2. Surgical treatment of DRUJ involvement is described in the extensor tendon section.
3. Partial arthrodeses include radiolunate and scaphoradiolunate fusions (Fig. 9-8). These procedures can prevent progression of collapse and should be reserved for patients with intermediate disease. Radiolunate fusions can be helpful in preserving function in patients with progressive ulnocarpal translocation.
4. Total wrist arthrodesis is the procedure of choice, with 90% to 95% good to excellent results. The optimum position for wrist fusion is 10 to 20 degrees of extension and neutral deviation. In cases requiring bilateral fusions, one side should be fused in neutral or slight flexion.

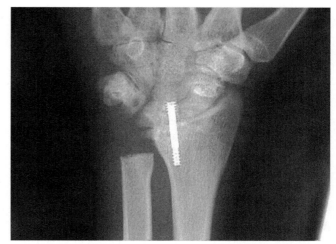

Figure 9-8 ◆ Patient with rheumatoid arthritis after radiolunate fusion and distal ulna excision.

5. Wrist arthroplasty is a motion-preserving procedure reserved for patients with good bone stock, minimal deformity, and intact extensors (Fig. 9-9). Biaxial prostheses are the implants of choice. Consider cementing only the distal stems. The distal end has a higher rate of loosening and must be cemented. The proximal portion is left uncemented because stress shielding is a major concern.

Metacarpophalangeal Joint

Characteristic deformities in the MP joint include ulnar deviation and palmar subluxation of the proximal phalanges (see Fig. 9-7B).

ETIOLOGY OF ULNAR DRIFT

1. Joint synovitis leads to stretching of the radial sagittal bands.
2. The extrinsic extensors then subluxate into the intermetacarpal sulcus, becoming ulnar deviators.
3. The MP collateral ligaments become lax because of joint synovitis.
4. Articular cartilage degeneration due to synovitis disrupts the bone congruity of the joint, leading to static joint imbalance.
5. The ulnar intrinsics contract and become an ulnar and volar deforming force.
6. Radial deviation of the wrist alters the vector of action of the extrinsic extensors and accentuates the ulnar direction of pull.
7. Synovitic MP joint distention stretches the accessory collateral ligaments and the membranous portion of the volar plate, causing the proximal portion of the flexor sheath to be displaced from the midline of the MP joint. In turn, the flexor tendons and flexor sheath shift ulnarly and volarly.

CLASSIFICATION (NALEBUFF) AND TREATMENT

1. Stage I: *synovial proliferation only.* Treatment is medical management and splinting.
2. Stage II: *recurrent synovitis without deformity.* The prophylactic procedure of choice is synovectomy if persistent pain and swelling are present in spite of adequate medical treatment for at least 6 months.
3. Stage III: *moderate articular degeneration, ulnar and palmar drift of the digits that is passively correctable.* In addition to synovectomy, soft tissue procedures including extensor tendon relocation, intrinsic releases, crossed intrinsic transfers, and radial collateral ligament reefing may be considered to address the deformities.
4. Stage IV: *severe joint destruction with fixed deformities.* The procedure of choice in these cases is silicone spacer arthroplasty in combination with extensor tendon relocation and radial collateral ligament reefing (Fig. 9-10). Surgical intervention should be reserved for patients with pain and functional disability. Reported arcs of motion achieved after silicone interposition arthroplasty range from 40 to 60 degrees. Although the gains in motion are not significant from preoperative measurements, it is thought that the arc of motion is displaced to a more functional position. Regression of the digits into the ulnarly deviated position is seen commonly; however,

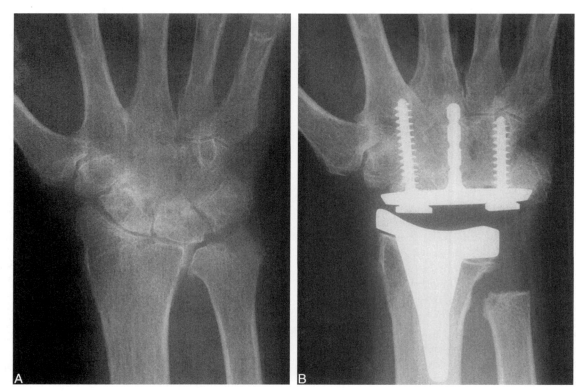

Figure 9-9 ◈ **A,** Preoperative radiograph of patient with rheumatoid arthritis. **B,** Universal total wrist arthroplasty functionally well at 3 years after surgery. (*From Adams BD: Total wrist arthroplasty. In Beredjiklian PK, ed: Seminars in Arthroplasty. Philadelphia, WB Saunders, 2000.*)

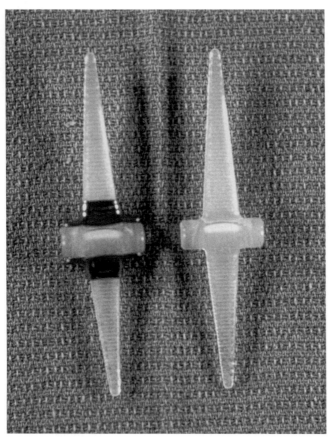

Figure 9-10 ✧ Swanson Silastic implants used for MP joint arthroplasty. The component on the left has titanium grommets in place.

the amount of the recurrence in deviation is typically less than 10 degrees. Complications include recurrence of deformity, implant fracture, and osteolysis.

Proximal Interphalangeal Joint

SWAN-NECK DEFORMITY (Fig. 9-11)

Swan-neck deformity is characterized by hyperextension at the PIP joint and flexion at the DIP joint. The PIP joint is often the site of *primary* involvement. Loss of the static (volar plate, collateral ligaments) and dynamic (FDS tendon) restraints due to synovial proliferation allows the extensor mechanism to act unopposed, leading to PIP joint hyperextension and a reciprocal DIP joint flexion deformity. Because the extensor mechanisms of the PIP and DIP joints are linked, PIP joint hyperextension results in a functional lengthening of the extensor mechanism. This relative lengthening creates an extension lag at the DIP joint. Decreased extension force of the DIP joint allows the FDP to flex the DIP joint unopposed, resulting in a flexion deformity of the DIP. Concomitant contracture of the intrinsic mechanism has also been implicated in this process. Similarly, the DIP joint can be the site of primary involvement, most commonly as a mallet finger caused by rupture of the terminal extensor tendon, which leads to PIP hyperextension due to extensor imbalance.

Classification and Treatment

1. Type I: *PIP joints flexible in all positions, independent of MP position.* In patients with mild deformity and minimal synovitis, splinting can be used to prevent PIP hyperextension or DIP flexion. In more severe cases, treatment should address the site of primary pathologic change. Surgical intervention to prevent PIP hyperextension (dermadesis, FDS tenodesis, Fowler's central slip [proximal] tenotomy) can correct the deformity. If the primary deformity is at the DIP joint, extensor tendon reconstruction or DIP arthrodesis can be performed.

2. Type II: *PIP joint mobility dependent on MP position.* The limitation of motion is directly related to intrinsic muscle tightness. With the MP joint in extension, flexion of the PIP joint is limited; conversely, with the MP joint in flexion, passive flexion in the PIP joint is increased. Involvement of the MP joint is considered the primary site of imbalance in type II deformities. Operative treatment of type II deformities not only should be directed at preventing PIP joint hyperextension but also should address the tightness of the intrinsic system, typically as intrinsic tendon releases. In cases of advanced rheumatoid involvement of the MP joint articular surface, arthroplasty and soft tissue balancing are necessary.

3. Type III: *PIP joints stiff in all positions, independent of MP position.* Significant loss of hand function is the result. Operative treatment should be directed at releasing soft tissue structures in the PIP joint. Capsular tightness can be relieved by manipulation of the PIP joint under digital block anesthesia. In addition, open capsular release including the collateral ligaments can be effective in improving joint motion. In addition to these releases, dorsal skin releases can be helpful in restoring PIP joint motion. Finally, mobilization of the lateral bands and translocation of these structures volar to the axis of rotation to the PIP joint may be necessary to regain flexion of the joint.

4. Type IV: *PIP joint stiffness with associated destruction of the articular surfaces.* Because of articular incongruity, arthrodesis and arthroplasty are the only options for treatment.

BOUTONNIÈRE DEFORMITY

Boutonnière deformity is characterized by flexion at the PIP joint and extension at the DIP joint. In contrast to swan-neck digits, the PIP joint is always the site of *primary* involvement. Because of synovitis in the PIP joint, the joint capsule and extensor mechanism become distended and weakened, resulting in elongation and attenuation of the joint capsule, the central slip of the extensor mechanism, and the transverse retinacular and triangular ligaments. The laxity of the soft tissue restraints about the joint eventually allows migration of the lateral bands volar to the axis of rotation of PIP joint motion. As the lateral bands migrate to this new position, the vector of force transmission is changed and they act to flex rather than to extend the PIP joint. With time, other periarticular soft tissue

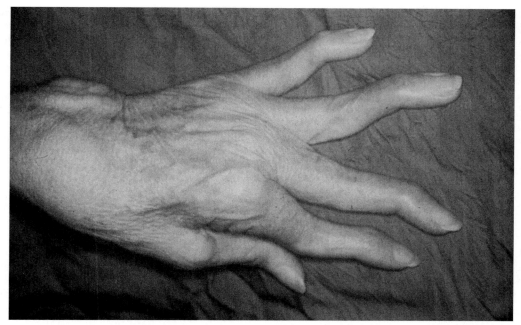

Figure 9-11 ◆ Patient with rheumatoid arthritis displaying swan-neck deformities of multiple digits.

structures, such as the volar plate and the collateral and oblique retinacular ligaments, become contracted and tether the lateral bands in their new position, leading to a static flexion contracture of the PIP joint.

There are several reasons that the DIP joint develops a reciprocal deformity. First, volar positioning of the lateral bands increases their ability to act as extensors at the DIP joint through the terminal tendon. Second, because extension of the PIP and DIP joints is linked, the flexion deformity of the proximal joint results in a *functional shortening* of the extensor mechanism, contributing to DIP hyperextension. Third, it is thought that contraction of the oblique retinacular ligament contributes to the deformity of the distal joint.

Classification and Treatment

1. Type I: *PIP joint deformity is passively correctable.* Deformity and functional impairment are minimal. It is characterized by 10 to 15 degrees of PIP joint flexion deformity. Flexion of the DIP joint improves as the PIP joint is flexed. Conservative treatment with splinting is indicated. For those with marked DIP hyperextension, Fowler's extensor (distal) tenotomy can restore the imbalance of the extensor mechanism.

2. Type II: *PIP joint deformity is moderate but passively correctable.* Deformity and functional disability are moderate. PIP joint flexion deformity reaches 30 to 40 degrees. MP joint hyperextension is usually present. Extensor mechanism reconstruction (imbrication of central slip and release/dorsal repositioning of lateral bands) in combination with Fowler's distal tenotomy can address the imbalance.

3. Type III: *PIP joint deformity is not passively correctable.* Deformity is severe, and there are fixed contractures. Soft tissue procedures are not effective in restoring function. Arthrodesis and arthroplasty are

the only options for treatment. Joint arthroplasty is best for the ring and small fingers (to restore grip) only if the patient has good bone stock and minimal extensor tendon dysfunction.

Thumb Deformities in Rheumatoid Arthritis

CLASSIFICATION AND TREATMENT

1. Type I: *Boutonnière deformity.* Boutonnière deformity is characterized by MP flexion and IP hyperextension. It is the most common thumb abnormality in RA. It is initiated by MP joint synovitis that dorsally attenuates the extensor pollicis brevis tendon. This displaces the extensor pollicis longus tendon ulnarward and volarly. Loss of dorsal support results in palmar subluxation of the proximal phalanx; hyperextension of the IP joint results from altered pull of the extensor pollicis longus tendon. Displacement of the extensor pollicis longus also results in thumb adduction. This deformity can be caused by a pathologic process in the IP joint, most commonly flexor pollicis longus rupture at the distal phalanx due to synovitis. It is divided into three clinical stages:

   a. Stage 1: *MP and IP joint deformities passively correctable.* Treatment is conservative with splinting and medication. Synovectomy of the MP joint and extensor realignment have a high recurrence rate.

   b. Stage 2: *MP joint deformity fixed, IP joint deformity correctable.* If the IP and CMC joints are minimally involved, MP arthrodesis is a good alternative. Otherwise, consider MP arthroplasty.

   c. Stage 3: *MP and IP joint deformities fixed.* Treatment is MP arthroplasty or fusion in conjunction with IP joint arthrodesis.

2. Type II: *Boutonnière deformity with CMC joint involvement.* Operative intervention including CMC hemiarthroplasty and MP joint fusion is the treatment of choice.

3. Type III: *Swan-neck deformity.* Swan-neck deformity is characterized by MP joint hyperextension, IP joint flexion, and metacarpal adduction. It results from synovial proliferation of the CMC joint that leads to dorsal and radial subluxation of the articular segment. As the joint subluxates, abduction forces are reduced and adduction contractures develop. Hyperextension of the MP joint develops if the volar plate is attenuated.
   a. Stage 1: *CMC joint synovitis, no MP joint involvement.* This stage is characterized by pain at the CMC joint and weak pinch; radiographic changes at the CMC joint may or may not be present. There is minimal deformity and no MP joint involvement. Consider convex condylar titanium hemiarthroplasty. In low-demand patients, concave Swanson toe implants may be used for hemiarthroplasty in addition to the convex condylar design.
   b. Stage 2: *CMC joint synovitis, MP joint extension deformity passively correctable.* Combine MP volar capsulodesis with hemiarthroplasty of the CMC joint.
   c. Stage 3 (advanced): *CMC joint destruction, MP joint extension deformity fixed.* Patients have weak pinch and difficulty grasping objects. Surgical treatment includes CMC hemiarthroplasty and MP fusion.

4. Type IV: *Gamekeeper's deformity.* Gamekeeper's deformity is characterized by radial deviation at the MP joint and adduction of the thumb metacarpal. Synovitis stretches the ulnar collateral ligament, leading to joint adduction. The CMC joint is unaffected. The treatment of choice is MP arthrodesis with adductor release of the metacarpal. If the MP joint is supple without significant arthritic changes, synovectomy with ulnar collateral ligament reconstruction may be an alternative.

5. Type V: *Swan-neck deformity with MP joint and CMC unaffected.* The MP joint volar plate stretches, leading to MP joint hyperextension. A secondary flexion deformity of the IP joint develops from increased tension on the flexor tendon. In contrast to type III, the CMC joint is uninvolved and the MP joint is the primary site of pathologic change. If no articular degeneration of the MP joint is present, volar capsulodesis may be sufficient to stabilize the joint. If joint degeneration is present, the MP joint must be fused.

6. Type VI: *Arthritis mutilans.* There is severe destruction at both the IP and MP joints. Bone destruction and resorption are common features. Treatment is by arthrodesis and soft tissue balancing whenever possible.

7. Patients with RA can develop a thumb adduction contracture due to CMC joint degeneration. Treatment should include CMC arthroplasty and web space deepening.

Juvenile Rheumatoid Arthritis

1. Juvenile RA is a chronic systemic idiopathic disorder affecting children and adolescents. It is the most common connective tissue disease in children, characterized by chronic synovial inflammation and hyperplasia. Girls are affected more commonly than are boys. In contrast to adult RA, deformities include ulnar deviation and flexion of the carpus and metacarpals and radial deviation and extension of the digits. Premature epiphyseal closure and diminished osseous growth are evident on radiographs. Rheumatoid factor is found predominantly in children older than eight years of age.

2. Three major subgroups exist: systemic, polyarticular, and pauciarticular (Table 9-2). Isolated digital swelling may be the initial presentation of juvenile RA. Patients who present with isolated digital swelling will most likely progress to the polyarticular disease.
   a. Still's (systemic, 25%): extra-articular manifestations such as rash, organomegaly, serositis, myalgia, hematologic changes, and arthritis.
   b. Polyarticular (30%): symmetric arthritis involving large and small joints (at least five). Hand involvement is most common in this type. Rheumatoid factor can be present or absent.
   c. Pauciarticular (45%): asymmetric arthritis involving four or fewer articulations, usually large joints.

3. The goals of treatment are to recognize the disease and to institute therapy to avoid other complications,

◆ Table 9-2						
TYPES OF JUVENILE RHEUMATOID ARTHRITIS						
Type	**Percentage**	**Joints**	**ANA**	**RF**	**Systemic Symptoms and Signs**	**Progress (%)**
Systemic—Still's	25	Many	–	–	Fever, rash, organomegaly	25
Polyarticular/RF–	15	Many	1/3	–	Mild fever	30
Polyarticular/RF+	15	Many	1/3	+	Mild	25
Pauciarticular I (F)	30	Large	+	–	Iridocyclitis*	15
Pauciarticular II (M)	15	Large	–	–	HLA-B27+, spondylitis	15

ANA, antinuclear antibodies; RF, rheumatoid factor; F, female; M, male.
*Slit-lamp examination is important to identify iridocyclitis, which is seen in the pauciarticular form.
From Stefko RM, Erickson MA: Pediatric orthopaedics. In Miller MD, ed: Review of Orthopaedics, 3rd ed. Philadelphia, WB Saunders, 2000, p 154.

such as iridocyclitis, which can lead to blindness if it is untreated. In half the patients, symptoms resolve without sequelae; 25% have slight residual disability, and 25% are significantly disabled.

4. Conservative splinting in a functional position will lead to autofusions in a functional position. Medical treatment with aspirin, gold, or other remissive agents is the standard of treatment.

5. Surgical treatment is preferably deferred until skeletal maturity is reached.

Gout (See Chapter 11)

1. Primary gout is idiopathic. Secondary gout results from disease processes that cause overproduction or underexcretion of uric acid. Examples include patients on hemodialysis, psoriasis, hemolytic anemia, hyperparathyroidism, and drug therapy (cyclosporine).

2. Diagnosis is made by identifying monosodium urate crystals on joint aspiration. Uric acid crystals are needle-like in shape and are negatively birefringent under polarized microscopy. Uric acid levels may be normal during an acute gouty attack. Peripheral joints of the hands and feet are first affected, presumably secondary to lower temperatures, which lead to precipitation of solubilized monosodium urate.

3. Patients have quick onset of a warm, erythematous, swollen joint. Joint inflammation can lead to gouty tenosynovitis and tendon rupture in some cases. Radiographic findings include soft tissue densities (tophi), intra-articular erosions at the joint margins, and extra-articular erosions (punched out appearance with overhanging lip). It may be confused with infection.

4. Acute attacks are treated with colchicine or indomethacin. Chronic treatment with allopurinol can decrease the frequency of gouty attacks.

5. Surgical treatment includes removal of gouty tophi, flexor and extensor tenosynovectomies, and arthrodeses of degenerative joints if bone stock is adequate.

Calcium Pyrophosphate Deposition Disease (Chondrocalcinosis, Pseudogout)

1. Calcium pyrophosphate crystals are deposited in cartilage. It is thought to be caused by increased calcium or inorganic pyrophosphate in cartilage, leading to crystal deposition.

2. Patients may present with morning stiffness, digital flexion contractures, and elevated sedimentation rate. It can mimic infection. Examination may show acute inflammation (usually less pain than with gout). Tendon ruptures may rarely occur from chronic inflammatory changes about the tendon.

3. Diagnosis is confirmed by joint aspiration and presence of crystals. In contrast to gout, calcium pyrophosphate crystals are rod shaped and weakly positively birefringent under polarized microscopy.

The classic radiographic appearance is calcification of knee menisci and the triangular fibrocartilage complex (Fig. 9-12). It is occasionally seen between the bones of the carpus.

4. Treatment is usually nonoperative; affected joints are immobilized during flare-up. No medication exists to remove crystals; however, intra-articular steroids and oral anti-inflammatories can be used to reduce inflammation. Colchicine can be used for chronic cases.

Systemic Lupus Erythematosus

1. Systemic lupus erythematosus is a systemic autoimmune disorder affecting women more often than men in a ratio of 5:1. Up to 90% of patients have hand and wrist involvement. Patients may present with rashes on the face and skin, Raynaud's phenomenon, synovitis, and ligamentous laxity. Antinuclear antibodies are present, and anti-DNA and anti-RNP antibody titers are also present.

2. In the digits, systemic lupus erythematosus presents as acute and tender swelling of the digital joints. In the wrist, dorsal subluxation of the DRUJ is common. Radiographs may show mild carpal translocation; however, most joints usually appear normal despite severe clinical deformity.

3. Treatment is primarily medical (steroids, NSAIDs, hydroxychloroquinine). Splinting of the thumb, digits, or wrist may be attempted, but often unsuccessfully. The wrist may be addressed surgically with distal ulnar arthroplasty and extensor tendon reconstruction. The carpus may be addressed with intercarpal or radiocarpal arthrodesis. Options at the MP joint include soft tissue procedures

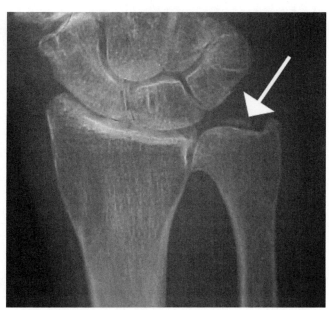

Figure 9-12 ◆ Radiograph of a patient with calcium pyrophosphate deposition disease. The classic radiographic appearance shows calcification of the triangular fibrocartilage complex.

(high failure rate due to soft tissue stretching), arthroplasty, and arthrodesis. At the IP joint level, arthrodesis remains the treatment of choice.

Scleroderma (See Chapter 4)

1. Scleroderma is also known as systemic sclerosis, a multiorgan disease also affecting the hand and wrist. Hand manifestations include Raynaud's phenomenon, digital tip ulcerations, MP joint hyperextension, PIP joint flexion contractures, thumb adduction contractures, septic arthritis, and calcific deposits. Diagnosis is mostly made with antinuclear and anticentromere antibodies.
2. Anticentromere antibody is found in most with the CREST form of the disease (calcinosis cutis, Raynaud's phenomenon, esophageal dysfunction, sclerodactyly, telangiectasia).
3. Treatments: Raynaud's phenomenon is treated conservatively with heated gloves and calcium channel blockers. Refractory Raynaud's phenomenon may be treated with periadventitial digital sympathectomy. Refractory fingertip ulcerations can respond to amputation. Arthrodesis can be performed for PIP contractures not responsive to splinting.
4. Calcinosis circumscripta (calcific deposits locally) may be treated with débridement. One must be careful with postoperative wound healing in these cases of débridement. PIP joint contractures with dorsal skin loss are best treated with shortening and fusion.

Psoriatic Arthritis

1. Patients present with a scaly erythematous rash that usually precedes joint involvement. Only 5% of patients with psoriasis develop arthritis; however, 90% of those will have involvement of peripheral joints. It is associated with HLA-B27, HLA-DR7, and HLA-DR4. Results of RA and antinuclear antibody tests are usually negative; however, the disease may assume a rheumatoid pattern.
2. Onychodystrophy (nail pitting), "sausage" digits, distal phalanx acrolysis, PIP fusions, MP erosions, and wrist autofusions may be seen. Patients may present with isolated tenosynovial swelling in the digits. Radiographic findings include bone destruction, joint widening, classic pencil-in-cup deformity, and "opera glass" hand (Fig. 9-13).
3. Nonoperative treatment includes methotrexate, NSAIDs, gold, antimalarials, sulfasalazine, and cyclosporine.

Classification and Treatment

1. Type I: *spontaneous ankylosis at the PIP and DIP joints, MP joint unaffected.* Functional loss is only mild. Spontaneous DIP joint fusion requires no treatment. If the PIP joint is autofused in poor position, consider osteotomy and arthrodesis.
2. Type II: *osteolysis.* Bone loss is common and seen at all joints. Functional loss may be severe. Arthritis mutilans is the most severe form. Fusion is required at every joint level. Rigid fixation and bone graft may be necessary in some cases.

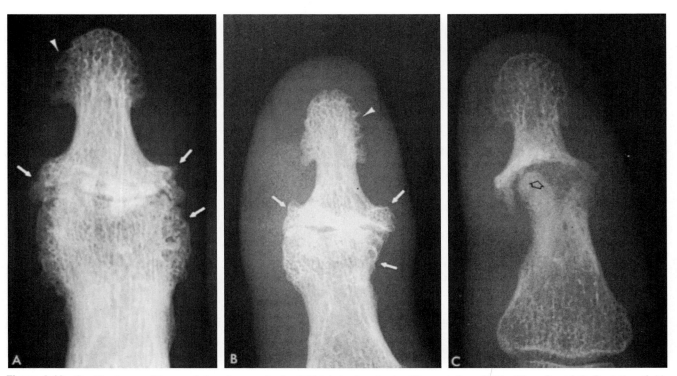

Figure 9-13 ❖ Classic pencil-in-cup deformity seen in the DIP joints of patients with psoriatic arthritis. (*From Resnick D: Psoriatic arthritis. In Resnick D, ed: Bone and Joint Imaging, 2nd ed. Philadelphia, WB Saunders, 1999.*)

3. Type III: *rheumatoid arthritis–like pattern with stiffness.* Tenosynovitis and tendon ruptures are less common than in RA. MP arthroplasty is indicated if extension is limited. IP joints may be treated with corrective osteotomy, arthrodesis, or arthroplasty.

Miscellaneous

1. Hemochromatosis. Can lead to joint destruction characterized by high serum ferritin levels. Typically affects MP joints. Also associated with chondrocalcinosis.
2. Diabetic cheiroarthropathy. Also known as diabetic hand syndrome. Patients present with limited joint mobility, flexion contractures of the interphalangeal joints. Splinting and surgery are typically unsuccessful in treating the contractures.

Bibliography

Bamberger HB, Stern PJ, Kiefhaber TR, et al: Trapeziometacarpal joint arthrodesis: a functional evaluation. J Hand Surg Am 17:605-611, 1992.

Brown FE, Brown ML: Long-term results after tenosynovectomy to treat the rheumatoid hand. J Hand Surg Am 13:704-708, 1988.

Burton RI, Pellegrini VD Jr: Surgical management of basal joint arthritis of the thumb. Part II. Ligament reconstruction with tendon interposition arthroplasty. J Hand Surg Am 11:324-332, 1986.

Carroll RE, Hill NA: Arthrodesis of the carpometacarpal joint of the thumb. J Bone Joint Surg Br 55:292-294, 1973.

Cobb TK, Beckenbaugh RD: Biaxial total-wrist arthroplasty. J Hand Surg Am 21:1011-1021, 1996.

Cohen MS, Kozin SH: Degenerative arthritis of the wrist: proximal row carpectomy versus scaphoid excision and four-corner arthrodesis. J Hand Surg Am 26:94-104, 2001.

Eaton RG, Lane LB, Littler JW, Keyser JJ: Ligament reconstruction for the painful thumb carpometacarpal joint: a long-term assessment. J Hand Surg Am 9:692-699, 1984.

Ertel AN: Flexor tendon ruptures in rheumatoid arthritis. Hand Clin 5:177-190, 1989.

Ertel AN, Millender LH, Nalebuff E, et al: Flexor tendon ruptures in patients with rheumatoid arthritis. J Hand Surg Am 13:860-866, 1988.

Imbriglia JE, Broudy AS, Hagberg WC, McKernan D: Proximal row carpectomy: clinical evaluation. J Hand Surg Am 15:426-430, 1990.

Kirschenbaum D, Schneider LH, Adams DC, Cody RP: Arthroplasty of the metacarpophalangeal joints with use of silicone-rubber implants in patients who have rheumatoid arthritis. Long-term results. J Bone Joint Surg Am 75:3-12, 1993.

Krakauer JD, Bishop AT, Cooney WP: Surgical treatment of scapholunate advanced collapse. J Hand Surg Am 19:751-759, 1994.

Mannerfelt L, Norman O: Attrition ruptures of flexor tendons in rheumatoid arthritis caused by bony spurs in the carpal tunnel. A clinical and radiological study. J Bone Joint Surg Br 51:270-277, 1969.

Millender LH, Nalebuff EA: Arthrodesis of the rheumatoid wrist. An evaluation of sixty patients and a description of a different surgical technique. J Bone Joint Surg Am 55:1026-1034, 1973.

Moritomo H, Tada K, Yoshida T, Masatomi T: The relationship between the site of nonunion of the scaphoid and scaphoid nonunion advanced collapse (SNAC). J Bone Joint Surg Br 81:871-876, 1999.

Naidu SH, Ostrov BE, Pellegrini VD: Isolated digital swelling as the initial presentation of juvenile rheumatoid arthritis. J Hand Surg [Am] 22:653-657, 1997.

Nalebuff EA, Garrett J: Opera-glass hand in rheumatoid arthritis. J Hand Surg Am 1:210-220, 1976.

Tomaino MM, Delsignore J, Burton RI: Long-term results following proximal row carpectomy. J Hand Surg Am 19:694-703, 1994.

Watson HK, Ballet FL: The SLAC wrist: scapholunate advanced collapse pattern of degenerative arthritis. J Hand Surg Am 9:358-365, 1984.

Watson HK, Hempton RF: Limited wrist arthrodeses. I. The triscaphoid joint. J Hand Surg Am 5:320-327, 1980.

10

✧ Rakesh Donthineni-Rao, MD

TUMORS

Introduction

Benign and malignant tumors present far less frequently in the hand than in the rest of the body. A thorough history and examination (including regional lymph node evaluation) are necessary for the accurate diagnosis of any neoplastic process. Plain radiographs help distinguish the lesion as a soft tissue tumor or a tumor arising in bone and detail the effect on the skeletal architecture, periosteal changes, type of matrix, and presence of a fracture. Technetium bone scans may be useful for identifying lesions outside the hand, such as a metastatic disease or polyostotic lesions. Magnetic resonance imaging (MRI) can be a useful tool in studying the extent of the tumor and the normal surrounding anatomy. Incisional biopsy (if indicated) should be well planned to prevent contamination of neurovascular structures. More important, contamination of soft tissues should be avoided so that limb salvage is not jeopardized. Incisions should be longitudinal and planned with the definitive surgery in mind. Inappropriately placed biopsies may lead to the need for soft tissue coverage or even unnecessary amputation. All tissue obtained during biopsy should be cultured, and all suspected infections should be assessed histologically. ("Culture all you biopsy, and biopsy all you culture.")

Skin Tumors

Repetitive trauma, chronic wounds, and exposure to ultraviolet rays or toxic chemicals increase the risk for development of a malignant neoplasm. For both suspected benign and malignant diseases, a thorough examination is warranted, including the regional lymph nodes.

Benign Tumors

FIBROUS TUMORS

Dermatofibroma

Dermatofibroma is also referred to as cutaneous fibrous histiocytoma. It is commonly present as painless, solitary, round, firm, well-circumscribed, slow-growing lesions. Nodules can be red or blue-black. The nodule consists of collagen and fibroblastic cells. These benign tumors may be confused with melanoma or a soft tissue

sarcoma, and pathologic evaluation of the excised nodule is necessary. Treatment includes excisional biopsy. Recurrence is rare.

Keratoacanthoma

Keratoacanthoma is a common benign skin tumor with potential for malignant transformation into squamous cell carcinoma. Keratoacanthomas occur much more frequently in men than in women, usually in their 70s. Sunlight appears to be the major contributing factor, and thus these lesions are most often found in the face, neck, and dorsum of the hands. The incidence of this lesion is higher in patients with xeroderma pigmentosa, in radiated tissue, and in scar tissue. Various chemical carcinogens have also been shown to contribute to its occurrence.

The lesions are characterized by rapid growth within 3 to 4 weeks, forming a papular, pink lesion of about 2 cm. A stable period follows the rapid onset and growth spurt. The central portion becomes a thick, scaly crater that can leave an ulcer (Fig. 10-1). The lesion then slowly regresses during 2 to 6 months, leaving a scar. Keratoacanthomas can be diagnosed on the basis of their history and clinical presentation, but treatment includes excisional biopsy with a small margin of normal tissue. Closure may require advancement or rotational flaps. Recurrence is rare.

It can be difficult to differentiate keratoacanthomas from squamous cell carcinoma histologically. Subungual keratoacanthoma has rapid growth, can involve the distal phalanx, and in many cases may not regress. Surgical excision is recommended, and close follow-up for recurrence is necessary.

Actinic Keratosis

Actinic keratoses are potential precursors of squamous cell carcinoma and present as scaly red patches. Like the keratoacanthomas, actinic keratoses are found in areas of skin chronically exposed to the sun, such as on the face and dorsal aspects of the hand. Up to 5% of the actinic keratoses may progress to squamous cell carcinoma. The incidence is higher in older individuals with fair skin and is directly related to cumulative sun exposure, and therefore reducing sun exposure can dramatically reduce the risk for actinic keratosis. Immunocompromised patients also have a higher risk for development of keratoses. Other risk factors are similar to those for keratoacanthoma.

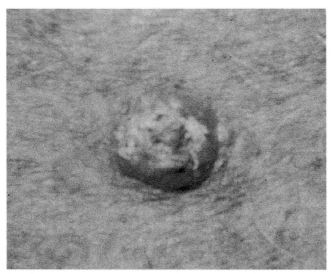

Figure 10-1 ◈ Clinical photograph of a keratoacanthoma revealing a small, raised lesion with a central crater that is scaly in nature.

Treatment includes excision. Excision allows evaluation of the tissue for possible conversion to squamous cell carcinoma, hence needing further care. Another common treatment is the application of topical 5-fluorouracil.

SWEAT GLAND TUMORS

Benign sweat gland tumors can be locally recurrent and can display malignant transformation. Histologic diagnosis can be difficult. Differential diagnosis includes giant cell tumor of the tendon sheath, basal cell carcinoma, squamous cell carcinoma, and metastatic malignant tumors.

Eccrine Poroma

Eccrine poroma presents as asymptomatic small masses. It is more frequently found in the extremities of older patients. Malignant transformation is possible and is manifested by pain and bleeding. Treatment includes excision with normal margins, and follow-up for recurrence is necessary.

Eccrine Spiradenoma

Eccrine spiradenoma may present as a single mass or multiple nodules. It can grow rapidly and has a tendency for local recurrence and malignant transformation.

GLOMUS TUMOR

Glomus tumors are typically found in the distal end of the extremities, under the nail (75%) and on the pulps of the fingertips. The tumors are composed of glomus bodies (whose function is to regulate skin circulation) and vascular and smooth muscle tissue. These tumors present as painful, deep red to blue nodules with hypersensitivity to cold, intermittent severe pain, and point tenderness. Nail ridging is common. The tumor may cause erosion of the distal phalanx. Multiple tumors occur in up to 25% of cases and present as persistent or recurrent pain after excision. MRI is helpful in the diagnosis.

Treatment is excisional biopsy by total nail plate removal, excision of the lesion from its capsule, and repair of the nail bed. Persistent pain after excision may be due to missed multiple lesions. Recurrence is rare.

Malignant Skin Tumors

Skin cancer is the most common type of cancer in the United States. Up to 50% of Americans who live to age 65 years will have skin cancer at least once. The most common malignant tumor of the hand is squamous cell carcinoma.

SQUAMOUS CELL CARCINOMA

Squamous cell carcinoma (SCC) originates from the keratinocytes of the epidermis and is the most common malignant tumor of the skin of the hand. SCC most often occurs on the dorsum of the hand and rarely on the volar aspect. It may present as a dry scaly erythematous lesion, although it is often noted as a slowly growing ulcer. Subungual SCC may present as a swelling with discoloration or even as a secondary infection of the nail bed. These lesions can be treated with disarticulation at the distal interphalangeal (DIP) joint.

SCC has a tendency to infiltrate the lymphatics and spread to the local lymph nodes. The regional lymph nodes should therefore be routinely examined. The overall metastasis rate for SCC is approximately 5%, but the rate for lesions originating in the hand is higher. SCC of the nail bed can be treated with excision, although if there is deep invasion, amputation is necessary. SCC can also arise at sites of chronic ulceration or inflammation, burn scars (Marjolin's ulcer), or sites of previous radiation treatment. These lesions behave more aggressively.

Localized SCC of the skin is a curable disease. Treatment options include cryosurgery, radiation therapy, electrodesiccation and curettage, Mohs' micrographic surgery, and excision. Each of these methods may be useful in specific clinical situations. Mohs' micrographic surgery has the highest 5-year cure rate for both primary and recurrent tumors in SCC. Lymphadenectomy is indicated when regional lymph nodes are involved. Radiation is often used with a good success rate in tumors that require extensive surgery. SCC requires close follow-up of patients for recurrence and lymph node involvement.

BASAL CELL CARCINOMA

Basal cell carcinoma (BCC) originates from the pluripotential epithelial cells of the deep layer of the epidermis and is the second most common malignant tumor of the skin of the hand. BCC rarely metastasizes, but it is locally an aggressive tumor and invades the underlying tissues. BCC presents as an asymptomatic nodular or nodular ulcerative lesion that is elevated from the surrounding skin and has a "pearly" quality with telangiectatic vessels (Fig. 10-2). Its incidence is directly related to sun exposure.

Although metastasis is rare, deep invasion of the tissues can result in significant local tissue destruction. Treatment options include cryosurgery, radiation therapy, electrodesiccation and curettage, and excision. Cryosurgery and electrodesiccation and curettage are typically used for removal of primary BCCs, although adequacy of treatment cannot be fully assessed immediately because the depth of microscopic tumor invasion is not visualized. Radiation therapy can be used for lesions that recur after surgical removal. Surgical excision offers the

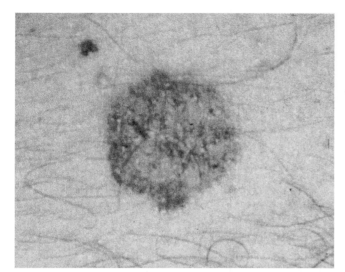

Figure 10-2 ◈ Clinical photograph of a basal cell carcinoma revealing a nodular lesion that is elevated from the surrounding skin.

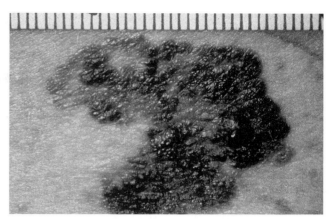

Figure 10-3 ◈ Clinical photograph of a malignant melanoma.

opportunity to remove the lesion with a margin and allows an assessment of the depth of tissue invasion. Long-term follow-up for recurrence is necessary. Cure rates of up to 90% can be achieved.

MELANOMA

Melanoma is a malignant tumor of melanocytes and the third most common malignant tumor of the skin of the hand (Fig. 10-3). These cells are derived from the neural crest. The mortality from melanoma has gradually increased during the last 2 decades and can be attributed to the increased exposure to sunlight. Melanoma can spread by lymphatics or by hematogenous routes and will spread to any organ, although the lungs and liver are common sites. Types of melanoma include lentigo maligna, superficial spreading, nodular, and acral-lentiginous melanoma.

The clinical staging of melanoma is based on the thickness or level of invasion into the skin, mitotic index, presence of lymphocytes within the tumor, number of regional lymph nodes involved, and ulceration or bleeding of the tumor. The depth of invasion affects the likelihood of metastases. The clinical staging uses the vertical thickness of the lesion in millimeters (Breslow's classification) and the anatomic level of local invasion (Clark's classification) as well as the regional and distant metastases. Elective regional lymph node dissection has shown no proven benefit for patients with a localized skin melanoma less than 1 mm in thickness. These patients can benefit from a sentinel node biopsy, and if it is proved to be involved, further lymphadenectomy is required.

Melanoma is curable if it is treated before the onset of the vertical growth phase with its metastatic potential. Melanomas that occur in younger patients and on the extremities have a better prognosis. The probability of tumor recurrence in 10 years is less than 10% for tumors less than 1.4 mm in thickness. For patients with tumors less than 0.76 mm in thickness, the likelihood of

recurrence is less than 1% in 10 years. Melanoma that has spread to distant sites is rarely curable with standard therapy.

Subungual melanomas can present as fungal infections, paronychia, or warts. The treatment of choice is wide resection with amputation and evaluation of the sentinel lymph node or lymphadenectomy.

MERKEL CELL CARCINOMA

Merkel cell carcinoma is a rare tumor that is associated with terminal axons in the basal layer of the skin. It is a neuroendocrine carcinoma of the skin and presents as a painless, indurated, solitary dermal nodule with red coloration. Lymph nodes are involved in more than 50% of the cases. It has a poor prognosis and should be treated aggressively with wide surgical excision and lymphadenectomy. There is a high metastatic rate and a local recurrence risk of 25%.

KAPOSI'S SARCOMA

Kaposi's sarcoma is a vascular tumor of lymphatic endothelial origin. It presents as painless red-blue plaques or nodules. These lesions are slow growing and respond to excision or radiation treatments. The diagnosis of acquired immunodeficiency syndrome should be considered in these patients.

MALIGNANT SWEAT GLAND TUMORS

This group of neoplasms includes clear cell carcinoma, digital papillary adenocarcinoma, and eccrine adenocarcinoma. These are aggressive lesions that commonly metastasize to regional lymph nodes and distant organs hematogenously. Treatment includes assessment of metastatic disease, aggressive surgical resection with wide margins, and lymphadenectomy.

Soft Tissue Tumors

Benign Tumors

GANGLION CYST

Ganglion cysts are the most common soft tissue tumors of the hand. They account for about 50% to 70% of masses. They present as a slow growing mass, often with accompanying cosmetic deformity, pain, and weakness.

The incidence is higher in women in a 3:1 ratio. Fluctuations in the size of the mass are common. There is rarely a history of trauma (10%). The ganglia are noted adjacent to joints and tendons. There may be osteoarthritic changes in the adjacent joints, although normal skeletal findings are common on radiographs. Malignancy has never been reported.

The capsule of the cyst consists of a relatively acellular fibrous wall, and there is no cell lining of the inner layer. The cyst contents are composed of thick mucinous fluid that includes glucosamine, hyaluronic acid, albumin, and globulin. The pathogenesis remains unclear; potential explanations include the herniation of joint lining into soft tissues with joint fluid extravasation and the mucoid degeneration of connective tissue.

Nonsurgical treatment is successful in most cases, particularly in children, where most ganglia resolve spontaneously. Needle aspiration with withdrawal of the fluid is diagnostic and can provide some pain relief, but recurrence is common (more than two thirds of the time). Surgical excision is the treatment of choice in patients with persistent symptoms and disability. Resection of the cyst and its stalk is often curative. The most common complication is recurrence, which is often related to incomplete removal of the stalk. Overall recurrence rates after surgical excision are about 5% to 10%. Volar wrist cysts have a higher recurrence rate than dorsal cysts do. Other postoperative problems include stiffness and nerve injuries.

Dorsal Wrist Ganglion

This is the most common ganglion cyst, accounting for about 70% of all wrist and hand ganglia. The cyst most commonly arises from the capsule over the scapholunate ligament (Fig. 10-4). Excision should include the pedicle and a portion of capsule. After initial postoperative splinting, motion of the wrist joint is allowed. Arthroscopic resection has also been reported as a treatment option. A 1-cm section of dorsal wrist capsule should be resected to prevent recurrence if it is treated arthroscopically.

Occult dorsal ganglia may present as dorsal wrist pain without a distinctly palpable mass. Compression of the posterior interosseous nerve has been implicated in the pathogenesis of the pain. The diagnosis can be confirmed by ultrasonography or MRI.

Volar Wrist Ganglion

These masses account for about 20% of hand and wrist ganglia. These ganglia arise most commonly from the capsule of the radiocarpal joint. They may also arise from the scaphotrapezial or pisotriquetral joints. The cyst is often adjacent to branches of the radial artery (Fig. 10-5). The patency of the radial and ulnar arteries must be assessed before surgery (Allen test). Radial sensory and lateral antebrachial cutaneous nerves must also be protected during the approach.

Volar Retinacular Ganglion (Flexor Tendon Sheath)

These lesions arise from the A1 pulley of the flexor tendon sheath. These lesions present as small, painful

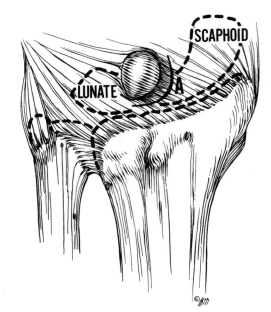

Figure 10-4 ❖ Dorsal ganglion cysts most commonly arise from the scapholunate interosseous ligament. A capsular incision (A) is made at the time of surgical excision. *(Illustration by Elizabeth Roselius, ©1999. Reprinted with permission from Angelides AC: Ganglions of the hand and wrist. In Green DP, Hotchkiss RN, Pederson WC, eds: Green's Operative Hand Surgery, 4th ed. New York, Churchill Livingstone, 1999.)*

masses on the palmar aspect, at the flexion crease of the metacarpophalangeal (MP) joint. The cyst is fixed to the tendon sheath and does not move with the tendon. Needle puncture is adequate in 70% of the cases, and 65% will resolve spontaneously. The ganglia can recur with this method alone, and recurrent cysts can be surgically excised.

Mucous Cyst

Mucous cysts are typically located on the dorsal aspect of the DIP joint. These are often related to degenerative changes in the joint. Pressure on the nail bed can cause grooving of the nail. In more severe cases, the skin may break down and the cysts become infected. Treatment options include aspiration and excision. If excision is performed, care is taken not to injure the nail matrix or extensor tendon. Associated osteophytes

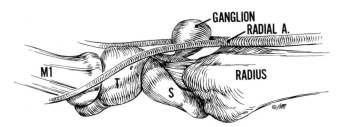

Figure 10-5 ❖ Volar ganglion cysts most commonly arise from the radiocarpal joint and are typically in anatomic proximity to the radial artery. M1, first metacarpal; T, trapezium; S, scaphoid. *(Illustration by Elizabeth Roselius, ©1999. Reprinted with permission from Angelides AC: Ganglions of the hand and wrist. In Green DP, Hotchkiss RN, Pederson WC, eds: Green's Operative Hand Surgery, 4th ed. New York, Churchill Livingstone, 1999.)*

should be removed to prevent recurrence. If degenerative changes in the articulation are severe, DIP joint fusion should be considered.

OTHER GANGLIA

Ganglia are also found about the proximal interphalangeal (PIP) joint, about extensor tendons, over the second and third carpometacarpal joints (carpal boss), at the volar carpus within the carpal tunnel, and within Guyon's canal. The ganglia within the carpal tunnel and Guyon's canal may present with nerve compression symptoms.

Intraosseous ganglia are common in the scaphoid and also the lunate, but they can occur in the other bones of the hand. The diagnosis is typically made incidentally on plain radiographs.

EPIDERMAL INCLUSION CYST

Epidermal inclusion cysts are slow-growing, painless lesions most likely resulting from the implantation of epithelial cells from trauma. They commonly occur in the distal aspect of the digits within the soft tissues or bone. The cyst may present as a lytic lesion of the distal phalanx. It is the most common lesion of the distal phalanx. Intralesional curettage or marginal resection is adequate treatment.

PYOGENIC GRANULOMA

Pyogenic granulomas are benign lesions that are often the result of trauma. They present as rapidly growing, pedunculated red masses that are friable and bleed easily. Small lesions can be treated with silver nitrate cauterization. Larger lesions and recurrent lesions should be excised surgically. These lesions are often confused with infections (see Chapter 11).

LIPOMA

This fatty tumor is common in the hand and the forearm. Lipomas can present in subcutaneous or intramuscular locations. They present as soft, nontender masses that have been long-standing or occasionally slow growing. If close to a major nerve, they may cause compression symptoms. Plain radiographs are typically normal. On MRI, lipomas appear as well-demarcated and homogeneous masses, bright on T1-weighted images and dark on T2-weighted images. Recurrences are rare after surgical excision.

Atypical lipomas represent a histologic variant that has a tendency for growth and displays a higher recurrence rate after excision. In spite of the local aggressiveness of these lesions, malignant transformation is rare.

LIPOFIBROMATOUS HAMARTOMA

Lipofibromatous hamartoma is a rare congenital anomaly involving peripheral nerves. It most commonly affects the median nerve. The involved nerve becomes enlarged, nodular, and tortuous. Histologic evaluation reveals fatty and fibrous tissue intimately associated with nerve fibers. For this reason, dissection from normal nerve tissue is difficult. The condition is commonly associated with macrodactyly (Fig. 10-6). Patients present with nerve compression symptoms. Treatment is directed at nerve decompression. Aggressive attempts at

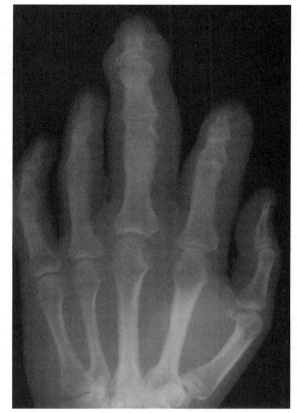

Figure 10-6 ◈ Anteroposterior radiograph of a hand in a patient with lipofibromatous hamartoma of the median nerve. Note the macrodactyly of the long finger.

excision may result in nerve dysfunction and require a nerve graft procedure.

GIANT CELL TUMOR OF TENDON SHEATH (PIGMENTED VILLONODULAR TENOSYNOVITIS)

Giant cell tumor of the tendon sheath is the second most common soft tissue tumor affecting the hand. Histologic evaluation reveals a single- or multiple-lobulated tumor containing multinucleated giant cells, histiocytes, and hemosiderin deposits, with varying degrees of fibrosis and cellularity. Patients present with a slow-growing, firm, nontender mass. The age range is 10 to 75 years. The volar aspect of the hand is affected more than the dorsal, and it is also more common in the distal part of the hand. Radiographs may show bone erosion in 10% of cases (Fig. 10-7). Joint involvement occurs 20% of the time. Surgical marginal excision is recommended, although the recurrence rate can be as high as 30% and usually reflects an incomplete removal. Recurrence is most common if the lesion is located in the DIP joint, if radiographic changes of osteoarthritis are present, in cases of previous recurrence, or if erosion of the bone is present. The recurrence rate is also higher for lesions in the distal part of the hand. Malignant transformation has not been reported.

SCHWANNOMA (NEURILEMMOMA)

This is a benign, slow-growing tumor of Schwann cells. It is the most common neoplastic lesion of

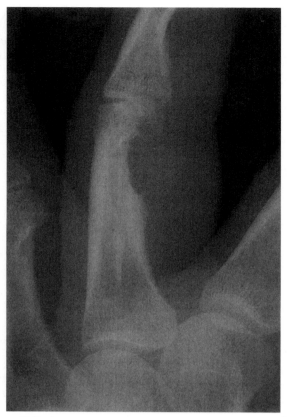

Figure 10-7 ❖ Oblique radiograph of a finger in a patient with giant cell tumor of the tendon sheath eroding into the proximal phalanx.

peripheral nerves. It forms a well-circumscribed mass within the nerve. Patients may present with peripheral nerve symptoms. It is often found on the flexor side of the hand and wrist; it is often found in the median nerve and also in the digital nerves. Radiographs may show surface erosion and scalloping if it is present on the surface of a bone, and MRI shows decreased signal on T1-weighted and increased signal on T2-weighted sequences. If it is symptomatic, careful enucleation from the nerve is possible without any permanent damage to the nerve. Recurrence is uncommon. Multiple schwannomas are associated with neurofibromatosis 2.

NEUROFIBROMA

Neurofibroma is a benign tumor of the nerve fibers containing Schwann cells, perineural cells, and fibroblasts. Solitary lesions are common, although multiple neurofibromas are associated with neurofibromatosis 1 (von Recklinghausen's disease). The tumor may be intimately involved with the nerve and can be difficult to excise. Nerve deficits are more likely with these tumors if surgery is attempted. Large neurofibromas or increased growth should raise the suspicion of malignant transformation and should be ruled out by multiple biopsies of a lesion.

GRANULAR CELL TUMOR

A tumor of Schwann cell origin, granular cell tumor presents as a nontender subcutaneous mass. Solitary or

multiple lesions can be found and may be associated with a nerve.

FIBROMATOSIS

Aggressive fibromatosis (extraskeletal desmoid tumor) has been reported in the upper extremity, although incidence is low in the distal forearm and hand. It presents as an enlarging mass with symptoms of local pressure. These tumors arise from fascial and musculoaponeurotic tissues. They lack a capsule and grow in an infiltrating manner into the surrounding structures. These lesions have a high recurrence rate. On MRI, the lesion appears dark on T1-weighted images and either dark or of intermediate signal intensity on T2-weighted images.

If the lesion is rapidly growing or symptomatic, options for management include surgical resection, radiation, and a combination of both. The risk of recurrence is about 30% after surgery alone, whereas for surgery and radiation, it is 6% in cases of negative margins. Reports detailing the use of low-dose chemotherapy seem to have beneficial effects, either by shrinking the tumor or by stabilizing the growth and decreasing symptoms.

Infantile Digital Fibroma

Infantile digital fibroma is a benign aggressive tumor affecting the fingers and toes. The majority of the cases occur in infants. The presentation is that of single or multiple, firm, nontender nodules that may be red. There is a tendency for occurrence in the distal part of the digit and at the level of interphalangeal joints. Local recurrence after excision is about 60%. The lesion may be confused with a malignant neoplasm, such as a fibrosarcoma, although it rarely has mitotic activity and lacks cytologic atypia.

Juvenile Aponeurotic Fibroma

This benign, locally aggressive fibrous lesion is commonly seen in children and adolescents. It presents as a painless mass on the palmar aspect of the hand and is closely associated with tendons and neurovascular structures. Excision is recommended for lesions affecting function. Recurrence rate is greater than 50%.

NODULAR FASCIITIS

Nodular fasciitis is a benign, reactive tumor of fibroblastic origin. Patients may have a history of trauma and note a rapidly growing tender mass. The imaging studies may suggest a sarcoma and it may be treated aggressively, although in the history, the growth rate is reported to be much faster than that of a true malignant neoplasm. Histologic examination should reveal the true diagnosis. Misdiagnosis for a high-grade sarcoma will lead to overtreatment. The condition is usually self-limited. It is more common in the forearm but can affect the hand.

VASCULAR MALFORMATIONS

Vascular malformations are much more common in the pediatric population and include hemangiomas. Hemangiomas are often seen on the dorsum of the hand and rapidly grow within the first 2 years and then undergo an involution in the following 3 years. In children,

70% of hemangiomas will involute by the age of 7 years. Malformations can continue to grow and are subclassified into capillary, venous, lymphatic, and arterial. The slow-flow vessels develop phleboliths, which can be seen on radiographs. Treatment is reserved for the symptomatic lesions and includes compressive dressing and excision.

See also Chapter 4.

Malignant Tumors

Primary malignant soft tissue tumors of the hand are typically soft tissue sarcomas. These are high-grade tumors with a propensity to metastasize to the lungs. Prognosis is dependent on the grade, the size, and the location (deep versus superficial) of the tumors as well as the presence of metastasis. The staging is based on the American Joint Committee on Cancer and the Musculoskeletal Tumor Society designation (Table 10-1). Tumors with a higher grade and larger size (>5 cm)

have a poorer prognosis regardless of histologic diagnosis or identification of cell origin.

Patients often present with an enlarging, painless mass with symptoms of compression of surrounding structures. The sarcomas may be mistaken for a benign mass, such as a ganglion cyst or a fibroma. Surgery is the main mode of treatment, and wide resection of the lesion including 1 cm of surrounding normal tissue can decrease the risk of recurrence. Because of the compact structure of the hand, involvement of major tendons and neurovascular structures is likely, and amputation may be necessary if a wide margin is not attainable. Difficult salvage situations occur when the tumor is in the carpal tunnel or in the proximal palm.

Patients with a large tumor may benefit from preoperative irradiation to reduce the size of the lesion before surgical excision. Patients with small high-grade tumors can also benefit from postoperative irradiation to reduce recurrence. Radiation treatment may have adverse long-term effects on tendon, joints, and other soft tissues. Preoperative irradiation increases the risk of wound complications to 30%. Brachytherapy is a method of delivering a higher dose of radiation by insertion of catheters into the surgical bed in the area of tumor resection.

The role of chemotherapy is controversial. Adjuvant chemotherapy should be considered for large high-grade sarcomas with metastatic disease along with surgical resection of the lesion and lung nodules.

EPITHELIOID SARCOMA

Epithelioid sarcoma is the most common soft tissue sarcoma of the forearm and hand. It typically presents as a small nodule on the volar aspect of the hand that gradually increases in size. It may be misdiagnosed as a benign lesion, scar tissue, or infection. It has a predilection to infiltrate locally and is also known to spread along fascial planes, tendons, and lymphatic channels. Close physical examination, diagnostic imaging, and even sentinel lymph node biopsy may be warranted to detect lymphatic spread. Epithelioid sarcomas are high-grade tumors with a high recurrence rate. Wide margin resection or amputation is necessary to achieve local control (Fig. 10-8). Chemotherapy should be considered for metastatic disease.

SYNOVIAL SARCOMA

Synovial sarcoma arises commonly about joints or tendons, and not necessarily from synovial tissue. It is a high-grade tumor, often being present as a small mass for years before changing its clinical behavior. Only about 25% of the lesions display calcifications on radiographic examination. It also has a propensity to metastasize to the regional lymph nodes. Histologic evaluation reveals a monophasic or a biphasic cell type; the biphasic type has a poorer prognosis (Fig. 10-9).

CLEAR CELL SARCOMA (MALIGNANT MELANOMA OF SOFT PARTS)

Clear cell sarcoma is an uncommon lesion of the hand. It has a high risk for local recurrence, and more than half the patients will have metastatic spread to the regional

---

◆ Table 10-1

STAGING SYSTEM OF THE MUSCULOSKELETAL TUMOR SOCIETY (ENNEKING SYSTEM)

Stage	GTM	Description
I-A	$G_1T_1M_0$	Low grade Intracompartmental No metastases
I-B	$G_1T_2M_0$	Low grade Extracompartmental No metastases
II-A	$G_2T_1M_0$	High grade Intracompartmental No metastases
II-B	$G_2T_2M_0$	High grade Extracompartmental No metastases
III-A	$G_{1/2}T_1M_1$	Any grade Intracompartmental With metastases
III-B	$G_{1/2}T_2M_1$	Any grade Extracompartmental With metastases

Grade system (G): low grade (G_1) and high grade (G_2). High-grade lesions are intermediate in grade between low-grade, well-differentiated tumors and high-grade, undifferentiated tumors.

Tumor size (T): Determined by specialized procedures, including radiography, tomography, nuclear studies, CT, and MRI. Compartments are used to describe the tumor site. Compartments are usually easily defined on the basis of fascial borders in the extremities. Of note, the skin and subcutaneous tissues are classified as a compartment, and the periosseous potential space between cortical bone and muscle is often considered a compartment as well. T_0 lesions are confined within the capsule and within its compartment of origin. T_1 tumors have extracapsular extension into the reactive zone around it, but both the tumor and the reactive zone are confined within the compartment of origin. T_2 lesions extend beyond the anatomic compartment of origin by direct extension or otherwise (e.g., trauma, surgical seeding). Tumors that involve major neurovascular bundles are almost always classified as T_2 lesions.

Metastases (M): Regional and distal metastases both have an ominous prognosis; therefore, the distinction is simply between no metastases (M_0) or the presence of metastases (M_1).

From Miller MD: Review of Orthopaedics, 3rd ed. Philadelphia, WB Saunders, 2000, p 380.

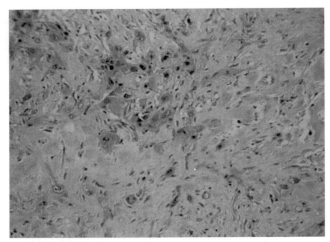

Figure 10-8 ◆ High-power micrograph of epithelioid sarcoma. Spindle cells and epithelioid cells are usually both present, but the proportion varies from tumor to tumor. Atypia may be minimal, moderate, or severe.

lymph nodes. Treatment includes wide resection and possibly adjuvant chemotherapy or radiotherapy.

FIBROSARCOMA AND MALIGNANT FIBROUS HISTIOCYTOMA

Although these tumors are not uncommonly found in the upper extremity, their occurrence in the hand is rare. These are high-grade tumors that can be differentiated histologically. Fibrosarcoma may be confused with infantile fibromatosis. Malignant fibrous histiocytoma can arise in the soft tissues or bone, where it often presents as a lytic lesion. Treatment of both entities includes wide resection and possibly adjuvant chemotherapy or radiotherapy.

DERMATOFIBROSARCOMA PROTUBERANS

This is a rare fibrohistiocytic tumor of low to intermediate malignancy that infiltrates surrounding tissues and

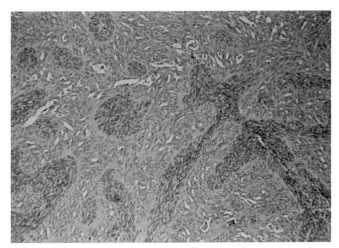

Figure 10-9 ◆ Low-power micrograph of synovial sarcoma. This lesion can present as biphasic or monophasic. The biphasic form is composed of both epithelial cell and spindle cell components. In contrast, the monophasic form can be epithelial cell or spindle cell type.

has a high capacity for local recurrence (~50%) and rare metastasis (~5%). It presents as a slow-growing cutaneous mass. Positive margins should prompt re-excision and adjuvant irradiation. Small areas of dermatofibrosarcoma protuberans may resemble fibrosarcoma because of the appearance and the higher mitotic rate but behave like dermatofibrosarcoma protuberans. Increased recurrence has been associated with likelihood of metastasis.

LEIOMYOSARCOMA

This lesion is a high-grade sarcoma rarely seen in the hand. It originates from the smooth muscle of vessel walls. Treatment includes wide resection and possibly adjuvant chemotherapy or radiotherapy.

LIPOSARCOMA

Liposarcoma is another rare lesion of the forearm and hand. Subtypes include well-differentiated (atypical lipoma), myxoid, round cell, pleomorphic, and dedifferentiated liposarcomas. They often present as slowly enlarging masses. The percentage of round cell type in a myxoid liposarcoma promotes it to a higher grade and also predicts a poorer prognosis. Myxoid liposarcoma can metastasize to extrapulmonary sites, such as spine and appendicular skeleton. Treatment includes wide resection and possibly adjuvant chemotherapy or radiotherapy.

MALIGNANT PERIPHERAL NERVE SHEATH TUMOR

Malignant peripheral nerve sheath tumor is a term used to encompass all the malignant tumors originating from nerve tissue. More than half of the cases arise in neurofibromatosis 1 (von Recklinghausen's disease). Wide surgical resection is the treatment of choice, although there is a high recurrence rate. These tumors are characterized by a poor response to adjuvant treatment.

RHABDOMYOSARCOMA

Rhabdomyosarcoma is a malignant soft tissue tumor of striated muscle. The incidence in the hand is rare. Histologic types include embryonal, alveolar, pleomorphic, and botryoid. The alveolar subtype is found in more than half of the cases in the extremities. This subtype often displays aggressive clinical behavior, with early metastatic evidence and high recurrence rates. Staging of the disease includes the site, involvement of the regional lymph nodes, metastasis, and surgical margins. Adjuvant chemotherapy and radiation treatment in addition to wide surgical resection can be helpful.

Bone Tumors

Benign Tumors

ENCHONDROMA

Enchondroma is the most common primary tumor of the hand skeleton; 35% to 50% of all enchondromas occur in the hand. The proximal phalanges are most commonly involved, followed by the metacarpals, the middle phalanges, and more rarely the carpal bones. Enchondromas are most commonly found incidentally but can present as localized swelling or as a pathologic fracture (Fig. 10-10). The common age at presentation is between 10 and 40 years. Radiographs typically reveal a lytic, expansile medullary lesion, with cortical thinning of the shaft and stippled calcification of the matrix (Fig. 10-11). On histologic examination, these are composed of mature cartilage tissue resembling articular cartilage surrounded by lamellar bone (Fig. 10-12). The appearance in the hand may be slightly more cellular and contain more atypia than enchondromas found in other parts of the body. Increased areas of myxoid matrix, increased cellular atypia, and intricate involvement of the marrow by the cartilage tissue are suggestive of a chondrosarcoma. Treatment includes a biopsy to confirm the diagnosis, followed by curettage. The lesions heal without bone graft after curettage, although autograft or allograft bone can be used. Pathologic fractured lesions are treated in the standard manner. After they have healed, curettage and bone grafting may be performed. The risk for malignant transformation in solitary enchondromas is less than 1%.

Multiple enchondromas occur in Ollier's disease (multiple enchondromatosis) and in Maffucci's syndrome. In both conditions, one side of the body is affected more often, and the enchondromas may continue to grow after puberty, unlike the solitary enchondromas that stabilize in size. The risk for malignant degeneration in Ollier's disease is about 25%. In Maffucci's syndrome, the multifocal enchondromas are

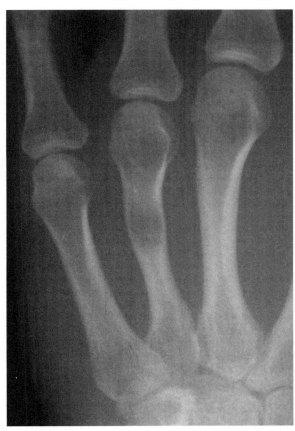

Figure 10-11 ✦ Anteroposterior radiograph of a hand in a patient with an enchondroma of the ring finger metacarpal shaft.

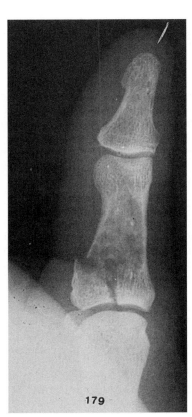

Figure 10-10 ✦ Anteroposterior radiograph of a thumb in a patient with an enchondroma of the proximal phalanx. Note the pathologic articular fracture extending into the MP joint.

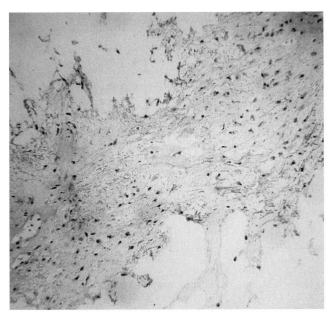

Figure 10-12 ✦ Low-power micrograph of enchondroma. These lesions are composed of mature cartilage tissue resembling articular cartilage surrounded by lamellar bone. Enchondromas of the bones of the hand are quite cellular.

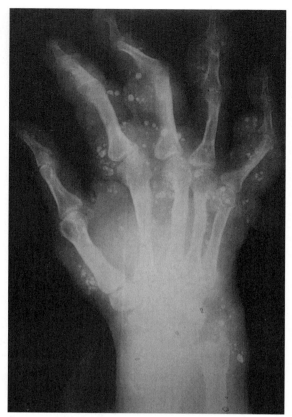

Figure 10-13 ◈ Oblique radiograph of a hand in a patient with Maffucci's syndrome. Note the multiple enchondromas and calcifications within hemangiomas.

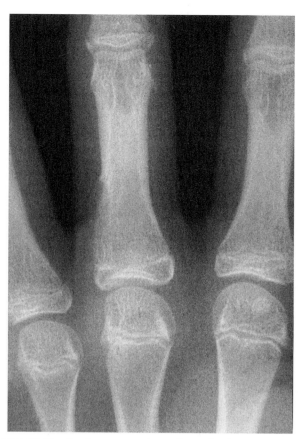

Figure 10-14 ◈ Anteroposterior radiograph of a patient with a periosteal chondroma of the proximal phalanx showing a well-circumscribed, crater-like surface lesion at the level of the metaphysis with overhang from periosteal calcification.

associated with soft tissue angiomatosis. Calcified thrombi within the angiomas can be seen on radiographs (Fig. 10-13). The risk for malignancy in Maffucci's syndrome reaches 100%; malignant degeneration of enchondromas affects more than 70% of patients.

PERIOSTEAL CHONDROMA

Periosteal chondroma is similar histologically to enchondroma except for the location, which is under the periosteum. These lesions typically present as a mass in the metaphyseal region of the phalanges. Radiographs show a well-circumscribed, crater-like surface lesion at the level of the metaphysis with overhang from periosteal calcification (Fig. 10-14). There may be punctate calcification within the matrix. The histologic appearance is similar to the enchondroma, but it may be confused with chondrosarcoma. Treatment involves curettage and close follow-up for recurrence, which is seen in less than 5% of patients.

CHONDROMYXOID FIBROMA

Chondromyxoid fibroma is a benign tumor with areas of cartilage and myxoid tissue in a background of fibrous tissue. It usually presents with localized swelling. Radiographs reveal a lytic lesion of the long bones surrounded by a sclerotic border. Biopsy, followed by thorough curettage to decrease recurrence, is recommended. Recurrence is variable in the hand.

FIBROUS DYSPLASIA

Fibrous dysplasia is a disease affecting the maturation of the bone, resulting in immature woven bone in a fibrous stroma. Fibrous dysplasia can present as a monostotic lesion or as polyostotic. The radiographic findings are those of an expanded diaphysis with a "ground-glass" matrix. Biopsy is recommended for diagnostic purposes in monostotic lesions.

OSTEOBLASTOMA

Osteoblastoma is commonly seen in the spine; less than 5% of these tumors present in the hand. This is a benign osteoblastic bone tumor consisting of a rich vascular stroma and osteoid surrounded by osteoblasts. Mitotic figures are not seen. It affects patients aged 10 to 25 years and presents as an expansile lytic lesion that is well circumscribed and with a broad osteosclerotic border. It is histologically similar to osteoid osteoma but larger (>2 cm in diameter). Recurrence after curettage is seen in almost one third of patients.

OSTEOID OSTEOMA

Pain is the usual presenting symptom, described as a dull ache, worse at night, and relieved with salicylates. Osteoid osteoma can cause clubbing if it is found in the distal phalanx. The lesions occur in the phalanges but may also occur in the carpus. The radiologic appearance

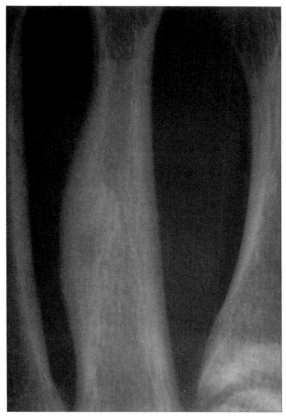

Figure 10-15 ◈ Anteroposterior radiograph of a hand in a patient with an osteoid osteoma of a hand bone revealing a small nidus (<2 cm) within cortical bone surrounded by a sclerotic reaction.

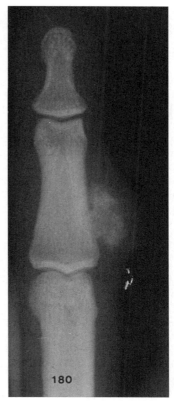

Figure 10-16 ◈ Anteroposterior radiograph of a patient with florid periosteal reaction of the middle phalanx.

is that of a small nidus (<2 cm) surrounded by a sclerotic reaction (Fig. 10-15). High levels of prostaglandins have been noted in the nidus, raising the possibility of inflammatory rather than neoplastic etiology of these lesions. The nidus may be present in the cortex or within the medullary canal. Treatment options include curettage or en bloc excision of the nidus, radiofrequency ablation, and long-term use of nonsteroidal anti-inflammatory drugs. Recurrence develops if the nidus is incompletely removed.

FLORID REACTIVE PERIOSTITIS AND BIZARRE PAROSTEAL OSTEOCHONDROMATOUS PROLIFERATION (NORA'S LESION)

Florid reactive periostitis and bizarre parosteal osteochondromatous proliferation are reactive bone-producing lesions of the small bones of the hands after trauma. These lesions are commonly found in the middle and proximal phalanges. They present as painful digital swelling. Florid reactive periostitis is an aggressive periosteal reaction associated with soft tissue swelling that may be confused with osteomyelitis or malignant neoplasia (Fig. 10-16). Histologic analysis of lesions of bizarre parosteal osteochondromatous proliferation reveals a hypercellular cartilage in a background of a fibrous matrix and bone trabeculae that can be confused with parosteal osteosarcoma. Bizarre parosteal osteochondromatous proliferation lacks cytologic atypia

and has no evidence of mitotic activity. Recurrence is rare after excision of florid reactive periostitis, but recurrence develops in up to 50% of cases of bizarre parosteal osteochondromatous proliferation.

OSTEOCHONDROMA

Osteochondroma is a rare lesion in the hand. Most originate from the site of tendon insertion or from the growth plate. It is formed of a bone prominence with a cartilage cap. There is a small chance of malignant transformation. It may cause growth or rotational deformity. *Acquired osteochondroma* (turret exostosis) is a reactive lesion on the surface of the bone that forms as a result of trauma. It develops as a well-delineated mineralized mass that fuses with the cortex. *Subungual exostosis* is found on the distal phalanx. It may be related to a history of trauma or infection. The presenting symptom is typically nail deformity. Nail removal and excision of the lesion are curative.

UNICAMERAL BONE CYST

Unicameral bone cyst is rare in the hand and forearm. It is often present as a result of a pathologic fracture. Radiographs reveal a lytic metaphyseal lesion with defined borders. These cysts can be treated with aspiration and corticosteroid injection or curettage and bone grafting.

ANEURYSMAL BONE CYST

These lesions present with pain and swelling and occasionally as a pathologic fracture. Frequency is higher in the metacarpals, although aneurysmal bone cysts can be found in the phalanges and also the carpals. Radiographs show an expansile lytic lesion within the bone. The expansion is asymmetric, with a thin rim of bone on the lesion and a sharp interface with the normal cortex. There is no mineralization of the matrix (versus enchondroma). The histologic appearance consists of fine septa separating cysts of blood. The solid portion of the lesion contains giant cells and macrophages with hemosiderin pigment. Aneurysmal bone cysts may be primary or secondary. Secondary aneurysmal bone cysts occur in a background of giant cell tumors or chondroblastomas. Treatment is by curettage and allograft, in combination with cryosurgery. The recurrence is as high as 40% and can be further managed by similar treatment.

GIANT CELL TUMOR

About 2% to 3% of the giant cell tumors occur in the hand. Giant cell tumor in the distal radius is the third most common location in the body. These lesions present with pain or as a pathologic fracture through the lesion. Radiographs reveal a lytic geographic tumor without any matrix calcification or periosteal reaction (Fig. 10-17). Cortical expansion and breakout into the soft tissue are not uncommon. Histologic examination reveals many multinucleated cells (giant cells) in a background stroma of bland cells.

Incisional biopsy is strongly recommended. Some authors have reported success with curettage, burring of the wall of the lesion, and adjuvant treatment (phenol or cryotherapy) for lesions of the bone of the hand. The void can be packed with allograft or polymethyl methacrylate. If there is soft tissue extension, resection with a margin is necessary to reduce recurrence. Wide excision of these lesions is associated with a lower risk of recurrence.

Although benign, these tumors are locally aggressive and have a 2% to 3% chance of metastasis to the lung. Giant cell tumor of the hand has a higher risk of recurrence (50%) and multifocal disease than does giant cell tumor of bones elsewhere in the body (18%). Because of the risk of metastasis, chest radiographs are strongly recommended. Distal radius tumors have been noted to have a higher recurrence rate with treatment by curettage and bone grafting. In these cases, especially if there is soft tissue extension, wide resection and reconstruction with osteoarticular allograft is recommended.

GIANT CELL REPARATIVE GRANULOMA

This is a benign reactive process that presents as a swelling or a pathologic fracture. The radiographs reveal a destructive bone process with thinned cortices. Histologic examination shows multinucleated giant cells in a fibrous background, with foci of hemosiderin. The treatment of choice is curettage and bone grafting. Recurrence rate is between 30% and 50%. Wide resection significantly reduces recurrence, although it is not the first choice for this benign disease. The radiographic and histologic picture is similar to giant cell tumor, aneurysmal bone cyst, and brown tumor

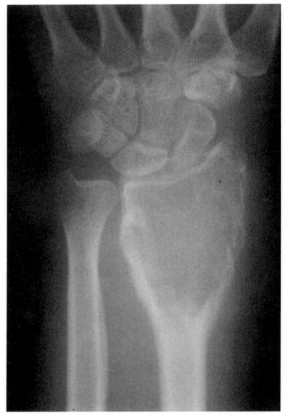

Figure 10-17 ❖ Anteroposterior radiograph of a patient with giant cell tumor of bone in the distal radius.

of hyperparathyroidism. Serum calcium and phosphate as well as parathyroid hormone determinations are recommended to rule out hyperparathyroidism.

Malignant Tumors

CHONDROSARCOMA

Chondrosarcoma is the most common primary bone sarcoma in the hand. Most arise de novo, but they may occur in a preexisting enchondroma. They are common in the metacarpals and the proximal phalanges. Presentation is that of a painful, slow-growing mass. Radiographs show a lytic lesion with matrix calcification and cortical expansion (Fig. 10-18). These tumors in the hand have a low tendency to metastasize. Surgical resection with wide margins is the treatment of choice. Diagnosis of a low-grade chondrosarcoma can be difficult because enchondroma of the hand displays more atypia and cellularity than does enchondroma elsewhere in the body. As for all sarcomas, staging studies should be performed before surgical resection with wide margins. Chondrosarcomas are not sensitive to chemotherapy and radiotherapy.

OSTEOSARCOMA

Osteosarcoma is a rare lesion of the hand. There may be preexisting diseases, such as Paget's disease, or a history of exposure to radiation. Pain and swelling are the presenting symptoms. Plain radiographs reveal a lytic

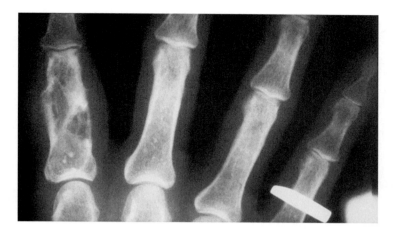

Figure 10-18 ◈ Anteroposterior radiograph of a patient with a chondrosarcoma of the proximal phalanx of the index finger revealing a lytic lesion with matrix calcification and cortical expansion.

lesion with periosteal reaction and new bone formation. There may be an associated soft tissue mass. Pathologic examination shows areas of atypia and mitosis with osteoid formation (Fig. 10-19). After confirmation by an incisional biopsy and staging studies, chemotherapy should be administered preoperatively and postoperatively. Wide resection or amputation is the treatment of choice. *Parosteal osteosarcoma* is a low-grade malignant neoplasm, and surgery is the mainstay of treatment.

Ewing's Sarcoma

Ewing's sarcoma commonly occurs in the first or second decades, although it is very rare in the hand. Pain and swelling are often the presenting symptoms. On radiographs, the appearance may be that of an aggressive, permeative lytic lesion with periosteal reaction (Fig. 10-20). Ewing's sarcoma often has a large soft tissue component. It is often misdiagnosed as osteomyelitis, which can adversely affect outcome. Incisional biopsy is strongly recommended. Surgery with wide margins should be attempted. Recurrence of Ewing's sarcoma has a poor prognosis for survival. If the margins of surgical resection are close or positive, irradiation of the tumor and surgical bed should be considered. Adjuvant chemotherapy administered preoperatively and postoperatively is controversial.

Metastatic Tumors

All of the bones in the hand can be involved in metastatic disease, although the distal phalanges are most commonly involved (Fig. 10-21). Metastasis from a lung primary is seen in up to 50% of the cases. Breast, renal, thyroid, colon, and other carcinomas can also be involved. The order of incidence of metastatic disease distal to the elbow is lung > breast > renal cell > colon carcinoma. Radiographs reveal a lytic lesion, which can be painful and swollen. It mimics an infection, and incisional biopsy is strongly recommended. Treatment is directed at palliation and preservation of function, usually through wide excision or amputation. For lesions involving the proximal phalanx, ray amputation can improve pain and maintain hand function.

Dupuytren's Disease

Introduction

Dupuytren's disease is characterized by fibrosis and contracture of the palmar fascia and resultant digital contracture. The cells responsible for the disease are the myofibroblast and the fibroblast-fibrocyte. The myofibroblast shares features with the fibroblasts and smooth muscle cells. It contains bundles of actin microfilaments (stress fiber) arranged parallel to the long axis of the cell. Myofibroblasts differ from smooth muscle cells by the presence of a well-developed Golgi apparatus and lack of a basal lamina. The microfilaments within the myofibroblasts are connected to the extracellular matrix and also to each other by fibronectin.

The presentation usually includes solitary or multiple painless nodules in the pretendinous bands of the palmar fascia of the ring and small finger rays, skin dimpling, and flexion contracture of the affected digits at the MP and interphalangeal joints. Web space

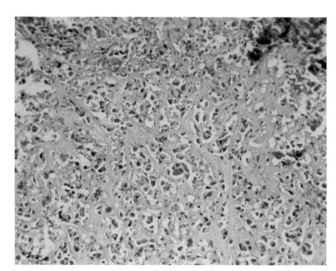

Figure 10-19 ◈ Low-power micrograph of an osteosarcoma. Note the areas of cellular atypia and mitoses and formation of immature osteoid.

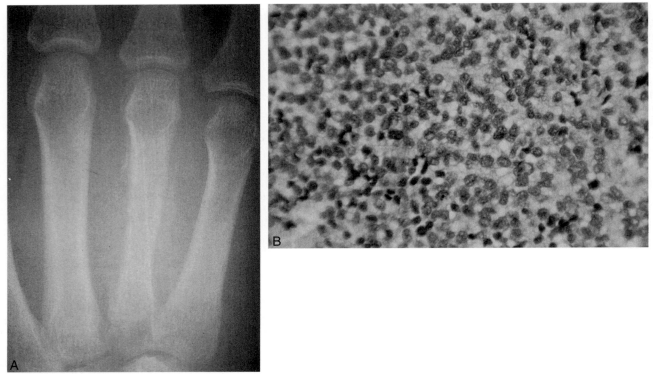

Figure 10-20 ◈ **A,** Anteroposterior radiograph of a patient with Ewing's sarcoma of the ring metacarpal. Note the aggressive periosteal reaction. **B,** High-power micrograph of Ewing's sarcoma revealing small, round neoplastic cells with large oval hyperchromatic nuclei. These cells have scant cytoplasm.

contractures can also occur, including the thumb-index web space.

The disease is divided into three stages:

1. Proliferative stage: the number of myofibroblasts increases significantly in the nodules and the cell-to-cell connections (gap junctions) also increase. This is a vascular stage.
2. Involutional stage: the myofibroblasts are smaller and aligned in the long axis (stress lines), and the ratio of type III collagen to type I is increased.
3. Residual stage: myofibroblasts and the nodules disappear, leaving a relatively acellular fibrotic tissue.

Incidence

The incidence of Dupuytren's contracture is high in patients of northern European descent and is uncommon in African and Asian countries. The incidence is higher in men, most commonly seen in the 40- to 60-year age range; less than 10% of patients are younger than 40 years.

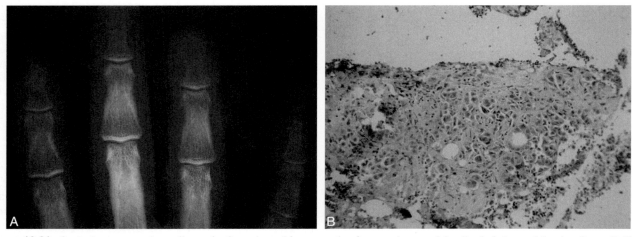

Figure 10-21 ◈ **A,** Anteroposterior radiograph of a patient with metastatic adenocarcinoma of the distal phalanx of the ring finger. **B,** High-power micrograph of adenosarcoma revealing a lesion composed of small glands that are lined by a single layer of hyperchromatic cells.

Dupuytren's contracture can be inherited as an autosomal dominant trait with variable penetrance, but most cases are sporadic. Dupuytren's diathesis is characterized by aggressive hand contracture (including knuckle pads), plantar fibromatosis (Lederhosen disease), penile fibrosis (Peyronie's disease), family history, and young age. Patients with diathesis have more severe disease, higher recurrence, and poor outcomes. Dupuytren's contracture has been associated with alcoholism, diabetes mellitus, epilepsy, smoking, and chronic pulmonary disease. An association between occupations such as manual labor and Dupuytren's disease has not been definitively proved. Patients with human immunodeficiency virus infection have a higher prevalence of the disease. Bilateral involvement is present in about 50% of the cases.

Etiology

The etiology of Dupuytren's disease has not been elucidated, and traumatic, occupational, and systemic etiologic factors have been proposed. The causation of the disease may be related to microvascular changes leading to hypoxia of the palmar tissues, with increased oxygen free radical formation. In vitro studies have shown that low concentrations of oxygen free radicals can stimulate fibroblast proliferation. Hypoxia also promotes angiogenesis and collagen synthesis, such as in wound healing. Factors associated with Dupuytren's disease include platelet-derived growth factor, a potent fibroblast mitogen that stimulates collagen synthesis (especially type III), promotes reorganization of cytoskeletal actin filaments, and induces formation of prostaglandins. Platelet-derived growth factor is known to be a stimulator of myofibroblasts in the proliferative and involutional stages of the disease. Transforming growth factor-β1 is another factor implicated in Dupuytren's disease that is responsible for fibrosis and tissue contracture in wound healing; it may play an important role in myofibroblast differentiation. Epidermal growth factor and basic fibroblast growth factor are also thought to be involved in the development of disease. Prostaglandin F_1 and F_2 and calcium channel blockers inhibit myofibroblast contracture, while serotonin and angiotensin induce contracture.

Pathoanatomy

The fascial components involved in Dupuytren's disease include the pretendinous and the spiral bands, the natatory ligament, the lateral digital sheet, and Grayson's ligaments (Fig. 10-22). Cleland's ligaments are not involved in Dupuytren's disease. Cords are defined as diseased palmar tissue that forms a longitudinal fibrous tether, which leads to digital contracture (Fig. 10-23). The cords that have been identified include the central cord, the abductor digiti minimi cord, the spiral cord, the retrovascular cord, the lateral cord, the natatory cord, and the first web's intercommissural cord. The central cord has no fascial precursor and is a continuation of the pretendinous band. The spiral cord arises from the pretendinous band, the spiral bands, the lateral digital sheaths, and Grayson's ligament.

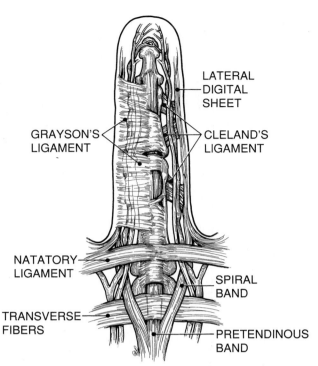

Figure 10-22 ◆ Parts of the normal digital fascia that become diseased. Grayson's ligament is shown on the left. It is an almost continuous sheet of thin fascia and is in the same plane as the natatory ligament. Cleland's ligaments are shown on the right. They do not become diseased. The lateral digital sheet receives fibers from the natatory ligament as well as the spiral band. The spiral bands pass on either side of the MP joint, deep to the neurovascular bundles, to reach the side of the finger. *(From McFarlane RM: Patterns of the diseased fascia in the fingers in Dupuytren's contracture. Br J Plast Surg 17:271-280, 1964.)*

It usually attaches to the middle phalanx and is often associated with severe PIP contractures. The pretendinous cord causes MP joint contracture, the spiral and central cords cause PIP joint contractures, the natatory cord predominantly causes web space contracture, and the retrovascular cord causes DIP and PIP joint contractures.

The spiral band passes beneath the neurovascular structures, bringing them to a more superficial level and making them susceptible to injury during surgery. In fact, the best predictor of superficial and central displacement of the neurovascular bundle is PIP joint contracture. A soft, pulpy mass between distal palmar crease and proximal flexion crease should alert the surgeon to digital nerve lying subcutaneously. The ulnar digital neurovascular bundle of the small finger is at risk when the abductor digiti minimi cord is excised.

Treatment

A nodule is occasionally painful, and a cortisone injection may be helpful. Enzymatic fasciotomy with clostridial collagenase injections has shown encouraging results particularly in dealing with MP joint flexion contracture. The injections tend to provide better results for contractures of the MP joints compared with the PIP joint. Small painless nodules and MP joint

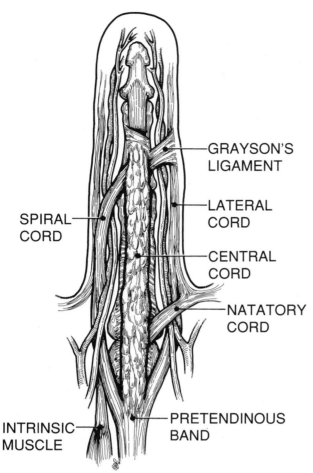

Figure 10-23 ◆ The change in the normal fascia bands to diseased cords. The pretendinous cord causes MP joint contracture, and the others cause PIP joint contracture. When the natatory cord is diseased, it becomes adherent to the pretendinous cord. As it is drawn proximally, it appears to bifurcate from the pretendinous cord. Grayson's ligament is diseased in two ways. On the right, it is shown simply thickened. On the left, it has contributed to the attachment of the spiral cord onto the flexor tendon sheath. (*Illustration by Elizabeth Roselius, ©1999. Reprinted with permission from McFarlane RM: Dupuytren's contracture. In Green DP, Hotchkiss RN, Pederson WC, eds: Green's Operative Hand Surgery, 4th ed. New York, Churchill Livingstone, 1999.*)

contractures of less than 30 degrees can be observed. Surgical indications include MP joint contractures of more than 30 degrees and any PIP contracture. Palmar fasciectomy (partial [most common] or complete) is the treatment of choice. Various types of incisions can be used for this purpose. Skin flaps must also be handled with care to help with wound healing and to decrease scar formation. Dermatofasciectomy may be used for patients with severe diathesis or recurrent disease. In these cases, the use of skin grafts is controversial, and the open (McCash) technique can give satisfactory results and greater total active digital motion compared to primary closure techniques. Palmar fasciotomy alone leads to recurrence, but it may give a temporary release for a severe PIP joint contracture. Risk of neurovascular injury is high if a percutaneous fasciotomy is attempted.

The need for amputation is rare, and it is usually performed for severe, long-standing contractures of the small finger. PIP joints with significant contracture may not be corrected by fasciectomy alone and may require check-rein ligament and accessory collateral ligament release.

Release of MP joint contracture often yields satisfactory results with excellent restoration of motion. Patients with PIP joint involvement and those with recurrent disease tend to have less successful surgical outcomes. In PIP joints with 60 degrees or more of flexion contracture, approximately 50% to 60% of the normal range of motion can be expected.

Hematoma formation is the most common complication and may lead to recurrence and reflex sympathetic dystrophy (RSD). Other complications include neurovascular injury, scar contracture, stiffness and RSD. Release of the carpal tunnel should not be performed concomitantly because of an increase in the incidence of a postoperative flare reaction and RSD. If patients develop a flare reaction, a therapy protocol including stress loading techniques is recommended. More than 80% of patients can expect a full recovery, although the recurrence rate is about 10% per year.

Bibliography

GANGLIA

Richman JA, Gelberman RH, Engber WD, et al: Ganglions of the wrist and digits: results of treatment by aspiration and cyst wall puncture. J Hand Surg Am 12:1041-1043, 1987.

Thornburg LE: Ganglions of the hand and wrist. J Am Acad Orthop Surg 7:231-238, 1999.

Westbrook AP, Stephen AB, Oni J, et al: Ganglia: the patient's perception. J Hand Surg Br 25:566-567, 2000.

SKIN TUMORS

Balch CM, Buzaid AC, Soong SJ, et al: Final version of the American Joint Committee on Cancer staging system for cutaneous melanoma. J Clin Oncol 19:3635-3648, 2001.

Greenlee RT, Hill-Harmon MB, Murray T, et al: Cancer statistics, 2001. CA Cancer J Clin 51:15-36, 2001.

Kirkwood JM, Ibrahim JG, Sondak VK, et al: High- and low-dose interferon alfa-2b in high-risk melanoma: first analysis of intergroup trial E1690/S9111/C9190. J Clin Oncol 18:2444-2458, 2000.

Lovett RD, Perez CA, Shapiro SJ, et al: External irradiation of epithelial skin cancer. Int J Radiat Oncol Biol Phys 19:235-242, 1990.

Manola J, Atkins M, Ibrahim J, et al: Prognostic factors in metastatic melanoma: a pooled analysis of Eastern Cooperative Oncology Group trials. J Clin Oncol 18:3782-3793, 2000.

Preston DS, Stern RS: Non-melanoma cancers of the skin. N Engl J Med 327:1649-1662, 1992.

Rayner CR: The results of treatment of two hundred and seventy-three carcinomas of the hand. Hand 13:183-186, 1981.

Shen P, Guenther JM, Wanek LA, et al: Can elective lymph node dissection decrease the frequency and mortality rate of late melanoma recurrences? Ann Surg Oncol 7:114-119, 2000.

Veronesi U, Cascinelli N, Adamus J, et al: Thin stage I primary cutaneous malignant melanoma: comparison of excision with margins of 1 or 3 cm. N Engl J Med 318:1159-1162, 1988.

Wagner JD, Gordon MS, Chuang TY, et al: Current therapy of cutaneous melanoma. Plast Reconstr Surg 105:1774-1799, 2000.

BONE AND SOFT TISSUE TUMORS

Athanasian EA, Wold LE, Amadio PC: Giant cell tumors of the bones in the hand. J Hand Surg Am 22:91-98, 1997.

Averill RM, Smith RJ, Campbell CJ: Giant cell tumors of the bones of the hand. J Hand Surg Am 5:39-50, 1980.

Brien EW, Terek RM, Geer RJ, et al: Treatment of soft tissue sarcomas of the hand. J Bone Joint Surg Am 77:564-571, 1995.

Carroll RE: Osteogenic sarcoma in the hand. J Bone Joint Surg Am 39:325-331, 1957.

Carroll RE, Berman AT: Glomus tumors of the hand: review of the literature and report on twenty-eight cases. J Bone Joint Surg Am 54:691-703, 1972.

Colon F, Upton J: Pediatric hand tumors: a review of 349 cases. Hand Clin 11:223-243, 1995.

Frassica FJ, Amadio PC, Wold LE, Beabout JW: Aneurysmal bone cyst: clinicopathologic features and treatment of ten cases involving the hand. J Hand Surg Am 13:676-683, 1988.

Frykman GK, Wood VE: Peripheral nerve hamartoma with macrodactyly in the hand: report of three cases and review of the literature. J Hand Surg Am 3:307-312, 1978.

Hays DM, Soule EH, Lawrence W, et al: Extremity lesions in the Intergroup Rhabdomyosarcoma Study (IRS-1): a preliminary report. Cancer 48:1-8, 1982.

Kerin R: Metastatic tumors of the hand. A review of the literature. J Bone Joint Surg Am 65:1331-1335, 1983.

Kneisl JS, Simon MA: Medical management compared with operative treatment for osteoid-osteoma. J Bone Joint Surg Am 74:179-185, 1992.

Kocher MS, Gebhardt MC, Mankin HJ: Reconstruction of the distal aspect of the radius with use of an osteoarticular allograft after excision of a skeletal tumor. J Bone Joint Surg Am 80:407-419, 1998.

Lucas GL, Sponsellar PD: Synovial chondrometaplasia of the hand: case report and review of the literature. J Hand Surg Am 9:269-272, 1984.

Meneses MF, Unni KK, Swee RG: Bizarre parosteal osteochondromatous proliferation of bone (Nora's lesion). Am J Surg Pathol 17:691-697, 1993.

Mohler CG, Jensen C, Steyers CM, et al: Osteosarcoma of the hand: a case report and review of the literature. J Hand Surg Am 19:287-289, 1994.

Muren C, Hoglund M, Engkvist O, Juhlin L: Osteoid osteomas of the hand. Report of three cases and review of the literature. Acta Radiol 32:62-66, 1991.

Nuyttens JJ, Rust PF, Thomas CR, Turrisi AT: Surgery versus radiation therapy for patients with aggressive fibromatosis or desmoid tumors: a comparative review of 22 articles. Cancer 88:1517-1523, 2000.

Okada K, Wold LE, Beabout JW, Shives TC: Osteosarcoma of the hand: a clinico-pathologic study of 12 cases. Cancer 72:719-725, 1993.

Steingberg BD, Gelberman RH, Mankin HJ, Rosenberg AE: Epithelioid sarcoma in the upper extremity. J Bone Joint Surg Am 74:28-35, 1992.

Takigawa K: Chondroma of the bones of the hand. A review of 110 cases. J Bone Joint Surg Am 53:1591-1600, 1971.

Vander Griend RA, Funderburk CH: The treatment of giant cell tumors of the distal part of the radius. J Bone Joint Surg Am 75:899-908, 1993.

Xarchas K, Papavassiliou N, Tsoutseos N, Burke FD: Rhabdomyosarcoma of the hand. Two case reports and a review of the literature. J Hand Surg Br 21:325-329, 1996.

Yuen M, Friedman L, Orr W, et al: Proliferative periosteal processes of phalanges: a unitary hypothesis. Skeletal Radiol 21:301-303, 1992.

DUPUYTREN'S DISEASE

Hill N, Hurst L: Dupuytren's contracture. Hand Clin 5:349-357, 1989.

Hueston J: Dupuytren's contracture. J Hand Surg Br 18:806, 1993.

McFarlane RM: Dupuytren's disease. J Hand Surg Br 21:566-567, 1996.

McFarlane RM, Ross DC: Dupuytren's disease. In Weinzig J, ed: Plastic Surgery Secrets. Philadelphia, Hanley & Belfus, 1998.

Mikkelsen OA: The prevalence of Dupuytren's disease in Norway. Acta Chir Scand 138:695-700, 1972.

Noble J, Arafa M, Royle SG, et al: The association between alcohol, hepatic pathology and Dupuytren's disease. J Hand Surg Br 17:71-74, 1992.

Rayan G, ed: Dupuytren's Disease. Hand Clinics, February 1999.

Sappino A, Schurch W, Gabbiani G: Biology of disease—differentiation repertoire of fibroblastic cells; expression of cytoskeletal proteins as marker of phenotype modulations. Lab Invest 63:144-161, 1990.

✧ Alexander M. Marcus, MD   ✧ Thomas R. Hunt III, MD

INFECTION

General Principles

Treatment Principles

Diagnosis of hand infections is based on a thorough history and physical examination supplemented by relevant tests. Critical facts to be garnered during the history include current symptoms; circumstances and time frame surrounding the onset and progression of the infection, including exposures, skin penetration, and results of previous treatments; presence of medical conditions that might compromise the patient's immune response; and whether the patient has had a similar infection previously that was cured or became quiescent.

Examination must take into account the anatomy of the hand and its effect on the presentation and severity of infections. For example, longitudinal swelling along the palmar aspect of a finger may be due to a septic flexor tenosynovitis compared with a less significant swelling along the dorsum of the same digit. Likewise, an insignificant-appearing laceration over the dorsal metacarpophalangeal joint region in someone who was in an altercation may indicate an intra-articular process.

There are several treatment principles that must be adhered to by the physician. **D**rainage and **D**ébridement, **I**mmobilization, **C**hemotherapy (antibiotics), and **E**levation (**DICE**) are critical to the successful eradication of a hand infection. Empirical antibiotics are chosen on the basis of expected pathogens (Table 11-1). The final antibiotic choice is determined by culture and sensitivity results. Daily soaks can help to encourage drainage. Appropriate tetanus prophylaxis should be given (Table 11-2).

Patient Medical Issues

DIABETES

Diabetes is a systemic disease that may cause diminished vascular perfusion, neuropathy, and impaired immune function. These factors can result in treatment delays, persistence of infection, and need for repeated débridements. Amputations are more often required in this population to control infection and tissue necrosis. Gram-negative and polymicrobial infections in the hand are more common in diabetic patients. Blood glucose levels should be closely monitored because extreme fluctuations may occur.

SYSTEMIC IMMUNOCOMPROMISE

Most hand infections in immunocompromised patients are caused by the same organisms seen in the general population. The infections tend to run unusually virulent courses. For example, in contrast to the self-limited course seen in most patients, herpetic whitlow in immunocompromised subjects tends not to resolve spontaneously, and antiviral agents are required for treatment in many cases.

INTRAVENOUS DRUG ABUSE

As with diabetic patients, there is a high incidence of gram-negative infections, although *Streptococcus* and *Staphylococcus* are still the most likely pathogens present in an abscess resulting from intravenous drug use.

Specific Infections and Locations

Generalized Processes

CELLULITIS

Cellulitis is a diffuse inflammatory disorder caused by leukocyte infiltration into infected soft tissues. It is characterized by erythema, swelling, and tenderness. No localized abscess or palpable fluctuation is present. However, cellulitis may extend from and be secondary to an underlying abscess and septic joint or bone infection. The possibility of a concomitant, deeper infection must be excluded as part of the evaluation process. If aspiration of a joint is needed, placement of the needle through cellulitic soft tissues should be avoided to preclude an iatrogenic infection of joints.

Diagnosis is usually made on physical examination. Results of laboratory studies, such as sedimentation rate and C-reactive protein level, are often elevated and can be used to follow the course of treatment. Most frequently, cellulitis is initiated by trauma to the skin and subcutaneous tissues. Other causes include chronic ulceration, lymphedema, and dermatitis. Group A beta-hemolytic streptococcus is the most common causative organism. *Staphylococcus aureus* is sometimes involved, especially in less severe cases.

Treatment of primary cellulitis includes antibiotics, elevation, and immobilization. If the organism and its sensitivities are known, antibiotics are directed accordingly. Otherwise, coverage for both *Staphylococcus* and *Streptococcus* is needed. For mild, early cases, oral

207

◆ Table 11-1

EMPIRICAL ANTIBIOTIC RECOMMENDATIONS FOR HAND INFECTIONS

Infection	Possible Organisms	Antibiotic Dosage	Alternative Antibiotic Dosage
Felon, paronychia	S. aureus, oral anaerobes	Dicloxacillin, 250-500 mg PO q6h, or Nafcillin, 1-2 g IV q4-6h, or Clindamycin, 150-300 mg PO q6h	Cephalexin, 250-500 mg PO q6h, or Cefazolin, 1 g IV q8h, or Erythromycin, 250-500 mg PO q6h
Flexor tenosynovitis	S. aureus, Streptococcus, gram-negative rods	Cefazolin, 1 g IV q8h	Nafcillin, 1-2 g IV q4-6h, or vancomycin, 1 g IV q12h, plus gentamicin,* or Imipenem, 0.5-1.0 g IV q6h
Herpetic whitlow	Herpes simplex virus	Consider acyclovir, 400 mg PO tid × 10 days	
Subcutaneous or deep space abscess	S. aureus, anaerobes, gram-negative rods	Cefazolin, 1 g IV q8h, or Ampicillin-sulbactam, 1.5 mg IV q6h	Nafcillin, 1-2 g IV q4-6h, plus gentamicin,* or Imipenem, 0.5-1.0 g IV q6h
Cellulitis, lymphangitis	Streptococcus, S. aureus	Dicloxacillin, 250-500 mg PO q6h, or Nafcillin, 1-2 g IV q4-6h, or Cephalexin, 1 g IV q8h	Cephalexin, 250-500 mg PO q6h, or Erythromycin, 250-500 mg PO q6h
IV drug abuse related	Gram-positive, gram-negative, or mixed or methicillin-resistant S. aureus	Nafcillin, 1-2 g IV q4-6h, plus gentamicin*	Vancomycin, 1 g IV q12h (for methicillin-resistant S. aureus), plus gentamicin,* or Imipenem, 0.5-1.0 g IV q6h
Human bite	S. aureus, E. corrodens, Streptococcus, anaerobes	Cefazolin, 1 g IV q8h, plus penicillin, 2-4 million U IV q4-6h, or clindamycin, 300 mg PO q6h, plus ciprofloxacin, 250-500 mg PO q12h, or trimethoprim-sulfamethoxazole (Septra DS) PO q12h	Nafcillin, 1-2 g, plus penicillin, 2-4 million U q4-6h, or Amoxicillin-clavulanate potassium, 250-500 mg PO q8h, or Ampicillin-sulbactam, 1.5 g IV q6h
Animal bite†	Gram-positive cocci, anaerobes, P. multocida	Cefazolin, 1 g IV q8h, plus penicillin, 2-4 million U IV q4-6h	Nafcillin, 1-2 g, plus penicillin, 2-4 million U q4-6h, or Amoxicillin-clavulanate potassium, 250-500 mg PO q8h, or Ampicillin-sulbactam, 1.5 g IV q6h
Diabetes related	Gram-positive cocci, gram-negative rods	Cefazolin, 1 g IV q8h, plus gentamicin*	Cefoxitin, 2 g IV q6h, or Ampicillin-sulbactam, 1.5 g IV q6h
Osteomyelitis	S. aureus, Streptococcus, (rarely) gram-negative rods	Cefazolin, 1 g IV q8h, plus gentamicin*	Nafcillin, 2 g IV q4h, or Vancomycin, 1 g IV q12h, or Clindamycin, 600-900 mg IV q8h, or Doxycycline, 100 mg PO q12h
Septic arthritis	S. aureus, Streptococcus (Neisseria gonorrhoeae)	Cefazolin, 1 g IV q8h, or Ceftriaxone, 1 g IV q24h (for N. gonorrhoeae)	Nafcillin, 2 g IV q4h, or Vancomycin, 1 g IV q12h, or Clindamycin, 600-900 mg IV q8h, or Doxycycline, 100 mg PO q12h
Traumatic, contaminated wound‡	S. aureus, Streptococcus, anaerobes, gram-negative rods	Imipenem, 0.5-1.0 g IV q6h	Cefazolin, 1 g IV q8h plus gentamicin*

*Loading dose, 2 mg/kg of body weight; then follow serum levels.
†Consider rabies prophylaxis.
‡Consider tetanus prophylaxis.
From Abrams RA, Botte MJ: Hand infections: treatment recommendations for specific types. J Am Acad Orthop Surg 4:219-230, 1996.

antibiotics are adequate. Oral antibiotics of choice are nafcillin, dicloxacillin, and cephalexin; erythromycin can be used for penicillin-allergic patients. If improvement is not noted in 48 hours or if the infection is more severe, intravenous antibiotics (cefazolin or vancomycin for penicillin-allergic patients) are initiated. The patient is observed closely in the hospital, and the possibility of a deeper infection is again considered. Once resolution is noted, oral antibiotics are given for 7 to 10 days.

SUBCUTANEOUS ABSCESS

A subcutaneous abscess typically occurs after a puncture wound or in response to a retained foreign body. Clinical findings include those described for cellulitis as well as an area of fluctuation. Treatment involves incision and drainage of the localized abscess and removal of any foreign material. Cultures are obtained before antibiotic administration, and the wound is packed open to encourage continued drainage. The hand is immobilized and elevated. The packing is removed 12 to 24 hours after incision and drainage, and whirlpools, soaks, or moist to dry dressing changes are started twice daily. The wound is allowed to close by secondary intention. Depending on infection severity, either oral or intravenous antibiotics are initiated. The most common causative organism is S. aureus. A first-generation cephalosporin is the antibiotic of choice. If the puncture wound occurred in a farm setting (or other contaminated environment), penicillin is added to cover clostridia.

◆ **Table 11-2**

SUMMARY GUIDE TO TETANUS PROPHYLAXIS IN ROUTINE WOUND MANAGEMENT, 1991

History of Absorbed Tetanus Toxoid (doses)	Clean, Minor Wounds		All Other Wounds*	
	Td†	TIG	Td†	TIG
Unknown or <3	Yes	No	Yes	No
≥3‡	No§	No	No‖	No

*Such as, but not limited to, wounds contaminated with dirt, feces, soil, and saliva; puncture wounds; avulsions; and wounds resulting from missiles, crushing, burns, and frostbite.

†For children <7 years old; DPT (DT, if pertussis vaccine is contraindicated) is preferred to tetanus toxoid alone. For persons ≥7 years of age, Td is preferred to tetanus toxoid alone.

‡If only three doses of *fluid* toxoid have been received, then a fourth dose of toxoid, preferably an adsorbed toxoid, should be given.

§Yes, if >10 years since last dose.

‖Yes, if >5 years since last dose. (More frequent boosters are not needed and can accentuate side effects.)

Td, tetanus and diphtheria toxoids; TIG, tetanus immune globulin (human).

Modified from MMWR Morb Mortal Wkly Rep 40(RR-10):1, 1991.

In diabetic patients and intravenous drug users, the organisms most commonly involved are *Streptococcus* and *Staphylococcus*. In addition to a first-generation cephalosporin, gram-negative coverage (gentamicin) must be provided.

OSTEOMYELITIS

Open fractures are the most common cause of osteomyelitis in the hand. The frequency ranges from 1% to 11% and is highly dependent on the degree of damage to the soft tissue envelope. Less frequently, bone infections are iatrogenic, caused by such procedures as open or percutaneous stabilization of closed fractures and placement of external fixator pins. On occasion, direct spread from a local soft tissue or joint infection or hematogenous spread can cause a bone infection. Bone infections may occur in patients with peripheral vascular disease or systemic illness such as diabetes, immune compromise, and intravenous drug or alcohol abuse.

Symptoms include persistent or recurrent swelling, erythema, pain, and sometimes drainage. Erythrocyte sedimentation rate, C-reactive protein level, and white blood cell count may be elevated. C-reactive protein level is more reliable than erythrocyte sedimentation rate for following the response to treatment. Radiographic changes include osteopenia and periosteal reaction (Fig. 11-1). These findings are usually not apparent when the patient first presents and tend to appear 2 to 3 weeks after the development of osteomyelitis. A sequestrum may be seen late. Sequential technetium-gallium scans and labeled white blood cell scans, such as indium-labeled leukocyte scans, are helpful in making the diagnosis. Magnetic resonance imaging may help define the presence and extent of the infection.

Antibiotics are sometimes used alone to treat osteomyelitis in its earliest stages. Most commonly, successful treatment is predicated on effective surgical débridement combined with intravenous antibiotics. If a sequestrum is present, débridement is required

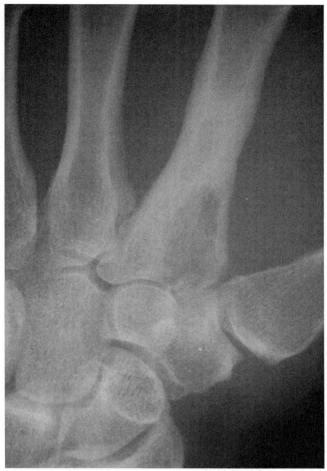

Figure 11-1 ◆ Anteroposterior radiograph of a hand depicting osteomyelitis of the index metacarpal base secondary to an external fixator. Note the osteopenia and periosteal new bone formation.

with removal of all necrotic bone. Antibiotic coverage is aimed initially at the most common organism, *S. aureus* (or another pathogen if the history indicates). It is then tailored according to culture results and clinical response. Once initial clinical improvement is documented, antibiotics are continued for 4 to 6 weeks on an outpatient basis, usually with a peripheral intravenous catheter. Normalization of the C-reactive protein level, wound status, and type of infecting organism are used to determine the length of antibiotic treatment.

In the case of an acute fracture with an associated infection and internal fixation in place, the fixation is maintained if the construct is stable and the fracture is not united. The internal fixation may be exchanged, or alternative fixation such as external fixation may be provided if the implant is not functional. If osteomyelitis develops in a healed fracture, the implant is removed and necrotic bone débrided. The goals of surgical management are to remove all necrotic tissue, to eradicate dead space, to provide healthy soft tissue coverage, to obtain fracture healing, and to restore function.

After the infection has been eliminated, reconstruction of bone defects may be required. Small defects less than 1.5 cm that are not required for structural stability may be treated with cancellous bone graft. Larger defects, in general greater than 1.5 cm and required for structural support, may require corticocancellous bone grafting after débridement or as a staged procedure. Staged reconstruction uses an antibiotic-impregnated polymethyl methacrylate spacer to fill dead space and local antibiotic. The second-stage reconstruction of the bone defect is considered when there is no evidence of persistent infection, which in general is 4 to 6 weeks after the first stage.

SEPTIC ARTHRITIS

As in other joints, septic arthritis in the hand can have permanent, detrimental effects if untreated. Cartilage destruction is mediated by bacterial toxins and enzymes produced primarily by the bacteria and the synovial and reticuloendothelial cells. Further damage occurs as the joint pressure increases, impeding synovial blood flow. A joint infection may be caused by direct trauma (see "Human Bites") as well as by local or hematogenous spread. In an adult, hematogenous spread most frequently occurs in an individual already weakened by systemic disease.

Patients with a septic joint complain of pain that is significantly aggravated by joint motion. Swelling, erythema, joint line tenderness, and severe pain with active and passive motion as well as with axial loading are classic findings on physical examination. Diagnosis is confirmed by joint aspiration. There is usually more fluid present than would normally be expected, and the aspirate is cloudy or thick. Fluid analysis indicates more than 50,000 white blood cells with an increased percentage of polymorphonuclear lymphocytes (>75%), decreased glucose levels (40 mg less than the fasting blood glucose level), and sometimes the presence of bacteria on Gram stain (Table 11-3). The fluid should be examined for crystals to rule out gout and pseudogout (see "Mimickers of Hand Infections"). However, the presence of crystals does not preclude a simultaneous septic process. Radiographs may reveal a foreign body or associated bone injury. In the early stages of an infection, radiographs may show a widened joint space. Late changes include loss of joint space due to the cartilage destruction.

S. aureus is the most common organism isolated in septic arthritis of the hand and wrist. *Streptococcus* species are the second most common pathogens isolated. In pediatric patients, *Haemophilus influenzae* should also be considered, but is rare since the advent of routine immunization.

The most common cause of atraumatic septic arthritis among patients younger than 30 years and sexually active patients is *Neisseria gonorrhoeae*. The disease is four times more common in women than in men and typically begins with low-grade fever, chills, and migratory polyarthralgia. In less than 50% of these patients does true septic monarticular arthritis develop.

Nongonococcal septic arthritis must be surgically decompressed in an urgent fashion to protect the integrity of the joint. The joint is thoroughly irrigated, necrotic tissue is débrided, and either the wound is left open or a drain is placed. Not infrequently, repeated irrigation is needed 48 hours later. Serial joint aspiration is not an effective method of treatment for septic arthritis in the joints of the hand.

Adequate irrigation can be accomplished arthroscopically for wrist joint infections. More severe infections are best eradicated by a formal open technique. The radiocarpal joint is drained from the dorsum, usually between the third and fourth extensor compartments. After irrigation and débridement, the wound can be left open to heal by secondary intention. If there is little concern for recurrent infection, the wound may be closed primarily to prevent articular desiccation.

The metacarpophalangeal joints are approached and drained through a dorsal longitudinally oriented incision just off the extensor tendon. The sagittal band is incised and the joint capsule is opened dorsal to the collateral ligament. The proximal interphalangeal joint may be released with a dorsal incision between the lateral band and central slip. The central slip must be protected to prevent a boutonnière deformity. Alternatively, the proximal interphalangeal joint may be drained by a midaxial incision. The joint is entered through the accessory collateral ligament. The distal interphalangeal joint may be released through a dorsal approach, incising the capsule adjacent to the terminal tendon while protecting the extensor mechanism to prevent a mallet deformity. Alternatively, a midaxial incision may be

◆ Table 11-3			
JOINT FLUID ANALYSIS			
Types of Arthritis	**White Blood Cell Count**	**Polymorphonuclear Leukocytes (%)**	**Other Joint Fluid Characteristics**
Noninflammatory	<500	25	Glucose and protein equal to serum values
Inflammatory	2,000–75,000	50	↓Glucose
			+Crystals (for gout and pseudogout)
Infectious	>50,000	>75	Thick or cloudy fluid
			↓Glucose
			↑Protein
			+Gram stain
			+Cultures

From Brinker MR: Basic science. In Miller MD, Brinker MR, eds: Review of Orthopaedics, 3rd ed. Philadelphia, WB Saunders, 2000.

performed as for the proximal interphalangeal joint. The thumb metacarpophalangeal and interphalangeal joints are approached in a similar fashion.

Whirlpools, in combination with gentle range-of-motion exercises, and moist to dry dressing changes are started 24 hours after surgery. If postoperative drainage is accomplished by a drain rather than an open wound, it is often left in place for 48 hours. The splint is discontinued as the wrist pain decreases with range of motion. Empirical antibiotics cover the common gram-positive organisms, unless circumstances indicate another likely pathogen. Intravenous antibiotics should be used until there are signs of clinical improvement. Intravenous or oral antibiotics are continued for 2 to 4 weeks.

Gram-negative rods, anaerobic organisms, polymicrobial infection, associated osteomyelitis or bacteremia, and longer duration of infection are associated with a worse outcome.

Arthritis caused by *N. gonorrhoeae* is usually treated nonsurgically. Intravenous ceftriaxone is the first line of therapy, sometimes accompanied by joint aspirations. After initial clinical improvement, oral antibiotics are used for an additional 7 to 10 days, depending on the severity of the infection.

NECROTIZING FASCIITIS

Necrotizing fasciitis is a severe, life- and limb-threatening infection of soft tissues often stemming from a small laceration or other insult to the extremity. Reported mortality rates range from 8% to 33%. Indigent patients who abuse intravenous drugs or alcohol are included in the at-risk population. A single organism, usually group A beta-hemolytic streptococcus, is identified in approximately 50% of cases. *S. aureus* and anaerobes may also be present.

This infection is extremely painful and rapidly progressive. It is characterized by poorly demarcated erythema, marked nonpitting edema, and shiny skin. Within a few days of onset, occlusion of the vessels supplying the skin results in patches of skin discoloration and bullae. At that point, necrotizing fasciitis begins to spread rapidly during a period of hours, dissecting along fascial planes and liquefying fat. Dissection along normally tough fascial planes in the digit is possible as well. Because skin and muscle are not primarily involved, the infection may extend well beyond the apparent zone of injury. Typical signs of infection may not be obvious early, although an increased white blood cell count is often present. As the infection develops, systemic effects occur, including disseminated intravascular coagulopathy and shock. The diagnosis should be suspected in patients with extreme pain, clinical examination findings consistent with cellulitis, and hemodynamic instability. Radiographs may reveal gas in the involved soft tissues.

Treatment is predicated on prompt recognition, early administration of antibiotics, and radical surgical débridement. The single most important factor affecting morbidity and mortality is early and adequate surgical débridement. Fibrinous, necrotic tissue, liquefaction of subcutaneous fat, and thin and watery, foul-smelling fluid ("dishwater pus") are characteristic surgical findings.

Multiple débridements are frequently required, and sometimes amputation is needed. Antibiotics should be started immediately, even before culture specimens are taken. Empirical antibiotics must include coverage of gram-positive organisms (cephalosporin), gram-negative organisms (gentamicin), and anaerobes (penicillin). Patients older than 50 years, with an underlying chronic illness or diabetes, and involvement of the trunk have the poorest prognosis.

GANGRENE

Gas Gangrene

Gas gangrene, or myonecrosis, is usually caused by a clostridial species, most often *Clostridium perfringens*. Clostridia are anaerobic, gram-positive rods. A low redox potential and low oxygen tension, such as is found with the combination of devitalized tissue and blood, provide the optimal conditions for clostridia to thrive and to produce toxins. Alpha toxin is primarily responsible for myonecrosis and hemolysis. Kappa toxin (destroys blood vessels), theta toxin (cardiotoxic), and others have local as well as systemic effects. Hydrogen sulfide and carbon dioxide are byproducts that help facilitate spread of the infection by dissection through soft tissue planes.

This infection often begins with an open wound associated with significant devitalized tissue, as would occur after a severe crush injury. Dirty wounds, especially from a farm injury, that are prematurely closed are at particular risk. Gangrene usually develops 1 to 4 days after the initial injury. The skin becomes edematous and bronze, and blebs and hemorrhagic bullae develop. Gram stain of the characteristic serosanguineous drainage reveals gram-positive rods. Pain increases quickly as the infection spreads, often within hours. Palpation of the soft tissues reveals crepitation caused by subcutaneous gas. This gas may be visible on radiographs. Septic shock can develop in a short period of time.

Wounds must be properly cleansed, with removal of all devitalized tissue, and left open to drain. Antibiotic prophylaxis is required for crush injuries associated with tissue necrosis and open fractures. In addition, in patients with wounds contaminated by soil, especially those with farm injuries, penicillin should be added to the drug regimen. Once myonecrosis has begun, treatment includes prompt, aggressive surgical débridement in combination with intravenous antibiotics, fluid management, and systemic support. Hyperbaric oxygen is an effective adjuvant therapy.

Diabetic Gangrene

Nonclostridial gangrene occurs most commonly in patients with diabetes. At greatest risk are those diabetic patients with renal failure and an arteriovenous fistula. These infections are primarily polymicrobial.

The most effective approach is prevention through vigilant surveillance and early diagnosis and treatment. Treatment of established gangrene involves surgical débridement and broad-spectrum antibiotics tailored appropriately when the causative organisms are identified (fungal cultures are always obtained). Amputation is sometimes necessary to eliminate the infection or because the remaining tissue does not allow a functional digit.

Specific Locations

FINGERTIP

Paronychia

Paronychia is an infection beneath the eponychial fold (Fig. 11-2). It begins with disruption of the seal between the eponychial fold and the nail, allowing bacteria, most commonly *S. aureus,* to enter. This disruption usually results from manicures, artificial nails, hang nails, or nail biting. The infection begins dorsal to the nail and may spread superficially around the nail to the other side (runaround lesion), or it may progress volar to the nail, spreading to involve the pulp (see "Felon"). Effective treatment for very early cases includes warm soaks and oral antibiotics. Drainage provides more definitive treatment and is performed when an abscess is noted. Under metacarpal block anesthesia, the eponychial fold is separated from the nail. If a subungual abscess is noted, the involved portion of the nail is removed (usually less than 25%) after it is carefully separated from the underlying matrix by a small elevator (Fig. 11-3). The area is fully decompressed and irrigated. Incisions in the eponychial fold are rarely

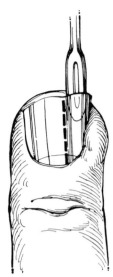

Figure 11-3 ◆ Surgical decompression of paronychia by elevation and removal of one fourth of the width of the nail plate. *(From Neviaser RJ: Acute infections. In Green DP, Hotchkiss RN, Pederson WC, eds: Green's Operative Hand Surgery, 4th ed. New York, Churchill Livingstone, 1999.)*

required and should be avoided. A sterile dressing is applied, sometimes with a thin slip of gauze to allow egress of purulent material. A protective splint may be used. The next day, the dressing is removed and twice-daily warm soaks are begun, followed by dry, sterile dressing changes.

Chronic paronychial infections result from repetitive and prolonged exposure to moisture. They are usually caused by *Candida albicans,* but atypical mycobacteria and gram-negative bacteria have been implicated. Inflammation and induration of the nail folds, retracted cuticles, periodic drainage, and nail grooving are characteristic findings. Patients are counseled to avoid moisture and to use antifungal agents. Secondary bacterial infections are common and may require removal of some of the nail or the entire nail in a manner as described before. Treatment of chronic paronychial infections can be frustrating because of recurrences. In refractory cases, débridement to remove the fungus and its byproducts followed by marsupialization is indicated. The procedure involves removal of a 3-mm-wide wedge-shaped piece of eponychium including skin and subcutaneous tissue proximal to the nail fold. The wound is allowed to heal by secondary intention.

Felon

A felon is a subcutaneous abscess in the fingertip. The fingertip is composed of a series of fascial septa running from the distal phalanx to the skin. These fascial bands define the poorly compliant compartments. An infection in this small, closed space results in rapid development of pain. Felons often follow a puncture wound or severe paronychia. The most common causative organism is *S. aureus.*

In the earliest cases, elevation, warm soaks, and oral antibiotics are effective. Surgical drainage is indicated when an abscess is evident. At this stage, treatment

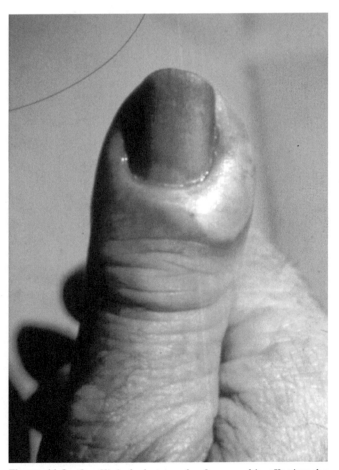

Figure 11-2 ◆ Clinical photograph of paronychia affecting the ulnar side of the nail fold.

needs to be relatively swift to prevent spread of the infection proximally to the distal phalanx, distal interphalangeal joint, or flexor sheath. If the infection is "pointing" on the volar surface, an oblique incision directly over that area on the digital pad is most effective. Otherwise, incisions over the volar, working surface of the digit are discouraged for fear of causing a neuroma and tender scar. The "workhorse" approach is through a midaxial, longitudinal incision on the ulnar side of the index, long, and ring fingers and on the radial side of the small finger and thumb (Fig. 11-4). Its exact position may be altered by the location of the infection. The incision is not carried around the tip of the digit because these "fish mouth" incisions can result in tip necrosis, especially in diabetic patients. Branches of the digital nerve are avoided while the pad is decompressed with a fine clamp or scissors, disrupting the fibrous septa so that all the small compartments of the fingertip can be decompressed. Care is taken not to probe into the flexor sheath and iatrogenically spread the infection. After irrigation, the wound is packed open and antibiotics are started. A protective splint is placed over the distal digit. The next day, the packing is removed and twice-daily soaks are begun.

Septic Flexor Tenosynovitis

Purulence within the flexor tendon sheath is one of the most dreaded hand infections. If left untreated, it can affect the precise gliding mechanism of the digit and cause tendon necrosis and rupture. *S. aureus* is the most common organism isolated, although *Streptococcus* and gram-negative organisms are also seen. A penetrating injury is the most common source of these organisms. Hematogenous spread can occur in gonococcal infections. Diagnosis is based on clinical criteria, specifically Kanavel's four cardinal signs (Table 11-4). Because contiguous spread is not uncommon, the anatomic relationship of the flexor sheaths to the deep spaces of the hand should be kept in mind in treating these infections (Fig. 11-5). The small finger flexor sheath becomes the ulnar bursa proximally, and similarly, the thumb flexor sheath is contiguous with the radial bursa.

◆ **Table 11-4**
KANAVEL'S FOUR CARDINAL SIGNS OF SEPTIC FLEXOR TENOSYNOVITIS
1. The finger rests in a flexed position
2. Tenderness over the course of the flexor sheath
3. Symmetric ("sausage-like") swelling of the finger
4. Pain with passive extension of the finger

The radial and ulnar bursae communicate at the level of the wrist in 50% to 80% of patients (see "Parona's Space"). The result may be a "horseshoe abscess."

Very early cases (<24 hours) can be treated nonoperatively with elevation, immobilization, intravenous antibiotics, and close observation. If improvement is not noted in 24 to 48 hours, surgical decompression is required. In fact, for most cases that present to the office or the emergency department, urgent drainage of the closed space is required. Two incisions are generally used, one oblique incision at the level of the distal palmar crease and a longitudinal midaxial incision at the level of the distal joint. The sheath is copiously irrigated in a flow-through manner. Care is taken to avoid extravasation of irrigant into the soft tissues. Excessive swelling of the digit can cause vascular compromise. On occasion, adequate irrigation of the sheath cannot be performed in this fashion because of loculation of pus or technical difficulties. In these cases,

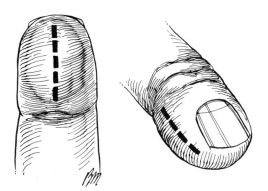

Figure 11-4 ◆ Preferred incisions for drainage of a felon. A longitudinal or slightly oblique volar incision may be used if the felon is "pointing" on the pad. The midaxial approach is the authors' preferred choice. (*From Neviaser RJ: Acute infections. In Green DP, Hotchkiss RN, Pederson WC, eds: Green's Operative Hand Surgery, 4th ed. New York, Churchill Livingstone, 1999.*)

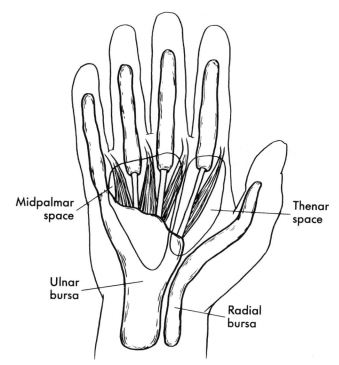

Figure 11-5 ◆ Flexor tendon sheaths and proximal extensions into the radial and ulnar bursae. Note the communication between the two bursae proximally at Parona's space. (*From Wright PE II: Hand infections. In Canale ST: Campbell's Operative Orthopaedics, 9th ed. St. Louis, Mosby, 1998; redrawn from Neviaser RJ, Gunther SF: Instr Course Lect 29:108, 1980.*)

the midaxial incision is extended and the sheath fully exposed. Brunner incisions over the volar digit risk coverage of the flexor tendons and make early motion more difficult and painful. If flow-through irrigation is achieved, a continuous postoperative irrigation system can be used. An angiocatheter is threaded into the theca through the proximal incision, checked for ease of irrigation, and sutured in place. A small Penrose drain is advanced into the tendon sheath through the distal incision to maintain adequate outflow. Sterile intravenous tubing connects the angiocatheter with a three-way stopcock. Fluff dressings are then applied with a resting hand splint. A bag of fluid and a syringe are attached to the remaining two ports of the stopcock. Postoperatively, 15 to 20 mL of fluid is flushed through the system four to six times per day for 48 hours. Irrigation is discontinued early if resistance is felt during fluid instillation or if the digit appears overly swollen or shows any sign of vascular compromise. The splint is removed in favor of whirlpools two to three times per day and functional rehabilitation. A resting hand splint is used until the infection clears.

Chronic tenosynovitis may result from infection by atypical bacteria, of which *Mycobacterium marinum* is the most common. Its clinical picture is quite different from acute septic tenosynovitis. This infection presents like rheumatoid tenosynovitis, with persistent or recurring synovitis of the finger. Usually, the digit or hand is chronically painful and swollen. A high index of suspicion in combination with tissue samples and mycobacterial cultures leads to the diagnosis (see "Mycobacterial Infection").

COLLAR-BUTTON ABSCESS

Patients with a collar-button or web space abscess present with abducted digits and pain, swelling, and erythema in the web space. The superficial transverse metacarpal ligament causes this abscess to assume a volar to dorsal hourglass configuration, hence the descriptive term collar-button abscess after the dumbbell-shaped old-fashioned collar buttons. This abscess forms from a distal palmar callus, blister, or fissure (often in laborers) or spreads from an infection in the proximal part of the finger. Because this infection is both volar and dorsal, two incisions are frequently needed. A transverse incision in the interdigital space causes web space contracture and should be avoided.

DEEP SPACE INFECTIONS

For deep space infections to be recognized and treated, it is critical to understand the anatomy of the potential spaces of the hand and their relationships to one another (Fig. 11-6). Infections are typically due to penetrating injury and can quickly spread to adjacent spaces. Urgent drainage, thorough irrigation, intravenous antibiotics, elevation, and immobilization are the critical components of successful management. The wound should be packed open, and 1 to 2 days later, soaks and rehabilitation are initiated. Each incision attempts to maximize surgical exposure while minimizing the possibility of surgical trauma to surrounding

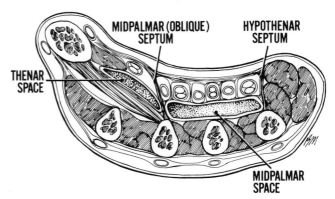

Figure 11-6 ◆ Potential midpalmar spaces. *(From Neviaser RJ: Acute infections. In Green DP, Hotchkiss RN, Pederson WC, eds: Green's Operative Hand Surgery, 4th ed. New York, Churchill Livingstone, 1999.)*

neurovascular structures and providing postoperative soft tissue coverage for tendons and nerves.

Midpalmar Space

The midpalmar space is defined by the long and ring finger metacarpals as well as by the second and third palmar interossei dorsally and the flexor tendons and lumbricals volarly. The fascia of the hypothenar muscles serves as the ulnar border, dividing the midpalmar space from the hypothenar space. The midpalmar septum, which runs vertically from the long finger metacarpal to the radial border of the long finger tendon sheath, acts as the radial border of the midpalmar space, dividing it from the thenar space. A midpalmar space infection usually follows penetrating trauma or contiguous spread from a long, ring, or (to a lesser extent) small finger flexor tenosynovitis. As with other deep space infections in the hand, marked dorsal hand swelling may divert the examiner's attention away from the palm, the true site of the infection. The midpalm is swollen, with loss of the normal palmar concavity in addition to tenderness and erythema. Passive motion of the long and ring fingers may be painful. Surgical débridement can be performed through transverse and oblique longitudinal incisions. A variety of incisions have been described (Fig. 11-7).

Thenar Space

The thenar space is bounded by the adductor pollicis dorsally, the index flexor tendon volarly, the midpalmar septum ulnarly, and the adductor insertion and thenar muscle fascia radially. The infection may extend from deep to the flexor tendons of the index finger over the adductor pollicis and first dorsal interosseous muscles, termed a dumbbell or pantaloon infection. Infection results from penetrating injuries or spreads from a septic process involving the index or thumb flexor sheath. In addition to erythema, tenderness, and swelling, patients present with a palmarly abducted thumb. Passive thumb adduction and opposition exacerbate the pain. Palmar, dorsal, and combined incisions for drainage have been described (Fig. 11-8). Release of the thenar space may require both volar and dorsal incisions to drain the dumbbell abscess fully. Incisions parallel to

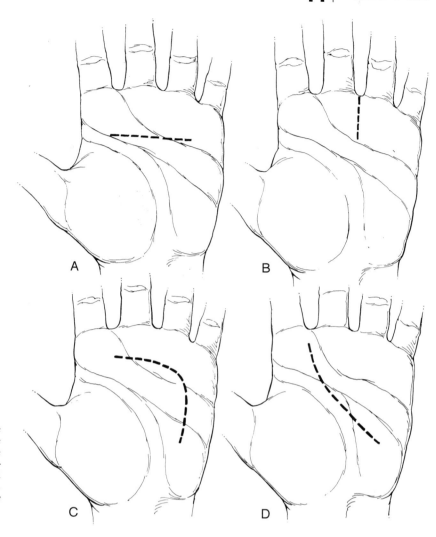

Figure 11-7 ◈ Surgical approaches for drainage of midpalmar space infections. **A,** Distal transverse incision. **B,** Approach to the midpalmar space through the lumbrical canal. **C,** Combined longitudinal and transverse approach. **D,** Longitudinal approach. *(From Neviaser RJ: Acute infections. In Green DP, Hotchkiss RN, Pederson WC, eds: Green's Operative Hand Surgery, 4th ed. New York, Churchill Livingstone, 1999.)*

the web commissure should be avoided to prevent web space contracture.

Hypothenar Space

Ulnar to the midpalmar space is the hypothenar space composed of the hypothenar muscles surrounded by their enveloping fascia. Hypothenar space infections are much less common than other deep space infections in the hand.

Parona's Space

Parona's space is the potential space bounded by pronator quadratus, digital flexors, flexor pollicis longus, and flexor carpi ulnaris. This space becomes infected by spread from either the radial or ulnar bursa and provides the "bridge" for development of a horseshoe abscess. A tender, erythematous fullness is palpable at the volar wrist crease level. Signs and symptoms of septic flexor tenosynovitis of the thumb or small finger and radial or ulnar bursa infection are likely (see "Septic Flexor Tenosynovitis"). Symptoms of median nerve irritation are frequently present. Incisions used for decompression are placed to protect the median nerve and its palmar cutaneous branch and to maintain

adequate postoperative soft tissue coverage for the median and ulnar nerves.

Dorsal Subaponeurotic Space

The dorsal subaponeurotic space is contained by the extensor tendons and fascia dorsally and the interosseous muscles and metacarpals palmarly. These are typically secondary to dorsal lacerations of the hand. In contrast to the other deep space infections, dorsal subaponeurotic space infections are accompanied by significant soft tissue swelling. Dorsal longitudinal incisions over the second and fourth metacarpals are used for drainage.

Atypical Organisms

Atypical organisms are defined as unusual organisms and opportunistic pathogens. There is more interest in these infections recently because of the growing numbers of immunocompromised patients.

ATYPICAL BACTERIAL INFECTIONS

Mycobacterial Infection

Mycobacterium tuberculosis infection can present as a nodular or pustular lesion that progresses to a draining

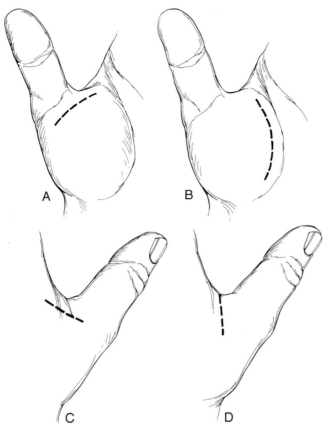

Figure 11-8 ◆ Surgical approaches for drainage of thenar space infections. **A,** Volar transverse approach, with digital nerves at potential risk. **B,** Thenar crease approach. **C,** Dorsal transverse approach. **D,** Dorsal longitudinal approach. *(From Neviaser RJ: Acute infections. In Green DP, Hotchkiss RN, Pederson WC, eds: Green's Operative Hand Surgery, 4th ed. New York, Churchill Livingstone, 1999.)*

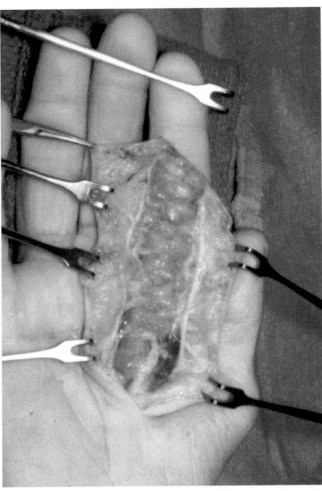

Figure 11-9 ◆ Severe tenosynovitis caused by a mycobacterial infection. *(From Wright PE II: Hand infections. In Canale ST: Campbell's Operative Orthopaedics, 9th ed. St. Louis, Mosby, 1998.)*

ulcer, unresponsive to routine antibiotics and wound care. It may arise as osteomyelitis, tenosynovitis, or dactylitis. Tubercular infections of the hand most commonly present as an extensor or flexor tenosynovitis; tubercular dactylitis occurs in children.

Atypical mycobacterial species include *Mycobacterium marinum, Mycobacterium kansasii, Mycobacterium terrae,* and *Mycobacterium avium-intracellulare. M. marinum* thrives in freshwater and saltwater environments. It is usually found in patients with injuries occurring around swimming pools, fish tanks, and fishing gear (see "Paronychia"). *M. kansasii, M. terrae,* and *M. avium-intracellulare* are frequently found in soil. These infections are uncommon, and when present, the hand is involved 75% of the time. Soft tissues, bones, and joints may be involved.

Because these infections are unusual, there are no pathognomonic physical findings, and onset is slow or prolonged. Mycobacterial infections are frequently missed and treatment is delayed. A chronically painful or swollen hand in a patient with progressive symptoms should raise suspicion, especially if the patient exhibits persistent or recurring tenosynovitis (Fig. 11-9) that worsens after a cortisone injection.

Work-up of a patient thought to have a mycobacterial infection includes examination for systemic disease, such as a chest radiograph and blood studies. Diagnosis requires tissue biopsy and culture. The tissue must be cultured on Löwenstein-Jensen medium at 32°C for *M. marinum* and 37°C for *M. tuberculosis.* Isolation of the bacteria may take 6 weeks. The organisms are fastidious, and false-negative results are common; therefore, multiple specimens are obtained. In addition, tissue samples should be sent for culture because swabs are often negative. At the time of biopsy, Ziehl-Neelsen staining is performed. A positive smear is consistent with acid-fast bacilli. All mycobacteria and nocardia are potentially acid-fast; therefore, a positive acid-fast stain is not solely consistent with a tubercular infection. Tissue is sent for histopathologic analysis, with granulomas representing the histologic hallmark of mycobacterial infections. In tuberculosis, the central portion of the granuloma is typically caseated.

Surgical débridement is an important component of the treatment. Synovial rice bodies are often found at the time of débridement. Frequently, extensive serial débridements are required in combination with long-term antibiotic administration. *M. tuberculosis* musculoskeletal infections are treated for a minimum of

9 months; chronic or complicated cases may require 18 months of therapy. Isoniazid, rifampin, streptomycin, ethambutol, and pyrazinamide may be used for tubercular infections. Minocycline is the antibiotic of choice for *M. marinum* infections, although combination therapy is often necessary and should be determined in conjunction with an infectious disease specialist.

Hansen's Disease (Leprosy)

Hansen's disease is a chronic infection caused by *Mycobacterium leprae*. The organism has a predilection for skin and nerve, particularly areas with lower temperature. Peripheral nerve injury is related to bacterial multiplication with the development of intraneural granuloma and perineural inflammation. This is characterized by patchy or regional anesthesia of thickened nerves (often the ulnar nerve at the elbow) and slightly hypopigmented macules. Patients with this infection may present to hand surgeons complaining of areas of diminished sensation, ulnar neuropathy symptoms, or disfiguring changes in the hands characteristic of leprosy and related to the neuropathy. The diagnosis is made by skin biopsy; acid-fast bacilli are found in skin slit smears. Nerve biopsy is performed only if the diagnosis is in doubt. There are two forms of the disease. The lepromatous form has symmetric involvement of the skin and nerves and has a poorer prognosis than the tuberculoid form, which has an asymmetric involvement.

Rifampin and dapsone are used to treat the disease. Treatment also includes splinting to prevent contractures and deformity. Precautions are taken to prevent injuries due to the insensate fingertips. The hands are kept warm. Surgical reconstruction may be required for ulnar and median nerve dysfunction. Tendon transfers are more difficult in these patients because of the progressive nature of the neuropathy, the poor sensation, and the limited available donor tendons. Management of the deformities is individualized.

FUNGAL INFECTIONS

Fungal infections in the hand may be broadly categorized into cutaneous, subcutaneous, and deep or systemic forms. Cutaneous lesions involve the skin or nails. Onychomycosis (tinea unguium) is a relatively common infection of the nail caused by dermatophytes such as *Trichophyton rubrum* and *C. albicans*. Individuals whose hands are constantly moist or wet are most susceptible. Early in the infection, there is thickening of the paronychium progressing to nail thickening, cracking, discoloration, and sometimes softening with eventual nail disintegration. This infection may be confused with nail deformities caused by psoriasis or vitamin deficiencies. Potassium hydroxide preparation of nail scrapings can confirm the diagnosis. Treatment consists of topical or oral antifungal agents. Unfortunately, onychomycosis is often refractory to treatment and has a high recurrence rate. In refractory cases, when the whole nail is involved or when a secondary bacterial infection is present, the nail is removed under a metacarpal block, and oral antifungal agents are used with an antibacterial medication if needed. Cure rates range from 57% to 80%.

Sporotrichosis is a subcutaneous infection caused by *Sporothrix schenckii*. The infection is found predominantly in people who work with plants, particularly roses. The rose thorn introduces the organism into the subcutaneous tissues. The initial papulonodular lesion ulcerates, and the infection spreads through lymphatic drainage. Regional lymph nodes enlarge and may ulcerate. Diagnosis is made by fungal culture. A saturated solution of potassium iodide is used as treatment. Itraconazole can also be used and is effective against lymphocutaneous disease. Even without the characteristic skin symptoms, sporotrichosis can become a deep infection and spread to bones and joints.

Deep fungal infections are usually coccidiomycosis, blastomycosis, or histoplasmosis. Opportunistic infections include aspergillosis, candidiasis, mucormycosis, and cryptococcosis. The route of inoculation is usually through the lungs with subsequent hematogenous spread. Treatment consists of amphotericin B and surgical débridement.

VIRAL INFECTIONS

Herpetic Whitlow

Caused by herpes simplex virus types 1 and 2, this infection is usually seen on the fingertips of young children or medical or dental personnel exposed to orotracheal secretions. Herpetic whitlow is characterized by vesicles (without pus) that coalesce into bullae, unroof, then ulcerate and eventually epithelialize. Systemic symptoms of fever, malaise, and lymphadenopathy are sometimes present. This painful infection begins 2 to 14 days after exposure and runs a self-limited course during several weeks. The patient is considered contagious until the lesions have healed. Immunosuppressed patients will experience a more prolonged course. These patients often require antiviral medication to resolve the infection. Recurrences are induced by a number of precipitants, especially stress, be it psychological or physical. Some patients may experience a prodrome of pain or paresthesias in the involved digit. Diagnosis is made by physical examination, culture of the fluid within the vesicles, analysis of the tissue with a Tzanck smear, and rise in antibody titers.

The treating physician can easily confuse herpetic whitlow with a paronychia or felon. Treatment of these pathologic processes is quite different. Herpetic whitlow subsides within weeks without specific medical or surgical therapy. If it is treated as a bacterial infection with incision and drainage, a superinfection is likely, and healing will be delayed. Herpes simplex infection is the most common infection in the hand in human immunodeficiency virus–positive patients.

Warts

Common warts (verruca vulgaris) and flat warts (verruca plana) are caused by human papillomaviruses. Common warts appear as a painless, raised, gray mass with an irregular surface. They are found alone or in groups that can coalesce into a larger wart. Treatment is usually sought for cosmetic reasons. There is a high rate of spontaneous regression, but it may take years. Although it is uncommon, physicians should look for signs of deeper spread or malignant transformation.

Treatment of patients with normal immune function is observation or topical therapies such as keratolytic agents.

Mimickers of Hand Infections

Several entities can mimic the infectious processes described and must be considered as part of the differential diagnosis.

CRYSTALLINE ARTHROPATHY

Gout and pseudogout (calcium pyrophosphate deposition disease) are inflammatory arthropathies that have a clinical presentation similar to that of septic arthritis. Involved joints are painful, erythematous, swollen, and tender. Differentiation is based on past medical history, radiographs, and especially arthrocentesis (see Table 11-3). The patient may have had similar "attacks" in the past, involving the metatarsophalangeal joint of the great toe or other joints. Chondrocalcinosis is sometimes seen on radiographs in patients with calcium pyrophosphate deposition disease. The triangular fibrocartilage of the wrist is a common location for ectopic calcification (Fig. 11-10). Under polarizing light, microscopic analysis of gouty joint fluid reveals monosodium urate crystals (strongly, negatively birefringent needle-shaped crystals), and aspirate from a joint with pseudogout shows calcium pyrophosphate crystals (weakly, positively birefringent rhomboid crystals). In both cases, the white blood cell count in the joint is moderately elevated, rarely reaching levels consistent with septic arthritis. A diagnosis of gout or pseudogout does not preclude a concurrent septic arthritis necessitating urgent surgical care (see "Septic Arthritis"). Therapy for crystalline arthropathy should include splinting and anti-inflammatory agents for symptomatic treatment until the acute episode subsides.

OTHERS

Pyogenic Granuloma

These lesions present as red, friable masses that can penetrate through the skin and can be prominent and dramatic in appearance (Fig. 11-11). Pyogenic granuloma may form in response to a penetrating wound or a retained foreign body. Treatment by cauterization with use of silver nitrate or surgical excision is curative.

Pyoderma Gangrenosum

This process is associated with several systemic diseases, such as ulcerative colitis and Crohn's disease. It presents as a small, painful ulcer that expands and undergoes central necrosis. Treatment includes biopsy, topical or systemic steroids, and evaluation for the systemic disease.

Neoplasia

Metastatic lesions to the hand can present with pain, inflammation, and ulceration similar to that seen in an infection.

Specific Sources

BITES

The hand is a common location of both human and animal bites. Bite wounds account for approximately 40% of hand infections. Management includes irrigation and débridement, prophylactic antibiotics, elevation, and immobilization. Wounds should be left open, and drainage should be encouraged with soaks or whirlpools.

Human Bites

Human bites most often occur when an aggressor strikes another individual in the mouth with a closed fist, a so-called fight bite. Direct contamination of the

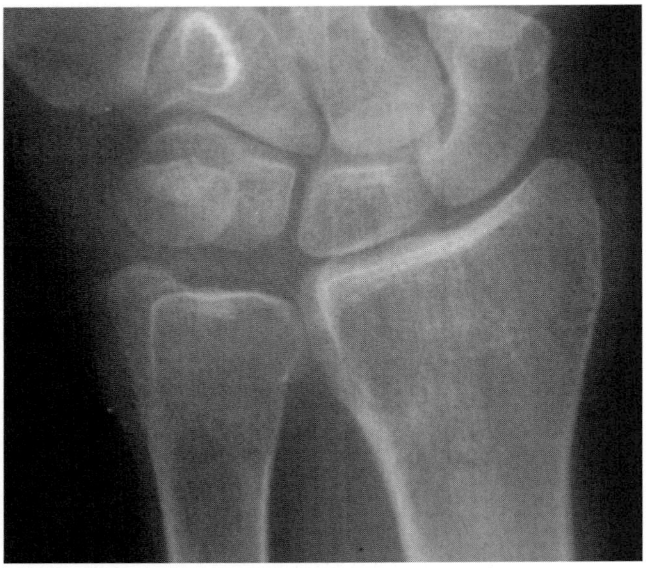

Figure 11-10 ❖ Anteroposterior wrist radiograph of a patient with pseudogout. Note the calcification of the triangular fibrocartilage.

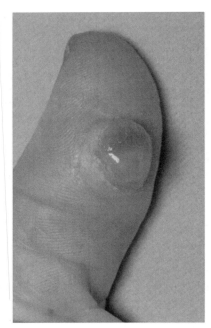

Figure 11-11 ❖ Characteristic appearance of a pyogenic granuloma involving the thumb.

metacarpophalangeal joint is common and communication of systemic infectious disease (e.g., HIV disease) is possible. Unfortunately, many patients who sustain a fight bite present more than 24 hours after the injury, once significant symptoms of an infection have developed. In all too many cases, even when presentation is timely, contamination of the joint goes unrecognized. A wound on the dorsum of the hand at the level of the metacarpophalangeal joint, no matter how small, should be considered a fight bite until proven otherwise (Fig. 11-12). When the zone of injury is explored with the joint in extension, distal tissues tend to glide proximally, sealing the joint. This makes it difficult to appreciate penetration of the joint capsule and creates a hospitable, anaerobic environment for bacterial growth (Fig. 11-13). Wound exploration is performed with the joint flexed as well as extended. In addition, injury to the extensor tendon can be missed because of proximal retraction of the site of injury with the digit in extension. Radiographs may reveal a fracture, cortical defect, or foreign body (e.g., a tooth).

Antibiotics should be administered after culture specimens are taken. Multiple organisms are often isolated from human bites. The most common organism cultured from human bites is *S. aureus* (alpha-hemolytic streptococcus is also common). *Eikenella corrodens* is cultured in 7% to 29% of human bites and must be cultured in 10% carbon dioxide medium and is susceptible to penicillin. *Bacteroides* species are the most common anaerobic bacteria cultured. Combination antibiotic treatment is necessary with ampicillin-sulbactam (Unasyn) administered intravenously or amoxicillin-clavulanate (Augmentin) administered orally. Other options for treatment include a combination of a cephalosporin and penicillin (intravenous or oral). For penicillin-allergic patients, a combination of clindamycin and a fluoroquinolone is typically effective. While tetracycline is effective against *E. corrodens*, it is avoided in children.

Animal Bites

Infections caused by animal bites commonly involve aerobic and anaerobic bacteria. Empirical antibiotics must cover both. In addition to more common pathogens, canine oral flora may contain *Pasteurella multocida, Streptococcus viridans,* and *Bacteroides* species. *P. multocida* is present in the mouths of 50% of domestic dogs and 65% of domestic cats and is the most common pathogen involved in infections. Special consideration should be given to rabies prophylaxis when the bite is inflicted by a bat, fox, skunk, coyote, raccoon, or bobcat or by a domestic animal exhibiting symptoms of rabies (Table 11-5). The frequency of the isolates from infections is as follows: alpha-hemolytic streptococcus, 46%; *P. multocida,* 26%; *S. aureus,* 13%; and anaerobes, 41%. Combination antibiotic treatment is necessary with ampicillin-sulbactam (intravenous) or amoxicillin-clavulanate (oral). Other options for treatment include a combination of a cephalosporin and penicillin (intravenous or oral). For penicillin-allergic patients, a combination of clindamycin and a fluoroquinolone is typically effective.

Dogs

Dog bites are the most common type of animal bite in the United States. The infection rate after a dog bite to the hand is approximately 30% or even higher for a severe contaminated crush injury. For most of these bites, the wound should be thoroughly irrigated, débrided, and left open. In the case of simple superficial bites treated acutely, the skin may be closed loosely. The most commonly isolated pathogen is alpha-hemolytic streptococcus. Prophylactic oral antibiotics such as amoxicillin-clavulanate should be given for these bites. In the case of established infection, treatment is similar to the treatment of human bites with antibiotics aimed at the relevant organisms and adjusted on the basis of culture and sensitivity results.

Cats

The organisms responsible for infection after a cat bite are similar to those mentioned for a dog bite. *P. multocida* is commonly cultured from cat bite wounds. Cat bites become infected more often (50% of cases) than dog bites do, partly because the puncture wounds are deeper and joints are more likely to be involved owing to the sharper, needle-like teeth of cats.

Cat-scratch disease occurs with a history of a scratch or a bite and usually presents in the pediatric population.

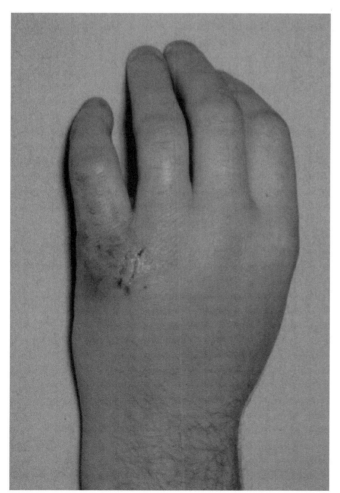

Figure 11-12 ◈ Typical appearance of a "fight bite." This laceration communicated with the small finger metacarpophalangeal joint.

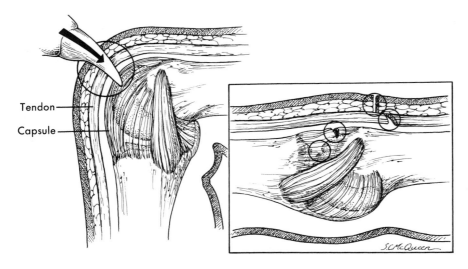

Tendon
Capsule

Figure 11-13 ◆ Schematic depiction of tendon and articular injury after a fight bite. The tendon retracts proximally with metacarpophalangeal joint extension, necessitating proximal exposure at the time of exploration. *(From Wright PE II: Hand infections. In Canale ST: Campbell's Operative Orthopaedics, 9th ed. St. Louis, Mosby, 1998.)*

It manifests itself as a small erythematous lesion, typically present for several weeks. *Rochalimaea henselae* is the infecting organism. Diagnosis is made by a combination of history, appearance, and regional lymphadenopathy as well as by a positive skin test result (presence of antibodies) or Gram stain showing the gram-negative, silver-staining bacilli. The disease is self-limited, but antibiotics are sometimes used.

OCCUPATIONAL INFECTIONS

Interdigital pilonidal cysts occur when a foreign piece of hair enters the web space and becomes secondarily infected. Barbers constitute an at-risk population (barber's interdigital pilonidal sinus), as do sheep shearers (shearer's disease). Milker's nodule (or granuloma) is caused by exposure to the poxvirus while handling a cow's udder during the milking process. Flat, reddish papules form. Within a week, these papules turn into reddish blue, firm, tender nodules surrounded by erythema. Lymphangitis is common. Spontaneous resolution of the lesion occurs within 1 to 2 months. Machine milking has made this a rare infection.

Fishermen can also be susceptible to algae infections, the most common being *Prototheca wickerhamii.* Algae infections respond to treatment with tetracycline. Freshwater catfish spine punctures involve envenomation and infection with aquatic organisms. Treatment should include spine removal, tetanus immunization, empirical antibiotic treatment, and wide débridement in cases with progressive necrosis.

POSTOPERATIVE INFECTIONS

Infections are unusual after elective hand surgery (1% to 7%; 0.47% deep infection rate after carpal tunnel release). When they do occur, they are most commonly caused by a gram-positive organism originating from

◆ **Table 11-5**

RABIES POSTEXPOSURE PROPHYLAXIS GUIDE—UNITED STATES, 1999

Animal Type	Evaluation and Disposition of Animal	Postexposure Prophylaxis Recommendations
Dogs, cats, ferrets	Healthy and available for 10 days' observation	Persons should not begin prophylaxis unless animal develops clinical signs of rabies*
	Rabid or suspected rabid	Immediate vaccination
	Unknown (e.g., escaped)	Consult public health records
Skunks, raccoons, foxes, and most other carnivores; bats	Regarded as rabid unless animal proven negative by laboratory tests†	Consider immediate vaccination
Livestock, small rodents, lagomorphs (rabbits and hares), large rodents (woodchucks and beavers), and other mammals	Consider individually	Consult public health officials. Bites of squirrels, hamsters, guinea pigs, gerbils, chipmunks, rats, mice, other small rodents, rabbits, and hares almost never require antirabies prophylaxis.

*During the 10-day observation period, begin postexposure prophylaxis at the first sign of rabies in a dog, cat, or ferret that has bitten someone. If the animal exhibits clinical signs of rabies, it should be euthanized immediately and tested.
†The animal should be euthanized and tested as soon as possible. Holding for observation is not recommended. Discontinue vaccine if immunofluorescence test results of the animal are negative.
From Talan DA, Moran GJ, Pinner RW: Update on emerging infections from the Centers for Disease Control and Prevention. Ann Emerg Med 33:590, 1999.

the patient's skin or scrubbed surgical personnel (their hands or their nasopharynx). Presentation is typically 3 to 7 days after surgery. The literature does not support the routine use of antibiotic prophylaxis in clean, elective hand procedures that last less than 2 hours.

The antibiotic chosen for prophylaxis should cover the organisms commonly involved in postoperative infections (*S. aureus* and *Staphylococcus epidermidis*) and have a low morbidity and expense. First-generation cephalosporins are favored for this purpose. Vancomycin is commonly used for patients allergic to cephalosporins or penicillin.

INFECTIONS IN POST-TRAUMATIC WOUNDS

The literature does not support the routine use of prophylactic antibiotics in healthy patients with uncomplicated soft tissue wounds without bone, joint, or tendon involvement that are treated acutely. No definitive studies exist concerning the use of antibiotics for more complex hand wounds that involve deeper tissues. The rate at which traumatic wounds become infected is dependent on injury factors such as the type and number of organisms introduced at the time of injury, the anatomic location of the wound, and the complexity of the injury. A wound with a high degree of tissue devitalization is more susceptible to infection.

Bibliography

GENERAL REFERENCES

Abrams RA, Botte MJ: Hand infections: treatment recommendations for specific types. J Am Acad Orthop Surg 4:219-230, 1996.
Jebson PJL, Louis DS, eds: Hand Infections. Hand Clinics 14, 1998.
Neviaser RJ: Acute infections. In Green DP, Hotchkiss RN, Pederson WC, eds: Green's Operative Hand Surgery, 4th ed. New York, Churchill Livingstone, 1999.
Ouellette EA: Infections. In Light TR, ed: Hand Surgery Update 2. Rosemont, Ill, American Academy of Orthopaedic Surgeons, 1999.
Patel MR: Chronic infections. In Green DP, Hotchkiss RN, Pederson WC, eds: Green's Operative Hand Surgery, 4th ed. New York, Churchill Livingstone, 1999.
Tetsworth KD: Infection. In Beaty JH, ed: Orthopaedic Knowledge Update 6. Rosemont, Ill, American Academy of Orthopaedic Surgeons, 1999.
Topper SM: Hand and microsurgery. In Miller MD, Brinker MR, eds: Review of Orthopaedics, 3rd ed. Philadelphia, WB Saunders, 2000.
Warner WC Jr: General principles of infection. In Canale ST: Campbell's Operative Orthopaedics, 9th ed. St. Louis, Mosby, 1998.
Wright PE II: Hand infections. In Canale ST: Campbell's Operative Orthopaedics, 9th ed. St. Louis, Mosby, 1998.

PROPHYLAXIS: SURGERY AND WOUNDS

Calkins ER: Nosocomial infections in hand surgery. Hand Clin 14:531-545, 1998.
Grossman JAI, Adams JP, Kunec J: Prophylactic antibiotics in simple hand lacerations. JAMA 245:1055-1056, 1981.
Hansen AD, Amadio PC, DeSilva SP, et al: Deep postoperative wound infection after carpal tunnel release. J Hand Surg Am 14:869-873, 1989.
Haughey RE, Lammers RL, Wagner DK: Use of antibiotics in the initial management of soft tissue hand wounds. Emerg Med 10: 187-192, 1981.
Hoffman RD, Adam BD: The role of antibiotics in the management of elective and post-traumatic hand surgery. Hand Clin 14:657-666, 1998.
Madsen MS, Neumann L, Andersen JA: Penicillin prophylaxis in complicated wounds of hands and feet: a randomized double blind trial. Injury 27:275-278, 1996.

Platt AJ, Page RE: Postoperative infection following hand surgery: guidelines for antibiotic use. J Hand Surg Br 20:685-690, 1995.
Roberts AHN, Teddy PJ: A prospective trial of prophylactic antibiotics in hand lacerations. Br J Surg 64:394-396, 1977.
Shapiro DB: Postoperative infection in hand surgery: cause, prevention and treatment. Hand Clin 10:1-12, 1994.
Thirlby RC, Blair J, Thal ER: The value of prophylactic antibiotics for simple lacerations. Surg Gynecol Obstet 156:212-216, 1983.
Turbiak TW, Reich JJ: Bacterial infections. In Rosen P, ed: Emergency Medicine: Concepts and Clinical Practice, 4th ed. St. Louis, Mosby, 1998.

PATIENT MEDICAL ISSUES

Ching V, Ritz M, Song C, et al: Human immunodeficiency virus infection in an emergency hand service. J Hand Surg Am 21:696-699, 1996.
Gunther SF, Gunther SB: Diabetic hand infections. Hand Clin 14: 647-656, 1998.
Pinzur MS, Bednar M, Weaver F, et al: Hand infections in the diabetic patient. J Hand Surg Br 22:133-134, 1997.

PARONYCHIA

Bednar MS, Lane LB: Eponychial marsupialization and nail removal for surgical treatment of chronic paronychia. J Hand Surg Am 16:314-317, 1991.

OSTEOMYELITIS

Barbieri RA, Freeland AE: Osteomyelitis of the hand. Hand Clin 14: 589-603, 1998.
Boutin RD, Brossmann J, Sartoris DJ, et al: Update on imaging of orthopaedic infections. Orthop Clin North Am 29:41-66, 1998.

SEPTIC ARTHRITIS

Murray PM: Septic arthritis of the hand and wrist. Hand Clin 14:579-587, 1998.
Scopelitis E, Martinez-Osuna P: Gonococcal arthritis. Rheum Dis Clin North Am 19:363-377, 1993.

NECROTIZING FASCIITIS AND GANGRENE

Ellis ME, Mandel BK: Hyperbaric oxygen treatment: 10 years' experience of a regional infectious disease unit. J Infect 6:17-28, 1983.
Fontes RA Jr, Ogilvie CM, Miclau T: Necrotizing soft-tissue infections. J Am Acad Orthop Surg 8:151-158, 2000.
Freeland AE, Senter BS: Septic arthritis and osteomyelitis. Hand Clin 5:533-552, 1989.
Gonzalez MH: Necrotizing fasciitis and gangrene of the upper extremity. Hand Clin 14:635-645, 1998.
Hart GB, Lamb RC, Strauss MB: Gas gangrene: a collective review. J Trauma 23:991-1000, 1983.
Hausman MR, Lisser SP: Hand infections. Orthop Clin North Am 23:171-185, 1992.
Tibbles PM, Edelsberg JS: Hyperbaric oxygen therapy. N Engl J Med 334:1642-1648, 1996.

SEPTIC FLEXOR TENOSYNOVITIS

Neviaser RJ: Closed tendon sheath irrigation for pyogenic flexor tenosynovitis. J Hand Surg 3:462-466, 1978.

MYCOBACTERIAL, FUNGAL, AND VIRAL INFECTIONS

Hitchcock TF, Amadio PC: Fungal infections. Hand Clin 5:599-611, 1989.
Hoyen HA, Lacey SH, Graham TJ: Atypical hand infections. Hand Clin 14:613-634, 1998.
Kozin SH, Bishop AT: Atypical *Mycobacterium* infections in the upper extremity. J Hand Surg Am 19:480-487, 1994.
Louis DS, Silva J Jr: Herpetic whitlow: herpetic infections of the digits. J Hand Surg 4:90-94, 1979.

MIMICKERS OF HAND INFECTIONS

Bennett CR, Brage ME, Mass DP: Pyoderma gangrenosum mimicking postoperative infection in the extremities. J Bone Joint Surg Am 81:1014-1018, 1999.
Louis DS, Jebson PJL: Mimickers of hand infections. Hand Clin 14:519-529, 1998.

BITES

Crown LA: Bites and stings. In Rakel RE, ed: Textbook of Family Practice, 6th ed. Philadelphia, WB Saunders, 2002.

Dire DJ, Hogan DE, Riggs MW: A prospective evaluation of risk factors for infections from dog-bite wounds. Acad Emerg Med 1: 258-266, 1994.

Dolan MJ, Wong MT, Regnery RL, et al: Syndrome of *Rochalimaea henselae* adenitis suggesting cat scratch disease. Ann Intern Med 118:331-336, 1993.

Faciszewski T, Coleman DA: Human bite infections of the hand. Hand Clin 14:683-690, 1998.

Goldstein EJC, Citron DM, Wield B, et al: Bacteriology of human and animal bite wounds. J Clin Microbiol 8:667-672, 1978.

Gonzalez MH, Papierski P, Hall RF Jr: Osteomyelitis of the hand after a human bite. J Hand Surg Am 18:520-522, 1993.

Patzakis MJ, Wilkins J, Bassett RL: Surgical findings in clenched fist injuries. Clin Orthop 220:237-240, 1987.

Snyder CC: Animal bite infections of the hand. Hand Clin 14:691-711, 1998.

Snyder CC, Leonard LG: Bites and stings of the hand. In Tubiana R: The Hand. Philadelphia, WB Saunders, 1988.

Zubowicz VN, Gravier M: Management of early human bites of the hand: a prospective randomized study. Plast Reconstr Surg 88: 111-114, 1991.

PEDIATRIC HAND SURGERY

Congenital Anomalies

Congenital anomalies affect 1% to 2% of newborns, and approximately 10% of these children have upper extremity abnormalities. The physician involved in the care of these children must possess a basic understanding of embryogenesis, limb formation, and inheritance patterns. The sequencing of the human genome and investigation into the molecular basis of limb development have provided new information about the etiology of limb malformation. This information has already had an impact on the ability to diagnose and to manage certain congenital differences.

Embryology

The majority of upper extremity congenital anomalies occur during embryogenesis, which commences with formation of the upper limb bud on the lateral wall of the embryo 4 weeks after fertilization. The limb bud develops by migration and multiplication of the dorsal somatopleure (ectoderm and underlying undifferentiated somatic mesoderm) from the 8th to 10th somites to the lateral wall.

The limb develops proximal to distal under the direction of distinct signaling pathways that function in synchrony to ensure proper limb growth (Table 12-1). A thickened layer of ectoderm, the apical ectodermal ridge (AER), concentrates over the limb bud; this acts as a signaling center to guide the underlying mesoderm to differentiate into appropriate structures. The AER secretes proteins, such as fibroblast growth factors, that influence the development of the underlying tissues. Complete removal of the AER during embryogenesis yields a truncated limb similar to a congenital amputation. Removal of the preaxial portion of the AER produces anomalies similar to radial deficiency. The AER also disperses around the hand paddle as embryogenesis progresses, which results in longitudinal interdigital necrosis between the digits. Failure of the ridge to separate is the most prevalent explanation for syndactyly. Within the posterior margin of the limb bud resides an additional signaling center, the zone of polarizing activity (ZPA). This center is responsible for anterior to posterior (radioulnar) development and orientation. The signaling molecule within the ZPA is the Sonic hedgehog compound. Transplantation of the ZPA or

the Sonic hedgehog molecule to the anterior part of the developing chick limb bud results in duplication of the elements along the radioulnar axis. This radioulnar replication offers a plausible explanation for the mirror hand deformity (Fig. 12-1). The Wnt (wingless type) signaling pathway resides in the dorsal ectoderm and secretes factors that induce the underlying mesoderm to adopt dorsal characteristics (known as dorsalization of the limb). In a mouse model, inactivation of the Wnt pathway prevents dorsalization of the limb and results in ventral pads on both sides of the foot. The AER, ZPA, and Wnt pathways are all necessary for normal limb development during embryogenesis, which is complete by the eighth week when all limb structures are present. The fetal period then commences with differential growth of existing structures and continues until birth. Hand dominance can be defined at the end of the first year of life.

Classification of Limb Anomalies

A valuable classification system should provide diagnostic, therapeutic, and prognostic information. Adequate detail must be included to separate different types of congenital anomalies without making the system overly complex. There are numerous classification systems for upper extremity limb anomalies based on embryology, teratologic sequencing, and anatomy. Embryologic classifications define the defect according to malformation during limb development. Teratologic sequencing grades congenital anomalies according to the severity of expression. Anatomic classifications rank the malformation

✧ **Table 12-1**

SIGNALING PATHWAYS DURING EMBRYOGENESIS

Signaling Center	Responsible Substance	Action
Apical ectodermal ridge	Fibroblast growth factors	Proximal to distal limb development, interdigital necrosis
Zone of polarizing activity	Sonic hedgehog protein	Radioulnar limb formation
Wnt pathway		Dorsalization of the limb

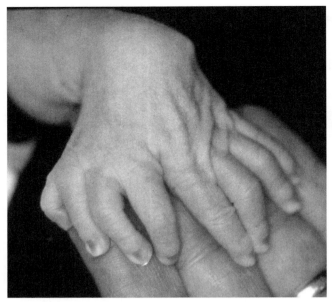

Figure 12-1 ❖ Mirror hand deformity attributed to transplantation of the zone of polarizing activity or the Sonic hedgehog molecule.

according to the degree of anatomic abnormalities or constellation of findings.

The most widely accepted classification of congenital limb anomalies is based on embryonic failure during development and relies on clinical diagnosis for categorization. Each limb malformation is classified according to the most predominant anomaly and placed into one of seven categories (Table 12-2). Varying degrees of damage within the limb bud explain the diverse clinical presentations of similar categories of embryonic failures. As our understanding of limb development advances, this classification system will most likely become outdated. Nonetheless, this scheme provides a useful framework to organize congenital anomalies of the upper extremity.

Failure of Formation

TRANSVERSE DEFICIENCIES

Group I is divided into transverse and longitudinal failures of formation. Transverse deficiencies are also called congenital amputations and are named according to the anatomic level of limb termination. The most frequent site of amputation occurs at the proximal third of the forearm and is referred to as a short below-the-elbow defect. Rudimentary digits or dimpling can be located on the end of the amputation stump and represent an attempt at limb recovery. These anomalies are usually unilateral, sporadic in occurrence, and rarely associated with other anomalies.

The most likely explanation for these deficiencies is disruption of the AER and subsequent limb truncation. A vascular insult to the AER during limb development appears probable. Early chorionic villous sampling and failed attempts at pregnancy termination by dilatation and curettage have been associated with transverse limb deficiencies, which lends further support to vascular disruption as an underlying cause.

The most important initial intervention is to provide the family with accurate information and resources. A prosthesis is initially fitted when independent sitting is achieved (usually 6 to 9 months of age) and consists of a passive device. Early fitting before 2 years of age increases the acceptance rate of upper limb prostheses. The other crucial variable that affects prosthetic wear is the family's acceptance and support. The child makes the transition to some form of body-powered prosthesis between 15 months and 2 years of age. The prosthesis of choice is a supracondylar socket, figure-of-nine harness, and voluntary opening terminal device. Myoelectric devices are usually introduced later (3 to 5 years of age) to ensure acceptance of a prosthesis and to encourage use of both a conventional and a myoelectric device. The conventional prosthesis is more durable and is often the preferred prosthesis for certain activities in adolescent and adult life. As the child develops and matures, prosthetic monitoring is necessary as the child's needs and expectations change (see Chapter 13).

Surgery is usually not indicated in short below-the-elbow transverse deficiencies. The stump is often well padded and can support a prosthesis without skin irritation or breakdown. On occasion, a small bone spicule or rudimentary nubbins can irritate the residual stump. Excision of the bone or removal of the nubbins can alleviate this problem. The use of limb lengthening for transverse deficiencies is controversial. At this level, an increase in limb length would not eliminate the use of a prosthesis, and the expected gains do not outweigh the risks. The Krukenberg procedure converts the forearm into a pincer apparatus by allowing the radius and ulna to function independently. This procedure is reserved for bilateral amputee patients with long forearms who are sight deficient and rely on sensory feedback for function. The Krukenberg procedure is also indicated for patients who reside in an impoverished country and who do not have access to prosthetic devices.

LONGITUDINAL DEFICIENCIES

Longitudinal deficiencies are designated according to bones that are partially or completely absent. In general, these deficiencies can be divided into radial (preaxial), ulnar (postaxial), and central forms. The central type includes deficiencies of the second, third, and fourth rays (digits and underlying carpus). There is considerable variability in the amount of insufficiency (i.e., phenotype), which is detailed in specific classification schemes based on teratologic sequencing and anatomic abnormalities.

Phocomelia

Phocomelia is another form of longitudinal deficiency characterized by an intercalary or intersegmental deficiency. The absent segment is variable but includes a portion of the limb between the shoulder and hand. In profound cases, the hand appears to be originating from the glenohumeral joint, producing an extremely shortened limb. Contemporary cases are usually sporadic

❖ Table 12-2

EMBRYOLOGIC CLASSIFICATION OF CONGENITAL ANOMALIES

Classification	Subheading	Subgroup	Category
I. Failure of formation	Transverse arrest		
	Longitudinal arrest	Radial deficiency	
		Ulnar deficiency	
		Central deficiency	
		Phocomelia	
II. Failure of differentiation	Synostosis		
	Radial head dislocation		
	Symphalangism		
	Syndactyly		
	Contracture	Soft tissue	Arthrogryposis
			Pterygium
			Trigger
			Absent extensor tendons
			Hypoplastic thumb
			Retroflexible thumb
			Camptodactyly
			Windblown hand
		Skeletal	Clinodactyly
			Kirner's deformity
			Delta bone
III. Duplication	Thumb		
	Triphalangism, hyperphalangism		
	Polydactyly		
	Mirror hand		
IV. Overgrowth			
V. Undergrowth			
VI. Constriction band syndrome			
VII. Generalized skeletal abnormalities			

in occurrence. Previously, thalidomide ingested during the first trimester of pregnancy was associated with phocomelia.

Radial Deficiency

Radial deficiency is a complex congenital anomaly that involves the entire limb and can be associated with systemic conditions (Table 12-3). The reported incidence varies between 1:55,000 and 1:100,000 live births. Radial deficiency is bilateral in 50% and slightly more common in boys than in girls (3:2). These children typically have normal intelligence. The majority of cases are sporadic without any definable cause. However, exposure to teratogens, such as thalidomide and radiation, can yield radial deficiencies. The incidence of radial deficiency within the same family is small, ranging from 5% to 10% of reported cases. Familial cases are often associated with Holt-Oram or thrombocytopenia absent radius syndrome (TAR—thrombocytopenia, Fanconi's anemia, absent radius [type IV], knee abnormalities).

The degree of deformity is related to the degree of AER malfunction, which explains the variable phenotype. The severity is graded I through IV and based on radiographic interpretation (Table 12-4). The observer must be aware that ossification of the radius is delayed in radial deficiency, and the differentiation between total and partial absence (types III and IV) cannot be established until approximately 3 years of age. A type I deficiency is the mildest expression characterized by mild shortening of the radius without considerable bowing. Minor radial deviation of the hand is apparent,

❖ Table 12-3

SYNDROMES ASSOCIATED WITH RADIAL DEFICIENCY

Syndrome	Characteristics
Holt-Oram	Heart defects, most commonly cardiac septal defects
TAR	Thrombocytopenia absent radius syndrome (Fanconi's anemia, knee abnormalities)
	Thrombocytopenia present at birth but improves over time
VACTERL	Vertebral abnormalities, anal atresia, cardiac abnormalities, tracheoesophageal fistula, esophageal atresia, renal defects, radial dysplasia, lower limb abnormalities
Fanconi's anemia	Aplastic anemia not present at birth; develops about 6 years of life
	Fatal without bone marrow transplantation
	Chromosome challenge test now available for early diagnosis

◆ Table 12-4		
CLASSIFICATION OF RADIAL DEFICIENCY		
Type	**Radiographic Findings***	**Clinical Features**

I
Short radius
	Distal radial epiphysis delayed in
	  appearance
	Normal proximal radial epiphysis
	Mild shortening of radius without bowing
		Minor radial deviation of the hand
		Thumb hypoplasia is the prominent
		  clinical feature requiring treatment

II† Hypoplastic	Distal and proximal epiphysis present Abnormal growth in both epiphyses Ulna thickened, shortened, and bowed	Miniature radius Moderate radial deviation of the hand

III†
Partial absence
	Partial absence (distal, middle, proximal)
	  of radius
	Absence of distal one to two thirds is
	  most common
	Ulna thickened, shortened, and bowed
		Severe radial deviation of the hand

IV† Total absence	No radius present Ulna thickened, shortened, and bowed	Most common type Severe radial deviation of the hand

*Because ossification of the radius is delayed in radial deficiency, the differentiation between total and partial absence (types III and IV) cannot be established until approximately 3 years of age.
†Centralization is indicated for types II, III, and IV.
Modified from Bayne LG, Klug MS: Long-term review of the surgical treatment of radial deficiencies. J Hand Surg Am 12:169-179, 1987.

although considerable thumb hypoplasia may be evident. A miniature radius with distal and proximal physeal abnormalities and moderate deviation of the wrist characterize a type II deficiency. A type III deficiency is partial absence of the radius, most commonly the distal portion, and severe wrist radial deviation. Complete absence of the radius is a type IV deformity and is the most common variant (Fig. 12-2).

Pathoanatomy

The most common type of radial deficiency (type IV) affects the entire limb. The scapula is often reduced in size, and the clavicle is shorter with an increased curvature. The humerus may or may not be shorter than expected; deficiencies of the capitellum and trochlea are common. Elbow motion is usually diminished more in flexion than in extension. The primary manifestations occur in the forearm segment and radial portion of the carpus and hand. The forearm is always decreased in length because the ulna is approximately 60% of the normal length at birth, and this discrepancy persists throughout the growth period. The ulna is thickened and frequently bowed toward the absent radius with an apex posterior direction. Forearm rotation is absent in partial or complete aplasia of the radius.

The wrist is positioned in radial deviation and will eventually develop a perpendicular relationship with the forearm (Fig. 12-3). This awkward position further shortens the limb and places the extrinsic flexors and extensors at a mechanical disadvantage. The articulation between the carpus and ulna is usually fibrous but can be lined by hyaline cartilage. Wrist motion is tangential and primarily occurs in the radial-ulnar and the flexion-extension planes. The carpal bones are delayed in ossification; the scaphoid and trapezium are often absent or hypoplastic. The status of the radial carpal bones is also related to the degree of thumb hypoplasia. The capitate, hamate, and triquetrum are usually present but may ossify late. The preaxial index and long fingers are often stiff and slender with limited motion at the metacarpophalangeal and interphalangeal joints. The postaxial ring and small digits are less affected.

The forearm demonstrates the most severe musculotendinous abnormalities, primarily in muscles that originate at or attach to the radius, such as the pronator

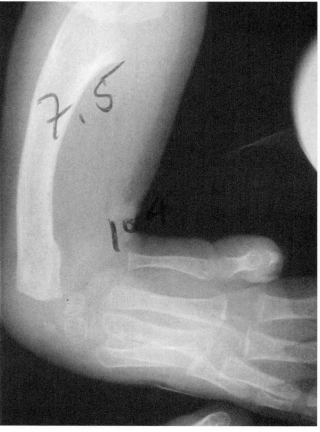

Figure 12-2 ◆ Complete absence of the radius is the most common type of radial deficiency.

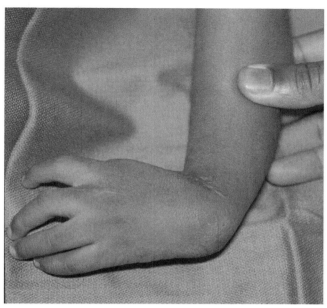

Figure 12-3 ❖ Severe radial deviation associated with complete absence of the radius.

teres, flexor carpi radialis, palmaris longus, flexor pollicis longus, pronator quadratus, and supinator. The radial wrist extensors (extensor carpi radialis longus and brevis) are frequently absent or fused. The extrinsic flexors and extensors of the fingers have abnormal origins and insertions. The flexor and extensor carpi ulnaris, as well as the interossei, lumbricals, and hypothenar muscles, are often normal. The abnormalities of the thumb muscles (extrinsic and intrinsic) are related to the degree of thumb hypoplasia.

The vascular anatomy demonstrates a normal brachial and ulnar artery. The radial artery is often absent, and the interosseous arteries are well developed. The ulnar nerve is normal, whereas the radial nerve usually terminates at the elbow. An enlarged median nerve substitutes for its absence and supplies a large dorsal branch for sensation to the radial aspect of the hand. This branch is positioned in the fold between the wrist and forearm, and an appreciation of this subcutaneous location is critical during surgical incision along the radial aspect of the wrist.

Goals, Indications, and Contraindications
The basic goals of treatment are to correct the radial deviation of the wrist, to balance the wrist on the forearm, to maintain wrist and finger motion, to promote growth of the forearm, and to improve the function of the extremity. The wrist assumes severe radial deviation, which shortens an already undersized forearm, places the extrinsic flexor and extensor tendons at an unfavorable angle, and creates tremendous functional deficits. The functional impairment is far greater in bilateral than in unilateral cases. The digital abnormalities also require consideration during formulation of a treatment plan because stiff fingers and a deficient thumb will hamper prehension and create an additional functional handicap. A hypoplastic or absent thumb also requires specific treatment because thumb function directly correlates with use of the extremity.

The radial deviation deformity is treated by a combination of nonoperative and operative management that begins shortly after birth. Passive stretching of the taut radial structures is instructed at the initial visit and performed at each diaper change and at bedtime. Splint fabrication is difficult in the newborn with a shortened forearm and is usually delayed until the forearm is long enough to accommodate a splint. Centralization remains the principal procedure to realign the carpus onto the distal ulna and is indicated in types II, III, and IV radial deficiencies in patients with a functional elbow joint. Surgical intervention is contraindicated for children with a limited life expectancy, in mild deformity with adequate support for the hand (type I), with an elbow extension contracture that prevents the hand from reaching the mouth, and for adults who have adjusted to their deformity.

The surgery is performed at about 1 year of age after extensive preoperative therapy to stretch the taut radial structures. Centralization is usually performed with two incisions. A zigzag radial incision is used for radial exposure and Z-plasty skin lengthening after centralization. The enlarged median nerve and its anomalous dorsal branch must be identified in the skinfold at the wrist. Aberrant preaxial musculotendinous units and anomalous contracted fibrous bands are identified and released to allow adequate passive correction of the carpus to a neutral position.

A second incision begins at the midline of the dorsal wrist and extends in an ulnar direction. The incision is elliptical to expose the carpus and excises the redundant skin and subcutaneous tissue. The carpus is reduced onto the distal ulna for centralization. Failure to achieve reduction requires repeated examination of the radial structures for any persistent contracted or fibrotic tissue. In severe cases, adequate reduction cannot be obtained and alternative measures are necessary. Surgical options include carpectomy, limited shaving of the distal ulna epiphysis, and application of an external fixator followed by postoperative distraction and delayed formal centralization. In fact, many cases of radial deficiency are treated with preliminary soft tissue distraction (i.e., external fixation) before centralization to facilitate carpal reduction.

The soft tissues are balanced by dorsal capsular reefing, distal advancement of the extensor carpi ulnaris insertion, and transfer of the flexor carpi ulnaris to the dorsum of the wrist. These techniques redirect the palmar and radial deviating forces to resist recurrence. The wrist is held in position by a Kirschner wire. Ulnar angulation of more than 30 degrees requires a diaphyseal closing wedge osteotomy performed at the apex of the deformity. The Kirschner wire is extracted 8 to 12 weeks after surgery. A splint is made and removed for exercises, with gradual weaning from the splint. A nighttime splint regimen is encouraged until skeletal maturity.

Numerous technical modifications and advancements have been proposed to sustain a well-aligned wrist position, including correction of the ulnar bow, radialization or overcorrection of the carpus, tendon transfer, capsular plication, and prolonged pin fixation. Even microvascular free toe transfer to support the radial side of the wrist with a growing part has been advocated. The toe proximal phalanx is fused to the base of the second metacarpal, and the proximal metatarsal is affixed to the side of the distal ulna. This joint transplantation avoids direct manipulation of the ulnocarpal joint, and growth is at a rate similar to that of the adjacent ulna. Unfortunately, no method reliably and permanently corrects the radial deviation, balances the wrist, and allows continued growth of the forearm. Currently, the maintenance of the carpus on the end of the ulna without sacrificing wrist mobility or stunting forearm growth remains a daunting task. Recurrence after centralization is the most common source of failure, and the cause appears multifactorial. Operative causes include inability to obtain complete correction at surgery, inadequate radial soft tissue release, and failure to balance the radial force. Postoperative reasons consist of early pin removal, poor postoperative splint use, and natural tendency of the shortened forearm and hand to deviate in a radial direction for hand to mouth use.

The management of recurrent deformity must be individualized to the patient and the specific deformity. The indications for a revision procedure have yet to be clearly defined. Surgery is offered to patients and family interested in correction of the deformity and willing to comply with an arduous postoperative course. Distraction histogenesis by an external fixator is usually part of the treatment regimen, and preoperative education is critical. This form of sophisticated treatment introduces additional complications, such as pin track infection, fracture of the regenerate bone, and digital stiffness, that require discussion before surgery. Chondrodesis or arthrodesis of the ulnocarpal joint can be considered in certain instances. Indications include a wrist with limited motion or a recurrence after revision surgery. The obvious downside to wrist fusion is a permanent loss of wrist mobility; careful assessment of hand use and compensatory motion is mandatory before this procedure. A functional evaluation by a therapist is a valuable preoperative tool. Painstaking measures should be taken to ensure that there will be no loss of function after wrist fusion.

Ulnar Deficiency

Ulnar deficiency is a failure of formation or longitudinal deficiency of the postaxial border of the upper extremity. Most cases are sporadic, nonhereditary, and without a definable cause. Ulnar deficiency is an uncommon anomaly, and the ratio between radial and ulnar deficiency ranges from 4:1 to 10:1. In contrast to radial deficiencies, ulnar deficiencies are associated with elbow deficiencies, musculoskeletal system anomalies (club feet, syndactyly), and not systemic abnormalities. The classification of this deficiency is based on the amount of ulna remaining and the degree of deformity (Table 12-5). A type I deficiency is a hypoplastic ulna with a proximal and distal epiphysis; a type II deficiency is absence of the distal or middle third of the ulna; a type III deficiency is total agenesis of the ulna; and a type IV deficiency is fusion of the radius to the ulna (i.e., radiohumeral synostosis). The wrist and hand deformities most commonly involve the ulnar carpus (pisiform, hamate, triquetrum) and ulnar digits. However, radial-sided deficiencies (e.g., thumb hypoplasia) can also occur in ulnar deficiency. Lower extremity anomalies occur in 45%.

The ulnar anlage is a remnant of the distal ulna made up of cartilage that has no growth potential. The anlage arises from the distal humerus or remaining proximal ulna and attaches to the ulnar carpus or distal radius. The anlage is most commonly present in types II and IV ulnar deficiency and may act as a tether to cause bowing of the radius, ulnar tilting of the radial physis, and ulnar deviation of the wrist. Progressive bowing of the radius and ulnar deviation of the wrist are indications of an anlage and warrant early resection. A static deformity indicates absence of an ulnar anlage and is treated by initial observation.

The deficient length of the ulna increases the load borne by the radius and may lead to radial head subluxation or dislocation. Symptomatic subluxation may require treatment. In a type I deformity, lengthening of the ulna can restore forearm integrity and preserve the

◆ Table 12-5		
CLASSIFICATION OF ULNAR DEFICIENCIES		
Type	**Grade**	**Characteristics**
I	Hypoplasia	Hypoplasia of the ulna with presence of distal and proximal ulnar epiphysis, minimal shortening
		Slight ulnar deviation of the hand
		Minimal bowing of the radius
II	Partial aplasia	Absence of the distal or middle third of the ulna
		Distal ulna anlage may be present and cause progressive ulnar deviation
		Stable elbow
		Progressive radial bowing
III	Complete aplasia	Total agenesis of the ulna
		Unstable elbow
		Radius relatively straight
		Severe deficiencies of the hand and carpus common
IV	Synostosis	Fusion of the radius to the humerus creates stable elbow
		Distal ulna anlage may be present and cause progressive ulnar deviation

radiocapitellar joint. In more severe deficiencies, the treatment is more difficult and depends on elbow stability, forearm integrity, and length of the ulna. A stable elbow and forearm with adequate proximal ulnar length can be treated by radial head resection. An unstable forearm and short proximal ulna may require creation of a one-bone forearm. The radius is transposed onto the ulna to restore forearm stability. This procedure results in loss of all forearm rotation, which may impair function.

In a type IV deformity, the extremity is often malpositioned and facing backward. The hand is pronated and rests on the flank (hand-on-flank deformity). This position prohibits use of the hand for activities of daily living. Corrective osteotomy through the radiohumeral synostosis can rotate the forearm and realign the elbow in a forward position. The goal is to place the hand in front of the trunk, forearm in midrotation, and elbow in flexion.

The hand deformities are the major predictor of function in ulnar deficiency. Ulnar-sided syndactyly is common, and separation with web space reconstruction is indicated. In addition, a thumb deficiency may be present, which limits prehensile activities. The thumb is treated according to similar principles for isolated thumb hypoplasia.

CENTRAL DEFICIENCY

Cleft hand is a longitudinal deficiency of the central rays of the hand (index, long, and ring), which differentiate at a separate time from the radial and ulnar rays (thumb and small). There are two types of cleft hand (typical and atypical) that possess separate features and require different treatment. In fact, there are major differences between typical and atypical cleft hand (also known as severe symbrachydactyly) that may warrant placement into different categories of embryologic malformation (Table 12-6). These findings suggest that typical cleft hand may result from fusion of digital rays rather than lack of constituents. In contrast, atypical cleft hand seems to be caused by necrosis of mesenchymal tissue (failure of formation) with attempts at regeneration.

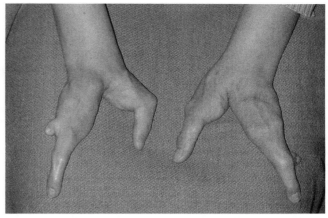

Figure 12-4 ❖ Bilateral typical cleft hand deficiency with large V-shaped defects.

The typical cleft hand has a V-shaped defect with a varying degree of long ray absence; most commonly, the phalanges are missing and the metacarpal is present (Fig. 12-4). This type is often bilateral and is usually inherited but may skip generations. There may be syndactyly of the ring-small or thumb-index web space, and associated foot involvement is common. The ring-small web space syndactyly is usually reconstructed before cleft closure. In contrast, concomitant release of a thumb-index syndactyly and closure of the cleft can be performed. This procedure uses the skin from the cleft as a random flap to reconstruct the first web space. The index digit is transposed to the long ray position to increase the breadth of the first web space and to facilitate cleft closure.

Surgical treatment of the V-shaped cleft involves closure of the defect to enhance grasp and to improve appearance. There is no urgency for cleft closure because hand development is not delayed and function is not seriously impaired. Therefore, closure is delayed until 2 to 3 years of age unless a concomitant thumb-index syndactyly is present. Closure of the cleft requires

❖ Table 12-6		
CHARACTERISTICS OF CLEFT HAND		
	Typical Cleft Hand	**Atypical Cleft Hand**
Clinical features		
Involvement	Bilateral	Unilateral
Inheritance	Familial	Spontaneous
Syndactyly*	Common	Rare
Associated with	No	Yes
Poland's syndrome		
Cleft lip, cleft palate	Yes	No
Anatomic findings		
Arterial supply	Ring finger may have three digital arteries	Vestigial supply to central digits
Tendon	Dual tendons to ring common	Minimal
Skeleton	Hypertrophy adjacent to cleft	Hypoplasia
Classification	Failure of differentiation or abnormal number of digits	Failure of formation
*Syndactyly is considered failure of differentiation and may indicate a parallel mode of occurrence.		

creation of a commissure by use of a local flap, removal of any intervening bones that block cleft narrowing, and reconstruction of the intermetacarpal ligament to prevent late splaying. The commissure flap can be created from a digit adjacent to the cleft. The deficient central ray metacarpals are removed at the base to facilitate closure. The digits bordering the cleft are approximated by construction of an intermetacarpal ligament or transposition of the index ray to the long position. Sutures placed between the metacarpals are insufficient to prevent delayed metacarpal divergence.

Atypical cleft hand is also known as symbrachydactyly and involves the central three rays (Fig. 12-5). This type of central deficiency is usually unilateral, sporadic, and without foot involvement. Atypical cleft hand is associated with Poland's syndrome, which is an ipsilateral chest wall deficiency (Fig. 12-6). The concept of teratogenic sequencing can be applied to the developing hand plate in an effort to explain the spectrum of deficiencies associated with symbrachydactyly. The concept begins with a brachydactylous hand that can progress into a variety of central defects culminating in a monodactylous or adactylous hand. The reduction usually starts at the long finger and proceeds in an ulnar direction or begins at the middle digit and progresses in a radial direction outward. The specific pathway of reduction and extent of progression will determine the ultimate deficit. Symbrachydactyly is more difficult to treat and requires individualized treatment. The goal is to create a functional pattern of grasp and adequate pinch. Many of these children are already proficient at these functions and do not warrant treatment. Surgery may be required to improve prehension; techniques include web space deepening, rotational osteotomy, tendon transfer, and digital lengthening. Formal closure of the cleft is contraindicated because it may have a detrimental effect on function.

Failure of Differentiation

Group II category infers failure of differentiation or separation of parts. This grouping implies development of all the necessary components but failure of arrangement into a proper finalized form. This failure of

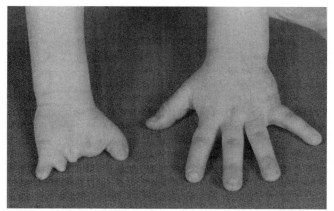

Figure 12-5 ❖ Atypical cleft hand or symbrachydactyly with suppression of the central rays.

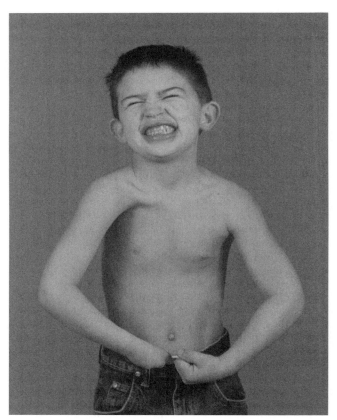

Figure 12-6 ❖ Ipsilateral absence of the sternocostal portion of the pectoralis major muscle, which is characteristic of Poland's syndrome.

differentiation can involve any tissue including skeletal, dermal, fascial, muscular, ligamentous, and neurovascular components of the limb. This category includes a heterogeneous group of disorders that are further subdivided according to anatomic abnormalities.

SYNDACTYLY

Syndactyly is the most frequent presentation of a group II anomaly. It is seen in 1 of 2000 births, more commonly in males, and 20% involve an autosomal dominant pattern of inheritance. Inheritable, spontaneous, and syndromic forms have been identified with various similarities and dissimilarities. Inheritable syndactylism is associated with genetic defects involving particular candidate regions on the second chromosome and transmitted as an autosomal dominant trait. The transmission occurs with incomplete penetrance and variable expressivity, which implies that syndactyly may skip a generation and not be present in full form. Familial syndactyly is also more prevalent in male offspring, which indicates a decreased penetrance in females.

In syndactyly, digital union is variable in extent and intensity, which guides the classification scheme. The basic terminology uses complete, incomplete, simple, and complex. The term *complicated* is a modifier that provides additional information about the pathoanatomy. The extent of syndactyly is incomplete if the skin bridge does not extend the full length of the

◈ **Table 12-7**

SYNDACTYLY CLASSIFICATION

Simple syndactyly (SS)	Standard (SSs)	Straightforward simple syndactyly of non-border digit; surgery can be delayed until 18 months of age
	Complicated (SSc)	Simple syndactyly associated with additional soft tissue interconnections, syndromes (e.g., Poland's syndrome, central deficiency), or abnormal bone elements (e.g., hypoplasia); treatment must be individualized, and beware of neurovascular anomalies
	Urgent (SSu)	Soft tissue syndactyly of border digits or digits of unequal length, girth, or joint level; requires early separation to prevent angular and rotational deformity of tethered digit
Complex syndactyly (CS)	Standard (CSs)	Complex syndactyly of adjacent phalanges without additional bone anomalies (e.g., delta phalanx, symphalangism)
	Complicated (CSc)	Complex syndactyly associated with additional bone interconnections (e.g., transverse phalanges, symphalangism, polysyndactyly) or syndromes (e.g., constriction band syndrome); treatment must be individualized, and digits may function better as a unit than as separate entities
	Unachievable (Csu)	Complex syndactyly with severe anomalies of the underlying bone structures that often prohibits formation of a five-digit hand without extensive surgical intervention

involved digits or complete when the connection encompasses the entire length. Complete syndactyly can also produce a shared or common fingernail (synonychia). The intensity of syndactyly is either soft tissue alone (simple) or in conjunction with bone (complex). Complex implies fusion of adjacent phalanges or interposition of accessory bones. Atypical forms of syndactyly also exist, which are labeled complicated and possess convoluted soft tissue abnormalities or an assortment of abnormal bones. Many of these atypical configurations occur in accordance with a variety of syndromes and defy standard terminology and classification. The term *complicated* can be incorporated into subtypes of simple and complex syndactyly to create a classification scheme that guides treatment (Table 12-7).

Simple syndactyly of any considerable degree warrants surgical reconstruction of the web space for improved function and appearance. The timing of release and technique of separation are both controversial but abide by certain guidelines (Table 12-8). Border digits (thumb-index and ring-small web spaces) have marked differences in their respective lengths and should be separated within the first few months of life (Fig. 12-7). This allows the thumb to participate in prehensile function and prevents tethering of the longer digit, which develops a flexion contracture and rotational deformity over time. In contrast, the long and ring fingers are of relatively equal length, and separation can be deferred until the child is older (between 12 and 18 months of age). This delay facilitates surgical reconstruction and

has a lower incidence of complications and unsatisfactory results (e.g., web creep). The need for supplemental skin graft is almost universal during release of complete syndactyly. The circumference of two digits separated is 22% greater than of those digits conjoined, and flap designs cannot mobilize additional skin. The skin graft should never be placed within the commissure to avoid interdigital contracture and motion-limiting scar. This requires design of a flap to recreate the commissure, which is usually based along the dorsum of the connected digits. The limiting structure in finger division is the distal bifurcation of the common digital artery.

Syndactyly of three or four adjacent digits creates additional difficulty and requires staged surgical procedures. Surgical reconstruction should include only one side of an affected digit at a time to avoid ischemia of the skin flaps or digit. Flap problems are more likely because frank digital ischemia is improbable without marked underlying arterial anomalies and inadvertent vessel injury.

Complex syndactyly adjoins the soft tissue and bone along a portion or the entire length of the adjacent digits. Complex syndactyly is associated with an increased incidence of neurovascular anomalies and is more challenging to treat, especially as the quantity of bone union intensifies. In addition, fusion of the distal phalanges creates a combined fingertip with a coalescence of the nail bed, which is difficult to reconstruct. Similar surgical principles are used during separation

◈ **Table 12-8**

SURGICAL GUIDELINES FOR SYNDACTYLY

Timing	Border digits and digits of unequal length early (3 to 6 months of age)
Commissure reconstruction	Avoid skin graft
Number of digits separated	Never operate on both sides of digit during a single setting
Skin graft	Almost always necessary, except in incomplete syndactyly
Dressings	Bulky dressings above the elbow reinforced with plaster

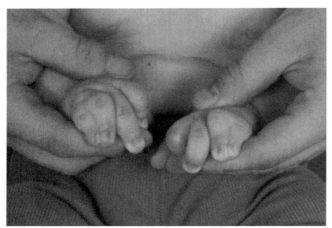

Figure 12-7 ◈ Bilateral ring-small complete syndactyly with flexion contractures of the ring fingers.

of adjacent digits. The neurovascular contribution to each digit must be defined. The proximal and distal extents of the bone connection are identified and probed for an interconnecting ridge or axilla that can guide division. Actual separation of the bone into individual components is usually accomplished with a knife blade. Separation of conjoined fingertips creates exposed bone and an absence of nail folds. Coverage requires coronal or palmar flaps to create a nail fold and to provide skin coverage without sacrificing width. Composite grafts harvested from the toes have also been used to provide pulp tissue and nail margins.

Complicated syndactyly is a broad category that encompasses many difficult forms of abnormal web space connection and bone abnormalities. Many of these cases are associated with a syndrome, most notably Poland's syndrome, amniotic disruption sequence, or acrocephalosyndactyly (Apert's syndrome). In certain instances of complicated syndactyly, the connected digits function better as a unit than as separate entities. This is particularly true in children with a normal thumb and a conglomeration of fingers with bizarre bone and joint abnormalities. Syndactyly separation is contraindicated because surgery may impair prehension and function.

Poland's syndrome is an ipsilateral anomaly of the chest wall and hand that frequently has syndactyly. The mild form is classically described as a small hand with incomplete simple syndactyly (symbrachydactyly) and an absence of the sternocostal portion of the pectoralis major muscle. This syndactyly is separated by use of the established principles for web space reconstruction (see Table 12-7). Hypoplasia as absence of the middle phalanges is common. More severe forms involve progressive bone reduction beginning in the central digits and resembling an atypical central deficiency or symbrachydactyly. Successive thumb and small finger involvement can occur, culminating in a complete deficiency of all digits. The proximal muscle deficiencies and breast underdevelopment can also progress to a hollow chest wall deformity with complete absence of the breast.

SYNOSTOSIS

Synostosis is a generic term that indicates an osseous union between bones that are normally separate. Synostosis can occur as an independent entity or as part of a more general condition (e.g., complicated syndactyly or ulnar deficiency). The most common deformity associated with fetal alcohol syndrome is radioulnar synostosis and capitate hamate fusion.

In general, surgical procedures aimed at restoration of forearm motion are universally unsuccessful and not recommended. Synostosis of the proximal radioulnar joint is a common problem. The synostosis can be isolated and complete (type I) or partial and associated with a radial head dislocation (type II). Proximal radioulnar synostosis can also occur with systemic conditions, such as trisomy (13 or 21) and fetal alcohol syndrome. Shoulder and wrist motions are able to compensate for lack of forearm rotation during many activities of daily childhood. A delay in presentation, therefore, is common until the complexities of daily activities amplify. Furthermore, an astute examination is necessary to discriminate intercarpal rotation from forearm rotation. The treatment depends on the position of the forearm synostosis. Mild degrees of pronation or supination are well tolerated, whereas extremes of position create functional handicaps. Deformities in excess of 45 degrees may require rotational osteotomy through the fusion mass to a more functional position. Caution must be used during correction of severe rotational deformities to prevent iatrogenic nerve injury, particularly of the posterior interosseous nerve.

RADIAL HEAD DISLOCATION

A radial head dislocation can occur in various directions. The most common route is posterior (65%), followed by anterior (18%) and posterolateral (17%). The differentiation between a congenital and a chronic traumatic dislocation may be difficult in a child (Table 12-9). In addition, there are other conditions, such as multiple hereditary exostosis and ulnar deficiency, that result in a shortened ulna. This disparity between the radius and ulna increases the load across the radiocapitellar joint and predisposes the radial head to subluxate or to dislocate.

The preferred treatment of congenital radial head dislocation remains observation until skeletal maturity. There are preliminary reports about surgical relocation of the radial head and annular ligament reconstruction. The ultimate outcome after relocation, however, still remains to be determined. Radial head excision after skeletal maturity provides consistent pain relief and improves appearance. Forearm and elbow motion will not change appreciably after radial head resection for congenital dislocation.

SYMPHALANGISM

Symphalangism is a longitudinal failure of joint differentiation that usually affects the proximal interphalangeal joint and results in synostosis. The finger is usually extended at the proximal interphalangeal joint without active or passive motion. The absence of skin creases (joint creases) across the affected joint is the classic

✦ **Table 12-9**

CONGENITAL VERSUS TRAUMATIC RADIAL HEAD DISLOCATION

	Congenital	Traumatic
Radiographic features		
Radial head	Dome shaped	Normal appearance
Capitellum	Hypoplastic	Normal
Ulnar variance	Positive	Often normal
Family history	Can be positive	Negative
Bilateral	50%	No

clinical sign. Initial radiographs demonstrate a joint space because the bridge across the joint is initially cartilaginous. Ossification of the connecting cartilaginous bar results in obliteration of the joint space and bone ankylosis over time. There is no reliable method to restore motion for symphalangism, and observation is warranted in cases without functional disability. Chondrodesis or arthrodesis can be performed to improve the position of the finger. A chondrodesis involves removal of the cartilage from the proximal interphalangeal joint surfaces and preservation of the underlying growth plate. A chondrodesis is preferred in a growing child, and arthrodesis is favored after skeletal maturity.

ARTHROGRYPOSIS

Arthrogryposis or arthrogryposis multiplex congenita is a syndrome of joint contractures that are present at birth and nonprogressive. The cause is not a malformation of the joint or limb during embryogenesis; rather, it is secondary to lack of motion during fetal life. There are multiple processes that can lead to lack of limb movement, including muscle abnormalities, nerve anomalies, restricted space within the uterus, vascular insufficiency, and maternal illness. The neuropathic form is by far more common and is often the result of degeneration of the anterior horn cells in utero. Presentation can be divided into three groups: group I, distal hand involvement only; group II, diffuse upper extremity involvement; and group III, upper and lower extremity involvement.

The multiple forms of arthrogryposis vary in presentation, severity, and number of involved joints. Amyoplasia (classic arthrogryposis) is the most common form characterized by symmetric positioning of the limbs. The upper extremities are postured with adduction and internal rotation at the shoulder, elbow extension, forearm pronation, wrist flexion, and hand ulnar deviation. The digits are postured in flexion and stiff. The thumb is flexed and clenched in the palm, which creates functional difficulties with activities of daily living. Additional clinical features include waxy skin devoid of skin creases, considerable muscle wasting, and paucity of subcutaneous tissue.

Arthrogryposis can be confined to the distal part of the extremities (distal arthrogryposis). The hand is flexed in a clenched fist posture with ulnar deviation of the fingers, which often overlap. This form of arthrogryposis has a relatively good response to early therapy and splinting. Arthrogryposis features can occur with many syndromes, including multiple pterygium syndrome, contractural arachnodactyly (Beals' syndrome), Freeman-Sheldon syndrome (whistling face syndrome), and Larsen's syndrome.

The treatment of patients with arthrogryposis is individualized to each child's needs. The traditional upper extremity goal is to achieve independent function for self-feeding and perineal care. The mainstays of early treatment are frequent passive movement of all involved joints and judicious use of splints. Static progressive splinting creates a low load and prolonged stretch and is efficacious for diminishing contractures. An increase in passive motion is beneficial for function and enhances the possibility of surgical reconstruction. Children with arthrogryposis develop adaptive maneuvers to accomplish many daily tasks. These positions may appear awkward but are functional for many activities of daily living. Surgical recommendations must consider the impact that the proposed procedure will have on adaptive maneuvers to ensure no degradation in function.

The shoulder often has limited motion and an internal rotation deformity. No reliable procedures exist to enhance shoulder mobility, although severe internal rotation can be treated by external rotation osteotomy. The lack of elbow flexion is incapacitating to function, especially hand to mouth activity. Early efforts to restore passive elbow flexion are critical and emphasized in therapy. Tendon transfer can treat passive flexion without active movement as long as viable donor muscles exist. Potential donor muscles include the pectoralis major, latissimus dorsi, triceps, and flexor-pronator mass. The selection of donor depends on numerous factors, such as muscle strength, excursion, and expendability. The use of upper extremity devices (e.g., crutches) for ambulation is a contraindication to triceps transfer. Unfortunately, the result after elbow flexion transfers for arthrogryposis is not as predictable as for other causes. This inconsistent outcome reflects the suboptimal motor function of the donor muscle.

Wrist flexion contractures are difficult to overcome because of the rigid posture and deficiency in active extension. A persistent wrist flexion deformity recalcitrant to therapy may require surgery to position the wrist better for function. Proximal row carpectomy is beneficial in young patients with mild to moderate flexion. In severe deformities, proximal row carpectomy often yields insufficient wrist extension. Alternative options for difficult deformities are a dorsal wedge midcarpal osteotomy and distraction histogenesis (e.g., Ilizarov device) to improve wrist extension. Irrespective of the procedure to reposition the wrist, a tendon transfer is essential to maintain wrist extension. The extensor carpi ulnaris is usually functional and is transferred to the dorsum of the wrist.

The thumb and fingers are commonly stiff and fixed in flexion, which creates a functional handicap. Surgical treatment aimed at restoration of supple finger motion is not successful. The thumb can be released from the palm to enhance prehension. The fingers can be realigned by osteotomy to position them better for function.

PTERYGIUM CUBITALE

Pterygium cubitale can occur as an isolated entity or as part of the pterygium syndrome, which involves webbing of the neck, axilla, knees, and digits. All structures about the elbow are involved, including the skin, subcutaneous tissue, muscle, and bone. Elbow flexion is usually present, but extension is severely limited and is seldom beyond 90 degrees. The underlying brachial and antebrachial muscles are atrophic or absent. Skeletal deformities include radial head dislocation, radioulnar synostosis, hypoplasia of the radius or ulna, and anomalies of the distal humerus. Surgical attempts to correct the deformity have resulted in recurrence and are not recommended. Release of the skin may improve the appearance but not the motion because the integument just conceals the fundamental problem.

TRIGGER DIGITS

Congenital trigger thumb is far more common than trigger finger. Bilateral involvement is present in approximately 30% of children. The diagnosis is often delayed because an infant postures the thumb in a position of flexion. A fixed flexion deformity of the thumb interphalangeal joint is most common. The cause is secondary to a nodular thickening of the flexor pollicis longus tendon and narrowing of the flexor sheath. This dichotomy prevents the flexor tendon from entering into the sheath, and palpation of the nodular thickening of the flexor tendon is readily apparent just proximal to the sheath.

Passive manipulation into extension may produce a noticeable click or pop. Splinting can be used to maintain this position but is not efficacious in the long term. Approximately one third of trigger thumbs diagnosed before 1 year may resolve, and a delay in surgery up to 3 years of age has no harmful effects. Therefore, a period of observation with or without splinting is often used in the child younger than 1 year. A delay in presentation, parental decision, or failure of spontaneous resolution requires surgical release of the first annular pulley with protection of the digital nerves.

Trigger fingers in children are less common and less straightforward. Triggering is not always secondary to a discrepancy between the flexor tendons and sheath. An abnormal relationship between the flexor digitorum profundus and superficialis tendons, proximal decussation of the superficialis tendon, nodular formation within the flexor tendons, and tightness of the second and third annular pulleys are potential reasons. Simple release of the first annular pulley may not resolve the triggering, and a more diligent search for alternative causes is warranted.

HYPOPLASTIC THUMB

Thumb hypoplasia is an entity different from partial thumb aplasia due to a transverse deficiency or amniotic disruption sequence. Hypoplasia of the thumb occurs in varying grades and most commonly is part of a radial deficiency. The underdeveloped thumb has been classified into five types, which guides treatment recommendations (Table 12-10). A type I deficiency represents the least involvement with generalized thumb hypoplasia without discrete absence of structures. A type II deficiency is more involved and characterized by thumb-index web space narrowing, thenar muscle absence, and instability of the thumb metacarpophalangeal joint. Type III hypoplasia possesses the intrinsic anomalies associated with a type II deformity plus additional skeletal and extrinsic musculotendinous abnormalities (e.g., flexor pollicis longus). Type III anomalies are divided into IIIA and IIIB, depending on the presence or absence of a stable carpometacarpal joint. Type IV deficiency represents a severe expression of thumb hypoplasia and denotes a *pouce flottant* or residual digit with two residual phalanges (Fig. 12-8). Type V is noted by complete absence of the thumb.

❖ Table 12-10

CLASSIFICATION OF THUMB HYPOPLASIA

Type	Findings	Treatment
I	Minor generalized hypoplasia	Augmentation
II	Absence of intrinsic thenar muscles	Opponensplasty
	First web space narrowing	First web release
	Ulnar collateral ligament (UCL) insufficiency	UCL reconstruction
III	Similar findings as in type II plus	
	Extrinsic muscle and tendon abnormalities	
	Skeletal deficiency	
	A: Stable carpometacarpal joint	A: Reconstruction
	B: Unstable carpometacarpal joint	B: Pollicization
IV	Pouce flottant or floating thumb	Pollicization
V	Absence	Pollicization

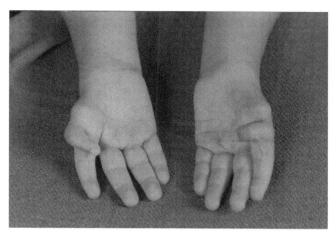

Figure 12-8 ◈ Bilateral type IV hypoplastic thumbs that were treated with ablation and pollicization.

REORGANIZATION IN POLLICIZATION

Structure	Pollicization Function
Distal interphalangeal joint	Interphalangeal joint
Proximal interphalangeal joint	Metacarpophalangeal joint
Metacarpophalangeal joint	Carpometacarpal joint
First dorsal interosseous	Abductor pollicis
First volar interosseous	Adductor pollicis
Extensor indicis proprius	Abductor pollicis longus
Extensor digitorum	Extensor pollicis longus

Pollex abductus is an anomaly that occurs most commonly in a hypoplastic thumb but also in thumb duplication. In this anomaly, flexor pollicis longus inserts in its normal position in addition to an abnormal connection to the extensor by way of a tendon that passes on the radial aspect of the digit. Contraction of the anomalous tendon will cause abduction of the thumb. In addition, an anomalous muscle arising from the flexor pollicis longus at the level of the metacarpophalangeal joint joining the index lumbrical (musculus lumbricalis pollicis) can contribute to the deformity.

The main distinction between a thumb that can be reconstructed and a thumb that requires ablation is the presence or absence of a carpometacarpal joint. A stable carpometacarpal joint provides a foundation for thumb reconstruction. An absent carpometacarpal joint negates the possibility of thumb reconstruction and is best treated by ablation and pollicization. The clinical differentiation between types IIIA and IIIB can be difficult. The child often helps discriminate between these types by pattern of use. An unstable thumb is not incorporated into pinch and grasp. Prehension develops between the index and long digits, and the index tends to pronate and rotate out of the palm. In equivocal cases, the decision may be further complicated by the ossification of the trapezium and trapezoid, which do not ossify until 4 to 6 years of age.

Thumb reconstruction in types II and IIIA requires addressing all elements of the hypoplasia. The adducted posture of the thumb is corrected with a web space deepening and reconstruction by Z-plasty or dorsal transposition flap. The metacarpophalangeal joint instability involves the ulnar side and is rectified by ulnar collateral ligament reconstruction. Transfer of the abductor digiti quinti or a flexor digitorum superficialis tendon for opposition augments the thenar hypoplasia. A type IIIA thumb also requires transfers to overcome the extrinsic musculotendinous abnormalities of extensor pollicis longus and flexor pollicis longus tendons.

Pollicization is the procedure of choice for types IIIB, IV, and V hypoplasia. This complex procedure involves neurovascular transposition of the index digit to the thumb position with reconstruction of the intrinsic muscles of the thumb (Table 12-11). The index digit must be rotated at least 120 degrees to attain proper orientation of the new thumb. The index must be shortened by removal of the diaphysis, and a metacarpal epiphysiodesis should be performed to prevent excessive length of the thumb. The neurovascular bundles must be carefully protected throughout the procedure. The proper digital artery to the radial side of the long digit is ligated to allow index finger transposition. Joint and tendon reorganization is necessary for pollicization.

The time to perform pollicization remains controversial, with a trend toward early surgery (6 months to 1 year of age) before the development of oppositional pinch. This early intervention avoids the occurrence of a compensatory side-to-side pinch pattern between adjacent fingers. The results of pollicization are directly related to the status of the transposed index digit and surrounding musculature. A stiff index finger will provide a stable thumb for gross grasp, but oppositional pinch is unlikely. In contrast, a mobile index finger transferred to the thumb position can provide stability for grasp and mobility for fine pinch (Fig. 12-9). The technical ability to restore bone alignment and intrinsic muscle function is integral for a successful outcome. The greatest improvement in function involves handling of large objects after pollicization. Unsatisfactory results require a stepwise approach to

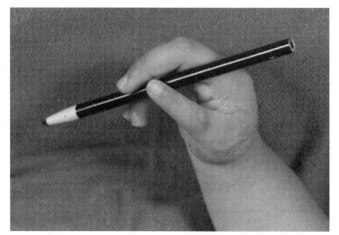

Figure 12-9 ◈ A mobile index finger can provide a pollicization that has adequate stability for grasp and dexterity for fine pinch.

◆ Table 12-12		
SOURCES OF FAILURE AFTER POLLICIZATION		
Type of Failure	**Etiology**	**Treatment**
First web space contracture	Insufficient first web space reconstruction or scarring	Web space deepening by Z-plasty or rotational flap
Stiffness	May be related to preoperative condition of index or be secondary to surgical complication	Innate stiffness of index is not correctable; surgical adhesions can be treated by tenolysis
Lack of opposition	Primary deficiency in intrinsic muscles; inability to reconstruct interossei at the time of surgery	Tendon transfer to enhance opposition
Malrotated	Technical error during thumb positioning or loss of fixation during postoperative care	Rotational osteotomy
Excessive length	Failure to ablate index metacarpal growth plate	Epiphysiodesis and ostectomy of metacarpal

analyze potential problems. Secondary reconstruction can rectify many of these problems and enhance function of the thumb (Table 12-12).

CLASPED THUMB

Congenital clasped thumb is caused by hypoplasia or absence of the thumb extensors. The diagnosis is often delayed because an infant frequently holds the thumb within the palm for the first few months. The clasped thumb rests in flexion and has an extension lag. Lack of metacarpophalangeal joint extension is most common and implies hypoplasia of the extensor pollicis brevis muscle-tendon unit. Simultaneous extension lag at the interphalangeal joint indicates a similar deficiency of the extensor pollicis longus. Initial treatment is splinting of the affected joint in extension for at least 3 months. Failure to achieve adequate active extension indicates extreme hypoplasia or absence of the tendons. A tendon transfer is indicated to restore active thumb extension. The extensor indicis proprius is a common donor tendon, although concomitant absence of this tendon has been reported in clasped thumb. An alternative donor tendon should be incorporated in the surgical plan if this situation is encountered.

CAMPTODACTYLY

Camptodactyly is a painless flexion contracture of the proximal interphalangeal joint that is usually gradually progressive (Fig. 12-10). Camptodactyly most commonly involves the small finger and is bilateral in approximately two thirds of the cases, although the degree of contracture is usually not symmetric. The metacarpophalangeal and distal interphalangeal joints are not affected, although compensatory deformities may develop.

Camptodactyly is divided into three categories. A type I deformity is the most common form and becomes apparent during infancy. The deformity is usually an isolated finding and limited to the fifth finger. This "congenital" form affects boys and girls equally. A type II deformity has similar clinical features, although they are not apparent until preadolescence. This "acquired" form of camptodactyly develops between the ages of 7 and 11 and affects girls more than boys. This type of camptodactyly usually does not improve spontaneously and may progress to a severe flexion deformity. A type III deformity is often a severe deformity that usually involves multiple digits of both extremities and is associated with a variety of syndromes, including craniofacial disorders, short stature, and chromosome abnormalities.

The exact etiology underlying camptodactyly remains unknown, and there is no consensus about the pathogenesis of the condition. Almost every structure about the proximal interphalangeal joint has been implicated as the principal cause of or a contributing factor to the formation of camptodactyly, including the skin, subcutaneous tissue, fascia, collateral ligaments, and musculotendinous anomalies. The most prevalent anomalies affect the flexor digitorum superficialis and intrinsic musculature (lumbricals and interossei). The flexor digitorum superficialis tendon has been noted to be contracted, underdeveloped, or devoid of a functional muscle. This abnormal musculotendinous architecture cannot elongate during periods of rapid growth (i.e., infancy and adolescence), which creates a tenodesis effect and a subsequent proximal interphalangeal joint flexion deformity. An aberrant lumbrical or interosseous muscle has also been implicated as the principal cause of camptodactyly, which creates an intrinsic minus deformity. In long-standing cases, radiographs are invariably abnormal with changes on both sides of the joint secondary to the prolonged flexion deformity.

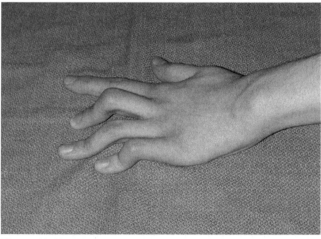

Figure 12-10 ◆ Camptodactyly of the long, ring, and small digits.

Conservatism is the tenet for treatment of mild camptodactyly. A contracture of less than 30 to 40 degrees does not create a functional handicap or interfere with activities of daily living. Static splinting at night is recommended to prevent progression of the deformity. The splint should be worn until the late teens or closure of the growth plate, which indicates cessation of longitudinal growth of the finger. The natural history of camptodactyly is no improvement or progression of the deformity in 80% of individuals. Severe involvement hinders various occupational and sporting endeavors and warrants treatment, although restoration of full motion is not a realistic goal.

A preliminary period of nonoperative treatment is always attempted to resolve any fixed flexion deformity, including stretching, splinting (static and dynamic), and serial casting. The extent of surgery depends on the degree of fixed flexion deformity. The procedure must evaluate all potential offending agents beginning at the skin and proceeding into the deeper tissues. The digit is explored for anomalous structures with specific examination of the intrinsic muscles and flexor digitorum superficialis. Any anomalous origin or insertion of the lumbrical or interosseous muscle is resected. The flexor digitorum superficialis tendon is identified and inspected. An anomalous flexor digitorum superficialis is released. A normal-appearing flexor digitorum superficialis can be transferred through the lumbrical canal to rebalance the proximal interphalangeal joint.

The outcome after surgery for camptodactyly is not always predictable and can be disappointing. Negative prognostic factors include contractures of more than 45 degrees and secondary bone changes. The principal problems are stiffness and loss of flexion, which impairs grasp and hand function.

WINDBLOWN HAND (CONGENITAL ULNAR DRIFT)

The windblown hand is characterized by ulnar deviation and flexion contractures of the fingers at the metacarpophalangeal joint. The etiology is related to the position of the extensor tendons, which are subluxated or dislocated into the valleys between the metacarpal heads. The thumb tendons may be involved, causing a fixed thumb-in-palm deformity. The deformities are present at birth and often progress with growth. The windblown hand is associated with craniofacial deformities (e.g., whistling face syndrome or Freeman-Sheldon syndrome) and may be related to arthrogryposis.

Treatment is notoriously difficult because of the considerable soft tissue anomalies. Release of the thumb web requires Z-plasty or dorsal rotation flap to overcome the narrowing of the web space. Flexor pollicis longus tendon lengthening and intrinsic release may be necessary to overcome severe contractures. The ulnar deviation and flexion contracture of the metacarpophalangeal joints also require an extensive release of the soft tissues. The extensor tendon hoods require centralization over the dorsal aspect of the metacarpophalangeal joints. In the untreated adolescent, a shortening osteotomy of the metacarpals is necessary to achieve satisfactory correction.

CLINODACTYLY

Clinodactyly refers to an angular deformity in the coronal plane. Although clinodactyly can occur in any digit, radial deviation of the small finger distal interphalangeal joint is most common. Clinodactyly is usually inherited as a dominant trait but can occur sporadically. There is a high incidence of associated anomalies (more than 30 syndromes), most notably Down syndrome. The critical factor in identifying clinodactyly may be the identification of any associated syndrome.

The primary complaint of the patient and family is often related to the appearance of the finger rather than a functional problem. The cause is usually secondary to an inclination of the middle phalanx articular surface. Radiographs are necessary to verify the inclination and to assess for other causes of digital angulation, such as a delta phalanx.

Conservatism and observation are the mainstays of treatment for simple clinodactyly. Mild and moderate distal interphalangeal joint angulation does not require surgery. Splinting is not recommended because the underlying deformity is a bone malformation. Corrective procedures are reserved for severe angulation with digital overlap during fist formation. An osteotomy of the distal phalanx realigns the joint surface and finger. A closing or opening wedge can be performed, with advantages and disadvantageous to each technique. The closing wedge is easier to perform but results in a shortened digit. The opening wedge lengthens the digit but is more difficult to perform.

KIRNER'S DEFORMITY

Progressive volar and radial angulation of the distal phalanx of the small finger is characteristic of Kirner's deformity. The deformity is more common in girls, is often bilateral, and does not begin until after 5 years of age. The primary complaint is often the appearance of the digit, which does not warrant treatment. Functional difficulties are limited to specific activities, such as playing a musical instrument or typing. Treatment for symptomatic deformity is multiple wedge osteotomies to correct the angulatory deformity.

DELTA BONE (DELTA PHALANX OR LONGITUDINAL BRACKETED DIAPHYSIS)

A longitudinal epiphyseal bracket (delta phalanx or longitudinal bracketed diaphysis) tends to occur in the phalanges. The longitudinal epiphyseal bracket represents a functioning physis and epiphysis along the side of the phalanx that courses in a proximal to distal direction. The surface overlying the longitudinal physis is covered by articular cartilage, and active enchondral ossification occurs along the involved side of the phalanx. The abnormal growth plate may bracket part of the phalanx or the entire phalanx. This orientation prevents appropriate longitudinal growth of the finger and may promote progressive angulation. Delta bones are seen most commonly in children with central polydactyly, and occasionally in patients with Carpenter's syndrome (obesity, cranial synostosis, clinodactyly).

The longitudinal epiphyseal bracket is highly variable in configuration. The ultimate shape of the phalanx and extent of the abnormal epiphysis and physis cannot be determined before ossification of the epiphysis. Serial radiographs will reveal the specific morphology of the bone and growth plate. The longitudinal epiphyseal bracket tends to be C shaped and situated along the shorter side of the bone. Magnetic resonance imaging can be used for early delineation of the shape and extent of the longitudinal epiphyseal bracket.

A longitudinal epiphyseal bracket can lead to progressive angulation of the digit over time. The rate of development and magnitude of the deformity are unpredictable. The ultimate deformity is related to the growth potential within the cells and the location of the bracket. Observation of the digit is the preferred initial treatment until progressive angulation is apparent or skeletal maturity is reached.

Multiple procedures have been proposed to correct the underlying physeal abnormality. These procedures are technically demanding, especially when the affected bone is small. As a general rule, the longitudinal epiphysis is cut and the growth plate along the convex side of the bone ablated. The horizontal portion of the epiphysis must be preserved to allow longitudinal growth. A closing or opening wedge osteotomy of the phalanx can be performed to realign the digit. A reversed wedge graft, which resects a wedge from the convex side and inserts the segment into the concave side, has also been described. The osteotomy must avoid the horizontal portion of the epiphysis to prevent closure of the growth plate and shortening of the digit.

A prophylactic procedure has been described for young children with progressive deformity. The longitudinal portion of the bracket is excised and a fat graft inserted to cover the ends of the split physis. Growth of the horizontal portions of the growth plate leads to a gradual correction of digital alignment.

Duplication

Duplication most commonly affects the ulnar (postaxial) or radial (preaxial) border of the hand. Postaxial or ulnar polydactyly demonstrates familial propagation and racial preference. The duplication is transmitted by an autosomal dominant pattern and occurs more commonly in black individuals. Preaxial duplication or radial polydactyly also demonstrates racial predilection toward white children, but it is usually unilateral and sporadic. Further subdivision into various categories has been performed according to extent of duplication. Genetic analysis of a particular form of polydactyly (ring finger duplication) combined with syndactyly (synpolydactyly) has been linked to a gene mutation (*HOXD13* gene), which is located on chromosome 2.

THUMB DUPLICATION

Duplication of the thumb (preaxial polydactyly) can be partial or complete and has been classified into various types, depending on the degree of skeletal replication (Table 12-13 and Fig. 12-11). In this classification, the extent of duplication is defined and whether the components are attached proximally (bifid) or completely separated (duplicated). Type IV is the most common

◆ Table 12-13	
CLASSIFICATION OF DUPLICATED THUMBS	
Type	**Duplicated Elements**
I	Bifid distal phalanx
II	Duplicated distal phalanx
III	Bifid proximal phalanx
IV	Duplicated proximal phalanx*
V	Bifid metacarpal phalanx
VI	Duplicated metacarpal phalanx
VII	Triphalangeal component

*Most common type.
Modified from Wassel HD: The results of surgery for polydactyly of the thumb. A review. Clin Orthop 125:175-193, 1969.

type of thumb duplication and constitutes about 50% of the cases.

Thumb duplication involves more than the bone elements; the parts may share common nails, tendons, ligaments, joints, and neurovascular structures. Treatment often requires use of portions of each component to construct a properly aligned and functional thumb. The treatment of type I and type II depends on the extent and size of each duplicated part. Asymmetric duplication is treated by ablation of the smaller thumb with transfer of the collateral ligament and centralization of the extensor tendon. Failure to restore stability by collateral ligament relocation will lead to persistent instability, and inadequate extensor and/or flexor tendon centralization will cause thumb deviation over time (Z-deformity). Symmetric thumb duplication can be treated by resection of the central portions of bone and nail from each component and approximation of the retained borders (Bilhaut-Cloquet procedure). This operation is difficult, and subsequent nail deformity and interphalangeal joint stiffness are common.

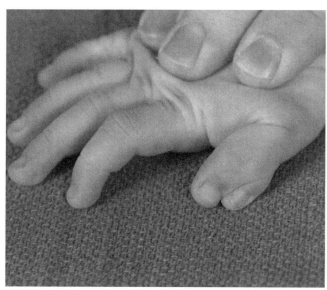

Figure 12-11 ◆ Preaxial or thumb duplication with distinct distal parts.

Type III and type IV duplication are treated with selection of a dominant thumb and ablation of the lesser counterpart. This decision is not always straight-forward and requires careful examination. If the components are equal, the ulnar thumb is preserved to retain the ulnar collateral ligament for pinch. The soft tissue from the ablated thumb is used to augment the retained thumb. The collateral ligament is retained with an osteoperiosteal sleeve from the deleted thumb and transferred to the preserved thumb. Articular surface modification and tendon realignment are necessary to optimize thumb function. Osteotomy or articular surface recontouring may be necessary to align the thumb correctly and to prevent progressive angulatory deformity. The thenar intrinsic muscles require transfer from the deleted thumb to the retained thumb. The treatment of type V and type VI duplication uses similar principles with the added complexity of additional intrinsic reconstruction.

The Z-deformity may develop, causing ulnar deviation of the thumb metacarpophalangeal joint and radial deviation of the interphalangeal joint. The most common cause is failure to centralize the flexor and extensor tendons due to the anomalous insertions of the tendons.

TRIPHALANGEAL THUMB

Triphalangeal thumb can develop as an isolated anomaly or occur with thumb duplication. The extra phalanx has a variable shape and directs treatment. A small and wedge-shaped middle phalanx causes deviation and requires excision with ligament reconstruction. A large and wedge-shaped extra phalanx produces deviation and excessive length. Excision of the phalanx can be performed, but subsequent instability is common. Fusion of the abnormal phalanx with the distal or proximal phalanx along with bone removal is a better option. The bone reduction shortens and realigns the thumb, and the arthrodesis eliminates the supernumerary joint.

POLYDACTYLY

Postaxial polydactyly is a common congenital anomaly that can occur as an isolated anomaly or as part of a syndrome (e.g., chondroectodermal dysplasia or Ellis–van Creveld syndrome). Isolated polydactyly is frequently inherited as an autosomal dominant disorder, but has a variable penetrance pattern. The supernumerary digit is either well developed (type A) or rudimentary and pedunculated (type B). A small nubbin or scrawny postaxial element (type B) can be safely removed by tying the base in the nursery. The digit will turn gangrenous and fall from the hand. A residual bump or nubbin is the most common complication. A large or robust digit (type A) requires formal surgical ablation (Fig. 12-12). The extra digit is removed, and any important parts (e.g., ulnar collateral ligament and abductor digiti quinti) are transferred to the adjacent finger.

MIRROR HAND

Mirror hand is a rare anomaly attributed to duplication of the ZPA signaling pathway or Sonic hedgehog

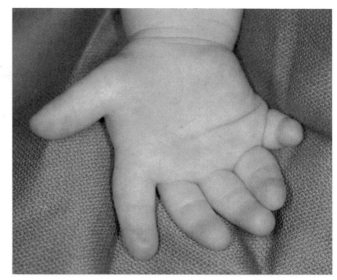

Figure 12-12 ◆ Type A postaxial polydactyly with a well-formed supernumerary digit.

molecule (see Fig. 12-1). The hand possesses eight digits and no thumbs. The ulna is duplicated (ulnar dimelia), which impairs forearm and elbow function. Treatment is to construct a thumb and to reduce the number of digits. Pollicization of one of the fingers combined with deletion of multiple digits provides a thumb and first web space.

Overgrowth

Overgrowth can present as diffuse hypertrophy of the entire limb or isolated enlargement of various parts (Fig. 12-13). This category is uncommon in occurrence but dramatic in presentation. Underlying causes of limb overgrowth (e.g., vascular abnormalities or malformations) must be considered during evaluation

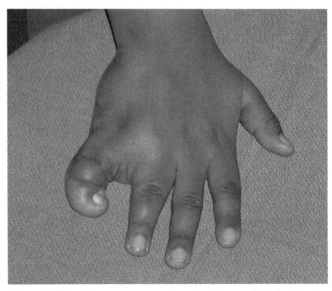

Figure 12-13 ◆ Isolated macrodactyly of the small digit with dramatic overgrowth.

of the patient. In addition, overgrowth can be a constituent of a variety of syndromes (e.g., neurofibromatosis or Klippel-Trénaunay-Weber).

MACRODACTYLY

Macrodactyly represents overgrowth of all structures of the involved digit and is different from an isolated enlargement of the bone (e.g., enchondroma) or vessels (e.g., hemangiomas). This disfiguring condition can affect one digit or multiple fingers. The radial fingers are more commonly involved than the ulnar. Macrodactyly is usually an isolated abnormality but can occur with neurofibromatosis or Klippel-Trénaunay-Weber syndrome (limb hypertrophy, hemangiomas, and varicose veins).

The etiology remains unknown, and static and progressive forms have been observed. Static macrodactyly consists of an enlarged digit that is present at birth and grows proportionately over time. Progressive macrodactyly is more common and begins in childhood. The involved digit increases in size throughout growth and stiffens during enlargement. Progressive growth persists until skeletal maturity and physeal closure.

Treatment of macrodactyly must address all constituents of the finger. The soft tissue component requires debulking to remove excessive fat, subcutaneous tissue, and skin. The procedure encompasses half of the finger at a time. Epiphysiodesis is indicated after the digit reaches the same length as the digit of the sex-matched parent. Simultaneous arrest of all the phalangeal growth plates is necessary to inhibit longitudinal growth. Circumferential growth continues and requires bone reduction procedures to narrow the width. Enlargement that is relentless and grotesque requires amputation.

Undergrowth

Undergrowth or hypoplasia can affect the entire limb or be isolated to a part and is subdivided according to anatomic locale. Undergrowth is prevalent in many disorders, including Poland's syndrome (symbrachydactyly) and radial deficiency (thumb hypoplasia).

Undergrowth can also be the predominant anomaly requiring classification. Brachydactyly is a hypoplastic digit that has the normal complement of bones (Fig. 12-14). The shortening usually occurs in the middle phalanx, and asymmetric shortening will lead to clinodactyly. Metacarpal shortening is uncommon and usually affects the ulnar digits (ring and small). This type of brachydactyly presents with absent knuckles of the ring and small fingers (knuckle, knuckle, bump, bump). A short fourth metacarpal may be associated with pseudohypoparathyroidism or pseudopseudohypoparathyroidism, and a short fifth metacarpal may be associated with cri du chat. Nonvascularized toe phalangeal transfers can be considered for the aphalangeal hand. After 1 year, one can expect an open physis in 94% of the transferred phalanges when the procedure is performed in a child younger than 1 year.

Symbrachydactyly is used to describe syndactyly accompanied by brachydactyly. It is usually sporadic without a family history and unilateral, with no involvement

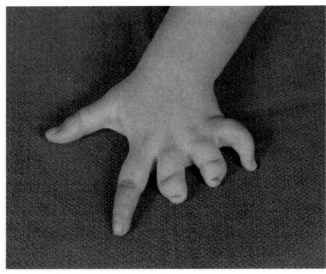

Figure 12-14 ◆ Undergrowth or brachydactyly of multiple digits.

of the feet. It is occasionally associated with Poland's syndrome.

The length and size discrepancy of the hypoplasia will not improve with growth, and the disparity may increase throughout childhood. Treatment depends on the degree of hypoplasia and quality of the adjacent digits. Mild hypoplasia requires no treatment; severe underdevelopment may warrant amputation. Digital lengthening can be useful to increase the length of a shortened digit. Brachydactyly secondary to short metacarpals is more amenable to distraction lengthening than are short fingers from small phalanges.

Amniotic Disruption Sequence

Amniotic disruption sequence or constriction band syndrome is a result of entrapment of developing embryonal tissue by fetal lining. This can be manifested as amputation of a part and most commonly affects the digits (hands or toes). The diagnosis of constriction band requires the presence of a constriction band either in the involved extremity or elsewhere. These deficiencies are not hereditary; the cause remains controversial, with both intrinsic and extrinsic theories. The intrinsic concept believes the amniotic bands represent a localized lack of mesodermal development, similar to a normal skin crease. The depth of the mesodermal defect determines the severity of clinical presentation. The extrinsic postulate reasons that either the amniotic membrane traps the developing hand or an amniotic band encircles the affected part, leading to a variable amount of injury (vascular insult). Currently, the extrinsic hypothesis is favored because amnion has been found in the constriction ring, and the bands tend to occur in a straight line across multiple digits. Amniotic bands can cause mild digital damage that initiates an embryonic repair process and yields a variable amount of circumferential stricture. Severe damage can lead to complete vascular ischemia and truncation of the affected part.

Clinical manifestations and treatment depend on the degree of involvement and most commonly include the presence of club feet (Fig. 12-15). Simple constriction rings may present as an appearance problem and are treated by elective band excision and Z-plasty. Deep circumferential rings can cause vascular insufficiency with cold intolerance, neurologic compromise, and tendon dysfunction. A more emergent band excision and Z-plasty are warranted. Multiple digital amputations require reconstruction or augmentation by a variety of techniques, including lengthening procedures and combining parts of adjacent digits. A pseudosyndactyly is often present and attributed to healing between the affected digits after injury induced by the amniotic band. The digits are connected, but a small cleft or web space remains and differentiates this coupling from true syndactyly. Treatment is separation of the pseudosyndactyly to enhance independent finger function. Neurovascular anomalies are common and require identification during release. Toe-thumb transfers usually have good functional outcomes due to intact proximal structures.

Madelung's Deformity

Madelung's deformity is related to a growth disturbance of the ulnar volar aspect of the distal radius physis. It occurs more often in girls and is most often bilateral. The deformity is usually not noticed until later in childhood. The radius is usually shortened, with the appearance of a volarly subluxated wrist and dorsally prominent distal ulna. A hereditary form has an autosomal dominant trait. A similar deformity may develop after infection, trauma, tumors, and other developmental syndromes. A variety of surgical procedures have been described for the deformity, including corrective osteotomy of the radius and arthroplasty of the distal radioulnar joint.

Generalized Skeletal Abnormalities

Group VII anomalies occur in conjunction with generalized skeletal abnormalities. Examples include dwarfism, Ollier's disease, Marfan's syndrome, and Ehlers-Danlos syndrome. The specific clinical findings depend on the underlying syndrome and phenotypic expression of the deformity. Systemic problems are common, and comprehensive evaluation is warranted.

Cerebral Palsy (see Chapter 13)

Cerebral palsy is an irreversible, static, perinatal brain injury that affects the musculoskeletal system. The extent and degree of involvement are extremely variable. Cerebral palsy can affect one side of the body (hemiplegia) or all four limbs (quadriplegia). The motor effect can range from flaccidity to spasticity to athetosis. Sensibility of the affected part is usually diminished, and the intelligence of the patient is unpredictable. These variations in presentation complicate the formulation of a generalized treatment plan and the assessment of a uniform outcome measurement. Early treatment relies on therapy to achieve developmental milestones. Physical therapy modalities are also useful to prevent joint contractures, and splints provide functional benefits. In appropriate candidates, surgery is performed during childhood and adolescence. Surgery is most beneficial in children who are less affected and have mild to moderate spasticity. Surgery is least helpful in children with severe involvement, uncontrollable spasticity, and athetosis. Realistic preoperative goals are paramount because surgery is reparative and not curative.

The characteristic posture of the extremity that can benefit from surgery is positioned with the shoulder internally rotated, elbow flexed, forearm pronated, wrist flexed, fingers flexed, and thumb within the palm. The goal is to rebalance the extremity by a combination of joint stabilization procedures, tendon lengthening techniques, and tendon transfers. The physical examination remains the basis to guide surgical treatment. The evaluation includes a determination of joint position and an inventory of muscle activity. The deforming forces (i.e., agonists) and antagonists about each deformity require assessment. Each muscle is assessed for volitional action, spasticity, and phasic activity. Muscles that exhibit continuous firing and scarce purposeful recruitment are not candidates for transfer and are better treated by release or lengthening. Muscles that possess volitional activity, have mild spasticity, and are expendable represent potential donor candidates for tendon transfer.

Adjunctive methods are available to supplement the physical examination before surgical reconstruction. Dynamic electromyograms are useful to identify spastic and flaccid muscles. The timing of muscle contracture during certain activities can also be delineated by electromyography. Temporary neuromuscular blockade of the agonists with botulinum toxin, phenol, or an anesthetic agent can provide additional information about the status of the antagonists.

Surgery is indicated to expand function, to enhance hygiene, and to improve appearance. The shoulder position is usually not a limiting factor with regard to function. Lengthening of the subscapularis and pectoralis major muscles, however, treats a severe internal

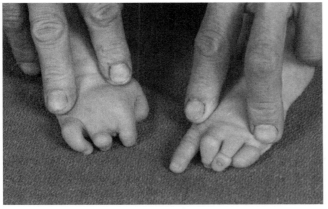

Figure 12-15 ◈ Various anomalies ranging from amputation to severe stricture secondary to amniotic disruption sequence.

rotation contracture. Deficient elbow extension decreases the available workspace and is detrimental to function. The amount of elbow flexion tends to increase during ambulation, which creates problems with balance. Treatment is directed at lessening the elbow flexion tone by lengthening the elbow flexors. The forearm pronation posture creates problems with feeding, perineal care, and bimanual activities. Surgical options are aimed at reducing the pronation force by a flexor-pronator slide or direct manipulation of the pronator teres and quadratus (lengthening, release, or rerouting).

The wrist flexion deformity directly impairs finger function and the ability to grasp and release. Wrist flexion deformities can be due to tight wrist flexors, capsular contracture, or weak wrist extensors. The wrist is treated by redirection of a flexion force to act as an extensor moment. Transfer of the flexor carpi ulnaris to the extensor carpi radialis brevis (Green transfer) is a common preference except in athetoid patients. Additional extension force can be obtained by transfer of the extensor carpi ulnaris to the midline. When passive digital extension is not possible during wrist extension, concomitant lengthening of the finger flexors is necessary to allow sufficient release of objects. Discrimination between flexor digitorum profundus and superficialis tightness is based on the distal interphalangeal and proximal interphalangeal joint tension. Augmentation of finger extension is better accomplished by an additional tendon transfer (for example, pronator teres) rather than by use of the extensor carpi ulnaris for both wrist and finger extension. Wrist fusion or proximal row carpectomy are reserved for adults with poor function or hygiene problems.

The thumb-in-palm deformity is extremely difficult to correct. An inventory of the thumb muscles often reveals spasticity of the intrinsic muscles (thenar and adductor pollicis muscles) and deficiencies within the extensor mechanism. Release of the thenar and adductor pollicis muscles from their origins allows these muscles to slide and diminishes their force. Augmentation of thumb extension and abduction is achieved by rerouting of the extensor pollicis longus tendon through the first dorsal compartment in patients with adequate passive thumb abduction and without adductor spasticity. Tendon transfers to the extensor pollicis brevis or abductor pollicis longus, flexor pollicis longus lengthening, and first dorsal interosseous lengthening are additional options. Thumb carpometacarpal joint arthrodesis is not an adequate surgical option.

Trauma

Trauma to the immature skeleton frequently involves the upper extremity. Fractures about the hand, wrist, forearm, and elbow are commonplace and require accurate diagnoses and treatment. The pediatric skeleton has certain distinct characteristics that require consideration during fracture management. First, sagittal and coronal plane remodeling can occur during growth. The amount of remodeling depends on the proximity of the fracture to the physis and the age of the child. This adjustment will not correct any malrotation, which

does not improve over time. Second, fracture readily separates the periosteum from the cortex and traps a subperiosteal hematoma. A portion of the periosteum often remains in continuity on the compression side of the fracture and limits displacement. This periosteum can help obtain and maintain a closed reduction of displaced fractures. Last, healing is quicker in children than in adults secondary to the abundant blood supply in growing bone. This property lessens the immobilization time required for fracture union. Growth plate fractures predominate and have been classified according to injury pattern (Table 12-14).

Hand fractures are common in children and involve the phalanges or metacarpals. Distal phalanx fractures are often crush injuries (e.g., car door) with considerable soft tissue injury. The priority of treatment is the loss of soft tissue and nail bed laceration. Soft tissue coverage principles are similar in children and adults, although young children (younger than 2 to 3 years) have an increased regenerative ability. In these instances, healing by secondary intention can cover small areas of exposed bone. Volar oblique injuries with considerable bone exposure require a local flap for coverage, such as thenar flap or cross-finger flap. The treatment of the underlying fracture depends on its location, amount of comminution, degree of stability, and status of the soft tissue envelope. In most instances, an external splint is adequate immobilization. A hyperflexion force can also damage the physis of the distal phalanx and create a Salter-Harris I, II, or III injury. As the fracture force propagates, the nail plate and matrix often avulse from beneath the eponychial fold. The child presents to the emergency department with the nail matrix above the nail fold, which is indicative of this injury. The germinal nail matrix must be placed back beneath the eponychium to permit nail growth. Fracture stabilization can be performed by external splint application or percutaneous longitudinal Kirschner wire fixation.

Proximal phalangeal fractures most commonly involve the border digits. An "extra-octave" fracture involves the small finger and is caused by an abduction force. The fracture pattern is often a Salter-Harris II fracture of the proximal phalanx with a small metaphyseal fragment. The small finger is positioned in abduction

❖ **Table 12-14**	
SALTER-HARRIS CLASSIFICATION OF GROWTH PLATE FRACTURES	
Type	**Characteristics**
I	Separation through the growth plate
II	Fracture through the growth plate that exits through the metaphysis, creating a metaphyseal fragment (Thurston Holland sign or fragment)*
III	Fracture through the growth plate that exits through the epiphysis
IV	Vertical split fracture that courses through metaphysis, growth plate, and epiphysis†
V	Crush injury

*Most common type.
†Physeal bar common.

and is tender over its base. A closed reduction is uniformly successful for re-establishment of bone alignment, followed by immobilization for 3 weeks. An abduction force can also injure the thumb and alter its stability. Because the collateral ligaments insert into the epiphysis of the proximal phalanx, fractures involving the ulnar epiphysis are similar to an adult skier's thumb. Therefore, a displaced fracture requires either closed or open reduction to restore bone alignment and joint stability.

Proximal phalanx fractures can also occur about the proximal interphalangeal joint. Extra-articular neck fractures can be particularly problematic and considerably displaced or rotated. A true lateral radiograph is mandatory to assess alignment. Closed reduction is applicable for fractures with mild displacement and angulation. Frequent monitoring is necessary to assess for loss of reduction. Open reduction is required for displaced fractures, with gentle handling of the fracture fragments and fixation with fine Kirschner wires. Overzealous periosteal stripping of the fracture fragment will lead to avascular necrosis of the condyles. Intra-articular fractures involve one or both condyles and are inherently unstable. The oblique fracture pattern is susceptible to displacement and joint incongruity. An undisplaced fracture can be treated by immobilization but must be observed closely. Any fracture displacement warrants closed reduction and percutaneous pinning. Open reduction is reserved for irreducible fractures that prohibit restoration of joint congruity.

Fractures of the metacarpals are less common than fractures of the phalanges, although the border digits still predominate. Small finger neck fractures are most prevalent and usually secondary to adolescent fighting. The amount of acceptable sagittal deformity remains controversial and ranges from 30 to 50 degrees. Rotational deformity requires closed reduction to prevent scissoring during fist formation. The thumb metacarpal base is also susceptible to fracture. An isolated metaphyseal or growth plate injury is common. A Salter-Harris III fracture is the pediatric equivalent of Bennett's fracture. The abductor pollicis and adductor pollicis muscles act as deforming forces on the untethered metacarpal. Closed reduction and percutaneous pinning are required to restore bone and ligament integrity to the metacarpal shaft.

Distal radius fractures are common in the pediatric population and have been divided according to type and location (Table 12-15). Physeal fractures can usually be treated by closed reduction and casting. The wrist must be radiographed once a week for 3 weeks to ensure preservation of alignment. Open reduction is reserved for irreducible fractures secondary to soft tissue interposition, which is usually a periosteal flap. Greenstick fractures are incomplete injuries and susceptible to repeated displacement. Closed reduction and casting are indicated for displaced or angulated incomplete fractures. The premise of fracture completion to decrease the incidence of redisplacement is controversial. Torus fractures are isolated compression fractures of the radius that occur 2 to 3 cm proximal to the growth plate. Point tenderness is universal, and

◆ **Table 12-15**

TYPES OF DISTAL RADIUS FRACTURES

Type	Characteristics
Physeal	Salter-Harris I or II with dorsal displacement plate
Greenstick	Incomplete fracture
Torus	Compression fracture 2 to 3 cm proximal to physis
Complete	Higher energy fractures, often involving distal radius and ulna

forearm rotation should be virtually painless. Short-arm cast immobilization is the treatment of choice. Painful forearm rotation and tenderness about the distal ulna are indicative of a pediatric Galeazzi fracture pattern. In these instances, the status of the distal radioulnar joint must be assessed, and long-arm immobilization is required. Complete fractures of the distal radius are associated with higher velocity injuries than are incomplete or compression injuries. A concomitant distal ulna fracture is common, and more soft tissue disruption is present. The skin must be inspected for small openings indicative of an open fracture. Any breach in the soft tissue envelope necessitates débridement. The bone injury often requires closed reduction and immobilization.

Gymnast wrist is a term used for stress-related changes of the distal radius physis. Repetitive injury can lead to early closure of the distal radius physis and ulnar overgrowth with an ulnar positive variance.

Frostbite may cause premature epiphyseal closure at 6 to 12 months from injury. The most common deformity involves radial deviation of the small finger distal interphalangeal joint. In addition to shortened digits, degenerative changes may occur about the affected joints.

Rotational finger deformities may be related to finger sucking. Significant deformities are treated with a metacarpal osteotomy in children older than 3 years.

Bibliography

Embryology

Bamshad M, Watkins WS, Dixon ME, et al: Reconstructing the history of human limb development: lessons from birth defects. Pediatr Res 45:291-299, 1999.

Beatty E: Upper limb tissue differentiation in the human embryo. Hand Clin 1:391-403, 1985.

Cohn MJ, Izpisua-Belmonte JC, Abud H, et al: Fibroblast growth factors induce additional limb development in the flank of chick embryos. Cell 80:739-746, 1995.

Riddle RD, Ensini M, Nelson C, et al: Induction of the LIM homeobox gene Lmx 1 by WNT7a establishes dorsoventral pattern in the vertebrate limb. Cell 83:631-640, 1995.

Riddle RD, Tabin CJ: How limbs develop. Sci Am 280:74-79, 1999.

Saunders JW Jr: The proximo-distal sequence of origin of the parts of the chick wing and the role of the ectoderm. J Exp Zool 108:363-403, 1948.

Classification

Buck-Gramcko D: Teratologic sequences. In Buck-Gramcko D, ed: Congenital malformations of the hand and forearm. London, Churchill Livingstone, 1998, pp 17-20.

Flatt AE: Classification and incidence. In Flatt AE: The Care of Congenital Hand Anomalies, 2nd ed. St. Louis, Quality Medical, 1994, pp 47-63.

Frantz CH, O'Rahilly R: Congenital skeletal limb deficiencies. J Bone Joint Surg Am 43:1202-1224, 1961.

Swanson AB: A classification for congenital limb malformations. J Hand Surg Am 1:8-22, 1976.

Failure of Formation

TRANSVERSE DEFICIENCY

Burton BK, Schulz CJ, Burd LI: Spectrum of limb disruption defects associated with chorionic villous sampling. Pediatrics 91:989-993, 1993.

Gonzalez CH, Marques-Dias J, Kim CA, et al: Congenital abnormalities in Brazilian children associated with misoprostol misuse in first trimester of pregnancy. Lancet 351:1624-1627, 1998.

Gover A, McIvor J: Upper limb deficiencies in infants and young children. Infants Young Children 5:57-71, 1992.

Hoyme HE, Jones KL, Van Allen MI, et al: Vascular pathogenesis of transverse limb reduction defects. J Pediatr 101:839-843, 1982.

Nathan P, Trung N: The Krukenberg operation: a modified technique avoiding skin grafts. J Hand Surg Am 2:127-130, 1977.

Scotland TR, Galaway HR: A long-term review of children with congenital and acquired upper limb deficiency. J Bone Joint Surg Br 65:346-349, 1983.

RADIAL DEFICIENCY

Bayne LG, Klug MS: Long-term review of the surgical treatment of radial deficiencies. J Hand Surg Am 12:169-179, 1987.

Bora FW Jr, Osterman AL, Kaneda RR, et al: Radial club-hand deformity. Long-term follow-up. J Bone Joint Surg Am 63:741-745, 1981.

Damore E, Kozin SH, Thoder JJ, Porter S: The recurrence of deformity after surgical centralization for radial clubhand. J Hand Surg Am 25:745-751, 2000.

Heikel HVA: Aplasia and hypoplasia of the radius. Studies on 64 cases and on epiphyseal transplantation in rabbits with the imitated defect. Acta Orthop Scand Suppl 39:1-155, 1959.

James MA, McCarroll HR, Manske PR: The spectrum of radial longitudinal deficiency: a modified classification. J Hand Surg Am 24:1145-1155, 1999.

Lourie GM, Lins RE: Radial longitudinal deficiency. A review and update. Hand Clin 14:85-99, 1998.

McCarroll HR: Congenital anomalies: a 25-year overview. J Hand Surg Am 25:1007-1037, 2000.

Vilkki SK: Distraction and microvascular epiphysis transfer for radial clubhand. J Hand Surg Br 23:445-452, 1998.

ULNAR DEFICIENCY

Miller JK, Wenner SM, Kruger LM: Ulnar deficiency. J Hand Surg Am 11:822-829, 1986.

Ogden JA, Watson HK, Bohne W: Ulnar dysmelia. J Bone Joint Surg Am 58:467-475, 1976.

Riordan DC: The upper limb. In Lovell W, Winter RB, eds: Pediatric Orthopaedics, vol 2. Philadelphia, JB Lippincott, 1978, pp 685-719.

Schmidt CC, Neufield SK: Ulnar ray deficiency. Hand Clin 14:65-76, 1998.

Swanson AB, Tada K, Yonenobu K: Ulnar ray deficiency: its various manifestations. J Hand Surg Am 9:658-664, 1984.

CENTRAL DEFICIENCY

Barsky AJ: Cleft hand: classification, incidence, and treatment—review of the literature and report of nineteen cases. J Bone Joint Surg Am 46:1707-1720, 1964.

Buck-Gramcko D: Teratologic sequences. In Buck-Gramcko D, ed: Congenital Malformations of the Hand and Forearm. London, Churchill Livingstone, 1998, pp 17-20.

Miura T, Nakamura R, Horii E: The position of symbrachydactyly in the classification of congenital hand anomalies. J Hand Surg Br 19:350-354, 1994.

Miura T, Suzuki M: Clinical differences between typical and atypical cleft hand. J Hand Surg Br 9:311-315, 1984.

Ogino T, Minami A, Kato H: Clinical features and roentgenograms of symbrachydactyly. J Hand Surg Br 14:303-306, 1989.

Snow JW, Littler JW: Surgical treatment of cleft hand. Transactions of the International Society of Plastic and Reconstructive Surgery, 4th Congress. Rome, Excerpta Medica, 1967, pp 888-893.

Failure of Differentiation

SYNDACTYLY

Bosse K, Betz RC, Lee YA, et al: Localization of a gene for syndactyly type 1 to chromosome 2q34-q36. Am J Hum Genet 67:492-497, 2000.

Eaton CJ, Lister GD: Syndactyly. Hand Clin 6:555-574, 1990.

Ireland DCR, Takoyama N, Flatt A: Poland's syndrome: a review of 43 cases. J Bone Joint Surg Am 58:52-58, 1976.

Kozin SH: Syndactyly. J Am Soc Surg Hand 1:1-13, 2001.

Richterman I, Dupree J, Kozin SH, Thoder J: Radiographic analysis of web height. J Hand Surg Am 23:1071-1076, 1998.

SYNOSTOSIS

Cleary JE, Omer GE: Congenital proximal radio-ulnar synostosis: natural history and functional assessment. J Bone Joint Surg Am 67:539, 1985.

Kozin SH, Thoder J: Congenital anomalies of the upper extremity. In Baratz ME, Watson AD, Imbriglia JE, eds: Orthopedic Surgery: The Essentials. New York, Thieme, 1999, pp 657-673.

Steel HH, Piston RW, Clancy M, Betz RR: A syndrome of dislocated hips and radial heads, carpal coalition, and short stature in Puerto Rican children. J Bone Joint Surg Am 75:259-267, 1993.

RADIAL HEAD

Campbell CC, Waters PM, Emans JB: Excision of the radial head for congenital dislocation. J Bone Joint Surg Am 74:726, 1992.

Sachar K, Mih AD: Congenital radial head dislocations. Hand Clin 14:39-47, 1998.

ARTHROGRYPOSIS

Ezaki M: Treatment of the upper limb in the child with arthrogryposis. Hand Clin 16:703-711, 2000.

Hall JG, Reed SD, Driscoll EP: Part I. Amyoplasia: a common, sporadic condition with congenital contractures. Am J Med Genet 15:571-590, 1983.

Weeks PM: Surgical correction of upper extremity deformities in arthrogryposis. Plast Reconstr Surg 36:459, 1965.

PTERYGIUM

Hall JG, Reed SD, Rosenbaum KN, et al: Limb pterygium syndromes: a review and report of eleven patients. Am J Med Genet 12:377-409, 1982.

TRIGGER

Cardon LJ, Ezaki M, Carter PR: Trigger finger in children. J Hand Surg Am 24:1156-1161, 1999.

Dinham DM, Meggitt BF: Trigger thumbs in children. J Bone Joint Surg Br 56:153-155, 1974.

Mulpruek P, Prishasuk S, Orapin S: Trigger finger in children. J Pediatr Orthop 18:239-241, 1998.

Rodgers WB, Waters PM: Incidence of trigger digits in newborns. J Hand Surg Am 19:364-368, 1994.

HYPOPLASTIC THUMB

Graham TJ, Louis DS: A comprehensive approach to surgical management of the type IIIA hypoplastic thumb. J Hand Surg Am 23: 3-13, 1998.

Kozin SH, Weiss AA, Weber JB, et al: Index finger pollicization for congenital aplasia or hypoplasia of the thumb. J Hand Surg Am 17:880-884, 1992.

Lister G: Reconstruction of the hypoplastic thumb. Clin Orthop 195:52-65, 1985.

Manske PR, McCarroll HR Jr, James MA: Type III-A hypoplastic thumb. J Hand Surg Am 20:246-253, 1995.

CLASPED THUMB

Mih AD: Congenital clasped thumb. Hand Clin 14:77-84, 1998.

CAMPTODACTYLY

Benson LS, Waters PM, Kamil NI, et al: Camptodactyly: classification and results of nonoperative treatment. J Pediatr Orthop 14:814-819, 1994.

McFarlane RM, Classen DA, Porte AM, Botz JS: The anatomy and treatment of camptodactyly of the small finger. J Hand Surg Am 17:35-44, 1992.

Senrui H: Congenital contractures. In Buck-Gramcko D, ed: Congenital malformations of the hand and forearm. London, Churchill Livingstone, 1998, pp 295-309.

Siegert JJ, Cooney WP, Dobyns JH: Management of simple campto-dactyly. J Hand Surg Br 15:181-189, 1990.

Smith PJ, Grobbelaar AO: Camptodactyly: a unifying theory and approach to surgical treatment. J Hand Surg Am 23:14-19, 1998.

Smith RJ, Kaplan EB: Camptodactyly and similar atraumatic flexion deformities of the proximal interphalangeal joints of the fingers. J Bone Joint Surg Am 50:1187-1203, 1968.

WINDBLOWN HAND

Zancolli E, Zancolli E Jr: Congenital ulnar drift of the fingers. Pathogenesis, classification, and surgical management. Hand Clin 1:443-456, 1985.

CLINODACTYLY

Ezaki M: Angled digits. In Green DP, Hotchkiss RN, Pederson WC, eds: Green's Operative Hand Surgery, 4th ed. New York, Churchill Livingstone, 1999, pp 517-521.

Poznanski AK, Pratt GB, Manson G, Weiss L: Clinodactyly, campto-dactyly, Kirner's deformity, and other crooked fingers. Radiology 93:573-582, 1969.

LONGITUDINAL EPIPHYSEAL BRACKET

Carstam N, Theander G: Surgical treatment of clinodactyly caused by longitudinally bracketed diaphysis. Scand J Plast Reconstr Surg 9:199-202, 1975.

Light TR, Ogden JA: The longitudinal epiphyseal bracket: implications for surgical correction. J Pediatr Orthop 1:299-305, 1981.

Vickers D: Clinodactyly of the little finger: a simple operative technique for reversal of the growth abnormality. J Hand Surg Br 12:335-345, 1987.

Duplication

THUMB DUPLICATION

Cohen MS: Thumb duplication. Hand Clin 14:17-27, 1998.

Ezaki MB: Radial polydactyly. Hand Clin 6:577-588, 1990.

Wassel HD: The results of surgery for polydactyly of the thumb. A review. Clin Orthop 125:175-193, 1969.

POLYDACTYLY

Muragaki Y, Mundlos S, Upton J, Olsen BR: Altered growth and branching patterns in synpolydactyly caused by mutations in HOXD13. Science 272:548-551, 1996.

Watson BT, Hennrikus WL: Postaxial type-B polydactyly. Prevalence and treatment. J Bone Joint Surg Am 79:65-68, 1997.

Overgrowth

Upton J, Coombs CJ, Mulliken JB, et al: Vascular malformations of the upper limb: a review of 270 patients. J Hand Surg Am 24:1019-1035, 1999.

Amniotic Disruption Sequence

Askins G, Ger E: Congenital constriction band syndrome. J Pediatr Orthop 8:461, 1988.

Foulkes GD, Reinker K: Congenital constriction band syndrome: a seventy year experience. J Pediatr Orthop 14:242-248, 1994.

Light TR, Ogden JA: Congenital constriction band syndrome. Yale J Biol Med 66:143, 1994.

Wiedrich TA: Congenital constriction band syndrome. Hand Clin 14:29-38, 1998.

Madelung's Deformity

Dobyns JH: Madelung's deformity. In Green DP, Hotchkiss RN, eds: Green's Operative Hand Surgery, 3rd ed. New York, Churchill Livingstone, 1993, pp 517-520.

Cerebral Palsy

Hoffer M, Perry J, Melkonian GJ: Dynamic electromyography and decision-making for surgery of the upper extremity of patients with cerebral palsy. J Hand Surg Am 4:424-431, 1979.

Manske PR: Cerebral palsy of the upper extremity. Hand Clin 6:697-709, 1990.

Waters PM, Heest AV: Spastic hemiplegia of the upper extremity in children. Hand Clin 14:119-134, 1998.

Trauma

Le TB, Hentz VR: Hand and wrist injuries in young athletes. Hand Clin 16:597-607, 2000.

Leclercq C, Korn W: Articular fractures of the fingers in children. Hand Clin 16:523-534, 2000.

Light TR, Ogden JA: Metacarpal epiphyseal fractures. J Hand Surg Am 12:460-464, 1987.

Salter RB, Harris WR: Injuries involving the epiphyseal plate. J Bone Joint Surg Am 45:587-622, 1963.

13

✧ Y. Leo Leung, MD ✧ Pedro K. Beredjiklian, MD ✧ David J. Bozentka, MD

REHABILITATION

Kinesiology

Hand

The spectrum of functional activities of the hand is extensive. In general, they can be grouped into non-prehensile and prehensile activities.

1. *Nonprehensile* activities include touching, feeling, pressing down, tapping with the fingers, vibrating the cord of a musical instrument, and lifting with the hand.
2. *Prehensile* activities involve gripping with the hand and are divided into precision and power grip.
   a. Precision grip
      i. *Palmar tip pinch* is used for fine motor functions without force, such as picking up a needle.
      ii. *Lateral pinch or key grip* involves contact of the pulp of the thumb with the lateral aspect of the corresponding finger. It provides a strong grip without precision.
      iii. *Palmar pad pinch* is a compromise between the other two grips and is therefore the preferred splinting position of the hand.
      iv. *The three-jaw chuck pinch* involves gripping with the thumb, index, and middle finger.
   b. Power grip
      i. The *hook power grip* involves flexion of the interphalangeal joints and minimal participation of the metacarpophalangeal joints to curve the fingers into the shape of a hook. It is useful in carrying objects with a handle (e.g., a briefcase).
      ii. In performing a *spherical grip,* the wrist is held in slight extension with the fingers wrapped around an object placed in the palm. The fingers are abducted and rotated, with the thumb providing a counterpressure to stabilize the object.
3. Grip strength can be tested by use of a Jamar dynamometer. The device has five settings, I through V (smallest to largest).
   a. Position I, the smallest setting, assesses intrinsic function.
   b. Position V, the largest setting, assesses the extrinsic flexor function.
   c. The maximal grip strength tested is at position II, in which both the intrinsics and extrinsic flexors are effective.
   d. Allows objective assessment of the patient's effort.

METACARPOPHALANGEAL JOINTS

The metacarpophalangeal (MP) joints are critical for finger function.

1. Contracture of the MP joint typically occurs in extension, as the collateral ligaments are relaxed in extension and taut in flexion.
2. As the MP joint goes into hyperextension as a result of a contracture, the interphalangeal joints tend to flex, and the digit can adopt an intrinsic minus position.
3. In a completely paralyzed hand, the MP joints are usually maintained in 45 degrees of flexion.

Wrist and Forearm

1. The prehensile force of the hand is greatest when the wrist is in 20 to 30 degrees of extension.
2. As the wrist assumes a flexed position, the extrinsic extensor tendons become taut and extend the MP joints through the tenodesis effect. This tenodesis effect limits grip strength.
3. Together with the wrist, forearm rotation governs the orientation of the hand by supination and pronation.

Elbow

1. The elbow acts primarily to position the hand in space.

Shoulder

1. The role of the shoulder is upper limb orientation, pointing the arm in the correct direction in space toward the desired object.

Orthotics

1. An orthosis can be defined as an externally applied device used to modify structural and functional characteristics of the neuromusculoskeletal system.

2. The goals of orthotics are the following:
   a. To immobilize or support.
   b. To apply traction.
   c. To assist a weakened muscle group.
   d. To substitute for absent motor function.
   e. To control movement.
   f. To allow attachment of assistive devices.
3. Orthoses can be static, dynamic, or functional.
   a. Static orthoses
      i. Static orthoses are rigid and give support without allowing movement.
      ii. A static orthosis can conform to rest a joint in a desired position.
      iii. When mild traction is needed, a nonconforming device can stretch a contracted joint or a muscle.
   b. Dynamic orthoses
      i. Dynamic orthoses permit a certain degree of movement under controlled conditions.
      ii. They are typically designed with some moving parts, such as elastic bands, springs, or hinges.
      iii. They can be used to neutralize a progressive deforming force (e.g., joint contracture), to allow controlled joint motion while preventing unwanted motion (e.g., after tendon repair or reconstruction), or to substitute for a weakened muscle (e.g., volar wrist splint in a patient with radial nerve palsy).
   c. Functional orthoses
      i. Functional orthoses help improve function, whether or not they allow motion or have moving parts.
      ii. They are commonly used in patients with permanent or slowly recovering conditions.
      iii. These devices usually require proper fabrication and fitting.
4. Factors to be considered in every orthotic prescription are sensation, weight or gravitational pull, comfort, simplicity, durability, utility, wear tolerance, and cosmesis.
5. Orthoses can be used in any of the upper extremity joints.

Shoulder Orthoses

1. The sling is the most common shoulder orthosis. It functions to support the upper extremity.
2. An airplane splint consists of a body piece that is connected by a static part to an arm support, holding the shoulder in the desired abduction and flexion.
3. A figure-of-eight orthosis pulls the shoulder upward and backward, decreasing tension and pain in the neck by supporting a drooping shoulder.
4. Dynamic orthoses are rarely indicated. They are often bulky, are cumbersome, and provide limited additional function.

Elbow Orthoses

1. Static orthoses are used to correct elbow flexion or extension contractures. They can be applied anteriorly or posteriorly or in the form of a three-point orthosis.
2. Static elbow-wrist orthoses are used to stabilize the forearm and to prevent supination and pronation.
3. Dynamic orthoses can be fitted to assist elbow flexion. Orthoses to assist in elbow extension are not usually necessary because this motion can be achieved by gravity.

Wrist Orthoses

1. These are the most frequently prescribed upper limb orthoses.
2. A simple wrist splint can be fashioned dorsally or volarly to provide wrist support.
3. Although commonly used, volar splints can obstruct the palm in gripping objects and cover up sensate skin.
4. Unless indicated, volar splints should not extend past the MP joints (distal palmar crease in the hand) to prevent extension contractures.
5. A volar splint should be about two-thirds the length of the forearm to have adequate mechanical leverage.
6. A dynamic orthosis can provide support and control flexion and extension while limiting radial and ulnar deviation. These splints can be used after arthroplasty, synovectomy, or fracture.
7. Specific splints for cervical cord injuries include the following:
   a. Wrist-driven flexor hinge hand orthoses are helpful in patients with active wrist extension.
      i. A three-jaw type of pinch is obtained by tenodesis effect.
      ii. It may be useful for C6 and C7 functional injuries.
   b. The ratchet hand splint is passively manipulated to achieve prehension in a patient who has no functional wrist extension but adequate elbow and shoulder function. This may be beneficial for the C5 functional level.

Hand Orthoses

1. Because most activities of daily living can be performed by one normal hand, patients often reject orthoses that do not significantly improve function.
2. Not every deformity requires orthotic correction.
3. Inappropriate splinting can interfere with residual hand function.
4. In splinting for extrinsic flexors or extensors, both the wrist and the fingers should be included.

Static Orthoses

1. Static devices can be used to hold the hand in a particular position or to immobilize a digit or a single joint.
2. For example, an MP extension block can be placed dorsally to prevent hyperextension of this joint in an intrinsic minus digit.
3. Static distal interphalangeal (DIP) joint extension splints are often used to treat extensor tendon injuries in the digits, such as mallet fingers.

Dynamic Orthoses

1. Dynamic MP joint flexion or extension orthoses can be made by modifying basic wrist-hand designs,

incorporating finger loops connected to rubber bands.

2. With the finger loops placed at the level of the proximal phalanges, these devices can help correct MP joint contractures.

3. Dynamic orthoses for interphalangeal joints can be fabricated in a similar fashion, keeping in mind that the MP joints or proximal interphalangeal (PIP) joints should be immobilized to maximize the pulling force at the distal segments.

Static Progressive Splints

1. These orthoses involve mobilization of the joints with inelastic splinting.

2. The splints maintain the tissues at end range under a low stress load. As the tissues lengthen, the splint is adjusted in small increments to maintain low-load prolonged stress at a newly established end range.

Prosthetics

Introduction

1. The ratio of upper to lower limb amputation is estimated to be 1:5.

2. Of upper extremity amputees, 60% are between the ages of 21 and 64 years.

3. The most frequent causes of upper limb amputation are trauma (approximately 75%) and malignant disease, followed by vascular insufficiency.

4. The most common level of amputation is transradial (57%). Transhumeral amputation accounts for 23% of all arm amputations.

5. Not surprisingly, the right arm is more frequently involved in work-related injuries.

6. The absolute surgical indication for amputation in trauma is ischemia in a limb with unreconstructible vascular injury.

7. Limb salvage in any situation should be based on providing an extremity that has sufficient sensation for protective feedback, has a durable soft tissue cover, and can be used to interact with the environment.

8. Amputation should never be viewed as surgical failure but rather as the means to return the patient to a more functional status.

9. The viability of soft tissue and the amount of skin coverage with adequate sensation usually determine the most distal functional level for amputation.

10. Bone prominences, scars, soft tissue traction, shear, and perspiration can complicate prosthesis use.

11. Early prosthetic fitting after arm amputation (within 1 to 3 months) is imperative for a successful prosthetic restoration.

12. In general, the more distal the amputation, the more functional the final outcome is.

13. When the dominant upper extremity is involved, the amputee often can transfer hand dominance to the contralateral limb.

14. The amputee rehabilitation program can be divided into eight stages (Table 13-1).

❖ **Table 13-1**

STAGES OF AMPUTEE REHABILITATION

1	Preamputation counseling
2	Amputation surgery
3	Acute postsurgical period
4	Preprosthesis fitting
5	Preparatory prosthesis fitting
6	Prosthesis fitting and training
7	Reintegration into the community
8	Long-term follow-up

Preamputation Counseling

1. Direct communication between all members of the surgical and rehabilitation teams with the patient and family is essential.

2. A complete discussion should include issues such as phantom limb sensation, prosthetic devices, prosthesis fitting and training, and the timing of these events.

3. A "pre-rehabilitation" program should include strengthening to the trunk and remaining upper limb musculature and stretching exercises to preserve range of motion of the involved glenohumeral, scapulothoracic, and elbow joints if they are present.

4. Relaxation techniques may be introduced as well.

Amputation Surgery

Digits

1. Finger amputation can occur at the DIP, PIP, or MP joint level or as a digital ray.

2. Distal tip amputation: see Chapter 3.

3. Amputation through the DIP joint
   a. If possible the head of the middle phalanx (including articular cartilage) should be preserved to improve healing and decrease inflammation. Otherwise, the middle phalanx should be shortened and contoured to allow soft tissue closure.
   b. The flexor digitorum profundus tendon should not be sutured to the extensor tendon to prevent the development of the quadriga effect (see Chapter 2).
   c. An amputation through the DIP joint (particularly the index finger) with retraction of the profundus tendon may lead to a lumbrical plus finger (see Chapter 2).

4. Amputation through the middle or proximal phalanges
   a. Active flexion of the PIP joint will be possible with an amputation distal to or through the insertion of the flexor digitorum superficialis.
   b. After an amputation through the proximal phalanx, flexion of the digit will occur through the intrinsic muscle attachments at the base of the proximal phalanx.
   c. Amputations near the MP joint may lead to functional difficulties (e.g., dropping small objects such as coins through the space left by

the missing digits). For this reason, ray amputations should be considered for these injuries, particularly for the ring and long fingers.

HAND

Ray Amputations

1. Ray amputation involves removal of the phalanges in addition to the corresponding metacarpal.
2. The base of the metacarpal may be preserved.
3. Ray amputation of the long or ring finger may benefit from transposition of the index or small finger, respectively, to take up the resultant gap.
   a. An alternative involves suturing the deep intermetacarpal ligaments of the adjacent residual metacarpals to close the resultant space.
4. After finger ray amputation, the grip strength and dexterity are generally equal for all four rays.
5. Quicker recovery is noted after primary ray amputation, although the final outcome is similar to that of secondary ray amputation.
6. The outcome of ray amputation is most highly influenced by the presence of a worker's compensation claim.

Transcarpal Amputations

1. These amputations are not commonly performed because of limited functional outcome.
2. Whereas reconstructive surgery for partial hand amputations may enhance function while preserving sensory feedback, that of the thumb should be carefully considered.
3. Although maintaining thumb length is important, many patients find that a thumb prosthesis alone provides adequate functional outcome.
4. A cosmetic prosthesis that shields sensate skin is likely to be discarded.

WRIST

Wrist Disarticulation

1. The distal radioulnar joint should be preserved in a wrist disarticulation to provide full forearm pronation and supination.
2. Sockets for this level of amputation are tapered and oval distally to provide rotational control.
3. The socket is attached to a triceps pad by flexible elbow hinges, and the harness is connected to the triceps pad (Fig. 13-1).

FOREARM

1. Transradial amputation is preferred in most cases to wrist disarticulation because it typically allows the highest level of functional recovery.
2. The resultant function of the amputation depends on the level of amputation and age of the patient.
3. The amputation can be performed at three levels.
   a. The *long* forearm residual limb is preferred when optimal body-powered prosthetic restoration is the goal. It is the ideal level for the patient who is anticipating a physically demanding lifestyle.
   b. The *medium* forearm residual limb is preferred when optimal externally powered prosthetic restoration is the goal. The relatively shorter

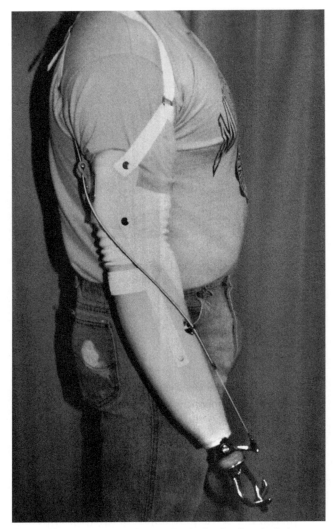

Figure 13-1 ◆ A definitive mechanical wrist disarticulation prosthesis with a triceps cuff, flexible elbow hinges, laminated socket, quick-disconnect/locking wrist, and stainless steel No. 7 hook. *(From Bowker JH, Michael JW, eds: Atlas of Limb Prosthetics: Surgical, Prosthetic, and Rehabilitation Principles, 2nd ed. Philadelphia, Mosby, 1992.)*

residual limb allows extra room for the battery and motor inside the prosthesis.
   c. The *short* transradial amputation can complicate suspension and limit elbow flexion strength and elbow range of motion. There is limited supination and pronation in a short below-elbow amputation, although flexion and extension are preserved.

ELBOW

Elbow Disarticulation

1. This procedure preserves the medial and lateral condyles of the distal humerus and therefore provides for prosthesis self-suspension through the bony anatomy, resulting in a less cumbersome socket.
2. The geometry of the distal humeral condyles adds rotational control to the connection between the prosthesis and the stump.

3. The lack of an anatomic elbow joint leads to additional mechanical effort and elevated cost for a proper prosthesis.
4. The length of the residual limb prevents the use of an externally powered elbow mechanism without significant alteration in the center of rotation of the elbow.

ARM

Transhumeral Amputations

1. Transhumeral amputations can be performed at three different levels as well (i.e., long, medium, and short residual limb).
2. Whereas all three levels require the same rehabilitation process and similar prosthetic components, the long residual limb permits optimal prosthetic restoration.
3. Amputations should be carried out at 7 to 10 cm proximal to the distal humeral condyles to accommodate a prosthetic elbow.

SHOULDER

1. Shoulder disarticulation and forequarter amputations are usually performed when no other option is available, typically in the setting of complex trauma or malignant disease.
2. With the number of joints involved and problems with securing a suspension, patients with these levels of amputation are the most difficult to fit with a functional prosthesis.
3. Greater success is noted in healthy, young male patients.

MUSCLE STABILIZATION

Stabilizing the distal end of a detached muscle can improve residual limb function and comfort.
1. *Myodesis* is the direct fixation of muscle or tendon to bone. The distal end of a muscle can be stabilized enough to counteract an antagonistic muscle group.
2. *Myoplasty* is the suturing of muscle to periosteum. This technique provides a less secure insertion than can be achieved by myodesis.

Acute Postamputation Period

1. The three major goals immediately after surgery are pain control with adequate analgesia, promotion of wound healing, and maintenance of range of motion and strength with appropriate therapy.
2. Postoperative wound management options include rigid plaster of Paris dressings, elastic bandage dressings, soft compressive dressings, and Unna bandages (Fig. 13-2).
3. Proponents of immediate prosthetic fitting advocate that it provides wound protection, edema control, and early shaping and shrinking of soft tissues while promoting early return to function.
4. Proper positioning and rehabilitation are essential in preventing elbow flexion contracture and shoulder abduction contracture, especially when wounds are close to or overlying these joints.

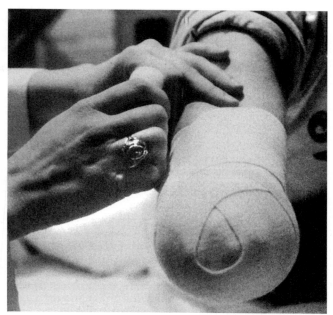

Figure 13-2 ◆ Figure-of-eight elastic bandage wrapping technique. (*From Bowker JH, Michael JW, eds: Atlas of Limb Prosthetics: Surgical, Prosthetic, and Rehabilitation Principles, 2nd ed. Philadelphia, Mosby, 1992.*)

5. Strengthening programs for proximal shoulder girdle muscles should be considered. Individual muscles to focus on include the trapezius, serratus anterior, pectoralis major, and residual deltoid and biceps.

Preprosthesis Fitting

1. Once wound healing occurs, a skin desensitization program including gentle tapping, massage, and soft tissue and scar mobilization should be initiated. Lubrication is recommended for the patient with a soft or elastic dressing.
2. The ideal elastic dressing involves the use of a figure-of-eight wrapping technique that extends over the proximal joint and is reapplied every 4 to 6 hours. Care is taken to avoid constricting circulation proximally, which would exacerbate swelling.
3. If a rigid dressing is used, it should be changed at a weekly interval to adjust for the reducing volume of the residual limb.
4. Virtually all amputees after surgery report feeling that all or part of the amputated limb is still present.
   a. This phenomenon is known as *phantom limb* sensation and is not always bothersome.
   b. Although the etiology is complex, surgeons should be aware of the observation that preamputation pain often ends in postoperative phantom pain.
   c. As many as 70% of patients perceive some form of pain in the first few months.
   d. Fortunately, such pain usually disappears or decreases to a level compatible with prosthesis fitting and daily activities.
   e. When pain persists for more than 6 months, the chance of spontaneous improvement is poor.

❖ Table 13-2		
ADVANTAGES AND DISADVANTAGES OF DIFFERENT UPPER EXTREMITY PROSTHESES		
Design	**Advantages**	**Disadvantages**
Passive or cosmetic	Lightweight Least harnessing Best cosmetic appearance	Least functional High cost if custom-made
Body powered	Most durable Moderate cost Moderately lightweight Provides sensory feedback to operating muscle groups	Most harnessing Least satisfactory appearance Most body movement required

Externally powered
  (myoelectric or switch control)
	Least body movement to use
	Enhances function in complex
	  prosthesis
	Moderate harnessing
		Heaviest
		Most expensive
		
		Most maintenance required
		Limited sensory feedback

f. Treatment includes prosthetic socket revision, desensitization techniques, transcutaneous nerve stimulation, neuropharmacologic agents, and mental imaging (i.e., the voluntary control of the phantom limb).

g. For severe cases, nerve blocks, steroid injection, or epidural analgesia can be helpful. Surgical management is far less successful.

h. Patients can also experience stump pain, which is localized pain at the amputation stump after the soft tissues are healed.

Preparatory Prosthesis

1. The use of the first prosthesis should be implemented as soon as the wound condition permits.
2. The first prosthesis is intended to promote residual limb maturation and desensitization; therefore, building up wear tolerance encourages the patient to become a successful functional user.
3. Because residual limb volume continues to fluctuate significantly, suction suspension or myoelectric control is not practical at this stage.

Prosthesis Fitting and Training

1. Upper extremity prostheses can be divided into three major groups: passive or cosmetic, body powered or conventional, and externally powered or electric.
2. The advantages and disadvantages of each are summarized in Table 13-2.
3. Difficulty in providing adequate body-powered control motions for more proximal joints is an indication for considering externally powered units.
4. Hybrid prostheses strive to achieve a compromise while maximizing the advantages of individual design. For example, a hybrid prosthesis with an electric elbow and a conventional terminal device, such as a hook, would minimize the effort needed to position the terminal device while reserving all body power for the operation of the hook.
5. The major advantage of a below-elbow myoelectric prosthesis over a standard below-elbow prosthesis is the increased ease of performing activities overhead and close to the body.

6. Cosmetic covers should be an integral part of the prosthesis. For many patients, this may be one of the most important measures of success of prosthetic restoration.
   a. These can be fabricated for a single digit, for the hand, or extending to the elbow (Fig. 13-3).
   b. Custom-made silicone components can provide excellent cosmetic appearance but can be expensive and difficult to maintain.
   c. Poorly manufactured gloves can stain easily.
   d. Digital prostheses after a digital amputation are most commonly used to improve appearance.
7. For bilateral amputees, the development of a dominant prosthesis should be encouraged.

Device Components

PROSTHETIC SOCKETS

1. The key functions of a prosthetic socket are comfortable total contact interface with the residual limb, efficient energy transfer from the residual limb to the prosthetic device, secure suspension, and cosmetic appearance.
2. Sockets are *custom made* by first obtaining a negative impression of the residual limb by plaster of Paris. This negative is then converted to a positive mold, often with clear thermoplastic material heated to 300° F or higher.
3. Provisional sockets are transparent to identify areas of excessive pressure with the residual limb inside the socket. Final modification by a prosthetist is essential to distribute pressure evenly throughout the entire surface of available soft tissues.
4. Computer-aided design and computer-aided manufacturing, when available, can be invaluable adjuncts to some of the more traditional socket fabrication steps.
5. Most upper extremity prosthesis sockets have two layers.
   a. The inner layer is closely contoured to fit the residual limb, whereas the external layer is used to generate the necessary length and shape to the socket.

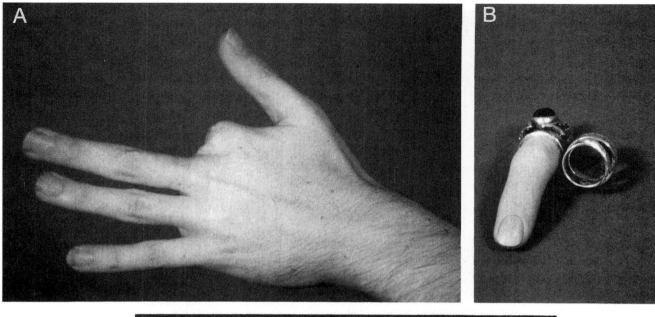

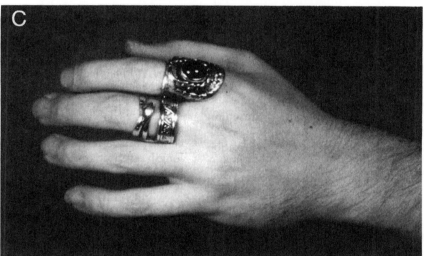

Figure 13-3 ❖ **A,** Short stumps present difficulties in good fixation of a digital prosthesis. **B,** Ornamental suspension rings. **C,** Prosthesis fitting with the use of rings worn on the involved and adjacent digits. *(From Bowker JH, Michael JW, eds: Atlas of Limb Prosthetics: Surgical, Prosthetic, and Rehabilitation Principles, 2nd ed. Philadelphia, Mosby, 1992.)*

  b. Velcro or some other removable fastener that requires only one hand to use usually holds the inner socket in place.
  c. Windows can be cut out in the exterior frame to make room for muscle expansion during contraction and to improve comfort and sensory feedback.
6. Socks can be used as an interface between the socket and the residual limb to protect the skin and to improve hygiene.
  a. Another advantage is that adding a variable number of layers can adjust for minor physiologic volume changes that occur in the amputated limb.

SUSPENSION SYSTEMS
1. The two main functions of a suspension system are to secure the prosthesis to the body and to provide control of the prosthesis.
2. The traditional suspension system is a figure-of-eight harness with a strap that suspends the prosthetic device over the shoulder.
3. The harness is a key component of the control mechanism that transmits body power to the terminal device or the elbow through cable connections.
4. For more proximal level amputations, a chest strap or shoulder saddle can be added to the suspension. These add to the stability of the prosthesis and its ability to carry heavier load.

Muenster Socket

1. This socket includes a self-suspension system and is an alternative for transradial amputees (Fig. 13-4).
2. This type of socket provides excellent suspension by encasing the distal humeral condyles.
3. The main disadvantage is the resultant limitation in elbow motion, which makes it less desirable in bilateral transradial amputations.

Suction Suspensions

1. These are used to eliminate the need for straps and harnesses.
2. The socket is made small enough to achieve an intimate fit between the residual limb and the socket, resulting in a tight seal.
3. A one-way valve permits air expulsion during donning.
4. The vacuum phenomenon therefore holds the prosthesis against the residual limb.
5. For this kind of suspension to work well, the residual limb must be mature and volume stable.
6. The patient should also have good contralateral upper extremity strength, endurance, and coordination to don the prosthesis independently.
7. Because direct contact of the residual limb and the socket is paramount, a sock cannot be used with suction suspensions.

Hypobaric and Semisuction Suspensions

1. These are transitions between no suction and full-suction suspension systems.
2. They use a silicone band on a sock with a one-way valve inside the socket.
3. During donning, air is expelled from inside of the socket. As the silicone band comes into contact with the socket, a seal is obtained.
4. Altering the thickness of the socks used can readily accommodate changes in residual limb volume that typically occur early in the rehabilitation process.

CONTROL MECHANISMS

1. When body power is used to activate the prosthetic device, a body harness with a cable system is typically implemented.

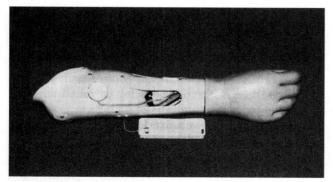

Figure 13-4 ◆ A transradial Muenster-style socket with attached fitting frame to hold electronic components in a preparatory/training electronic prosthesis. *(From Bowker JH, Michael JW, eds: Atlas of Limb Prosthetics: Surgical, Prosthetic, and Rehabilitation Principles, 2nd ed. Philadelphia, Mosby, 1992.)*

2. The patient needs to be able to coordinate movements that generate enough strength to control the terminal device or the prosthetic elbow.
3. The body movements most commonly employed are scapular abduction, chest expansion, shoulder depression-extension-abduction-flexion, and elbow flexion-extension.
    a. For a below-elbow prosthesis, the primary motion to operate the terminal device is glenohumeral flexion and scapular abduction.
    b. For an above-elbow prosthesis, the motion required to lock and unlock the prosthetic elbow is shoulder extension and abduction with scapular depression.
        i. Flexion of the prosthetic elbow with the elbow unlocked is performed with shoulder flexion or scapular abduction.
        ii. Terminal device control for an above-elbow prosthesis with the prosthetic elbow locked is also performed with shoulder flexion or scapular abduction.
4. A poorly adjusted harness, short residual limb, stump pain, joint contractures, or suboptimal sockets can affect force transmission.
5. Ideally, a separate cable-harness pair controls each joint in the prosthesis.

Externally Powered Prostheses

1. These use batteries and electrical motors to generate motion.
2. In general, these prostheses can provide greater prehensile forces.
3. When used in an elbow unit, they may provide more elbow function, especially in short transhumeral amputations.
4. Electric control switches can be activated with residual limb movements inside the socket that depress an on-off switch.
5. Other triggering mechanisms include a chest strap, waist belt, and figure-of-nine harness.

Myoelectric Prostheses

1. Myoelectric controls make use of the electrical signals generated during muscle contractions to control the flow of current from the battery to the motor.
2. A snug fit is required for accurate detection of electric activities by the reference electrodes inside the socket.
3. Ideally, muscles in the more distal portion of the residual limb should be used.
4. Multichannel components can distinguish slow, gentle muscle contractions from fast, strong ones and produce different prosthetic motions.
5. New technology allows the implementation of a proportional control that senses the strength of the muscle contraction and produces a corresponding output.
    a. For example, the Liberty Mutual or Boston elbow (Liberty Mutual, Boston, Mass) will flex or extend faster in direct proportion to the increasing amplitude of the muscle contraction.

6. The Utah elbow (Motion Control, Salt Lake City, Utah) is the most sophisticated and expensive of the current myoelectric systems.
   a. This system uses two sets of electrodes managed by a microprocessor to generate both elbow and terminal device functions.
   b. A free-swing mode can mimic the pendulum motion of the arm during normal walking.
   c. It is made from modular components.
7. The major disadvantages of myoelectric prostheses as noted in Table 13-2 are their cost, weight, and maintenance needs.
8. Myoelectric prostheses are most successful in patients with mid forearm amputations.

Specific Devices

A prescription for an upper extremity prosthesis should correctly describe the terminal device, joint components, choice of socket, method of suspension, and control system.

TERMINAL DEVICES

1. Terminal devices attempt to replace the complex mobility and dexterity of the human hand.
2. These can be classified into prosthetic hands or hooks.
   a. Prosthetic hands provide a three-jaw chuck pinch when closed and are more cosmetic in appearance.
   b. Prosthetic hooks simulate the hook power grip by virtue of their shape. They provide a lateral or tip pinch during opening and closing of two identical hooks placed next to each other.

Voluntary Opening Terminal Devices

1. These are maintained in a closed position by rubber bands or springs until a pull on a body-powered cable system opens them (Fig. 13-5).
2. The maximum closing strength of the device is determined by the number and tension of rubber bands present, which has to be overpowered by muscle strength through the harness-cable system during opening.
3. The patient can gauge the amount of prehensile force by exerting a pull on the terminal device to counteract part or all of the predetermined closing tension.
4. It is the most common terminal device prescribed because of its practicality.
5. No voluntary intention is required to sustain the grip as the terminal device is used to hold an object (Table 13-3).

Voluntary Closing Terminal Devices

1. These are kept open by a spring.
2. To close the device for grasping, the patient pulls on the harness that is connected to the terminal device through a cable.
3. These systems provide more proprioceptive input from the terminal device to the body through the cable and harness connection.
4. Although it is more physiologic than the voluntary opening terminal device, the disadvantage is apparent during prolonged grasping, when constant pulling is required.
5. In addition, the patient must be strong enough to overcome the tension that maintains that terminal device in an opened position to close it.

PROSTHETIC WRIST

1. Wrist units provide a receptacle for the terminal device to sit and position the terminal device for functional activities.
2. The most commonly used prosthetic wrist allows passive pronation and supination.
3. Spring-assisted rotation mechanisms are available for bilateral amputees.
4. Also indispensable for bilateral upper extremity amputees is a mechanical spring-assisted wrist flexion unit. Without this unit, it is difficult for the

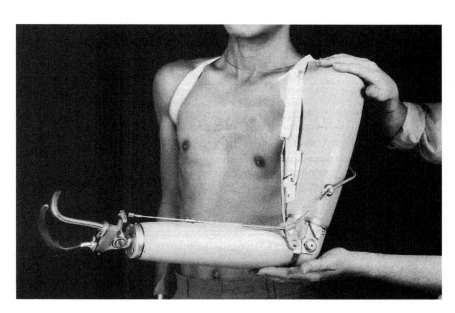

Figure 13-5 ◆ Terminal device operation. *(From Bowker JH, Michael JW, eds: Atlas of Limb Prosthetics: Surgical, Prosthetic, and Rehabilitation Principles, 2nd ed. Philadelphia, Mosby, 1992.)*

◆ **Table 13-3**

DIFFERENCES IN VOLUNTARY OPENING AND VOLUNTARY CLOSING TERMINAL DEVICES

Voluntary Opening	Voluntary Closing
Most commonly prescribed	Best for handling crushable objects
Resting position is closed	Resting position is variable
Less conscious effort required	More conscious effort required
Grip strength set by rubber bands or spring	More bulky and expensive
No voluntary control over amount of closing force	Not as durable as voluntary opening hooks

patient to reach the midline of the body, which makes grooming, feeding, personal care hygiene, and buttoning of a garment impossible.

5. A quick-disconnect wrist can be installed for rapid exchange of different terminal devices.

PROSTHETIC ELBOW

1. Prosthetic elbow joints can be passive, body powered, or externally powered.
2. The body-powered and externally powered prosthetic elbow joints are controlled by a cable system or electrical signals, respectively.
3. A locking mechanism for the elbow joint that is manually applied by use of the contralateral hand, the chin, or the ipsilateral shoulder through a cable fixes the joint at the desired angle achieved by one of the control mechanisms described before (e.g., figure-of-eight harness).
4. For transhumeral amputees, a turntable can enhance the internal and external rotation function of the arm.
5. For elbow disarticulations, the anatomy of the residual distal humerus provides rotational control as long as the shape of the prosthetic socket conforms to that of the medial and lateral condyles.
6. Polycentric elbow joints or a split socket with step-up hinges can be used to provide additional flexion at the price of less flexion power.

PROSTHETIC SHOULDER

1. Shoulder units for shoulder disarticulation or forequarter amputations add passive positioning of the prosthetic limb in flexion-extension and abduction-adduction.
2. Sockets extend onto the thorax to suspend and stabilize the prosthesis.
3. The socket is more extensive for forequarter amputations, in which the scapula is missing.
4. Open-frame sockets can be used to reduce weight and to promote air ventilation.

Prosthetic Training

1. Prosthetic training is an integral part of the rehabilitation process and focuses on education of the patient about prosthetic management.

2. The patient should learn the basic principles behind the function, care, and maintenance of each of the components in the prosthesis.
3. Independent donning and doffing of the prosthesis should be practiced.
4. Skin care and inspection techniques are also critical aspects of prosthetic care.
   a. Initially, the patient should not wear the prosthesis for more than 15 to 20 minutes without checking the skin.
   b. This duration can gradually be increased to an entire day within the first week with adequate skin tolerance.
5. For the prosthesis to be functional, the patient must be proficient in opening, closing, grasping with, releasing, transferring objects with, and positioning the terminal device.
6. Bimanual activities, such as grooming, dressing, feeding, driving, and special bathroom techniques, should be part of the training process for the bilateral amputee.
7. Foot skills should be reviewed and a lower extremity mobilization program initiated.
8. The goals for externally powered devices are similar. However, the training is more complex and probably requires more time.

Reintegration into the Community

1. This is best accomplished as a gradual process during a course of weeks or even months.
2. The entire process can be initiated early with the supervision of the rehabilitation team during organized outings, recreation trips, part-time work, or attending school.
3. The patient can return to work whenever it is safe to do so.
4. Modified duty should be provided initially. However, the patient should *not* be discouraged from returning to his or her premorbid functional level.
5. Realistic goals for the unilateral transradial or transhumeral amputees include independence in all activities of daily living, most household activities, driving, and most occupations.
6. A typical patient with a transradial amputation can be expected to lift 20 to 30 pounds; a transhumeral amputee should be able to lift 10 to 15 pounds.
7. For the bilateral amputee, after assisted donning of the prosthesis, realistic goals are independence in most activities of daily living, household activities with limitations, driving with a spin ring, and most types of sedentary work.
8. Strong magnetic fields or large electric currents at the workplace may interfere with myoelectric devices without special shielding material.

Long-term Follow-up

1. After completion of a rehabilitation program, patients are observed every 3 months for the first 18 months or more frequently if problems arise.

2. After this critical period, follow-up can be more spread out. The aim is assessment of the need for maintenance and the overall functional level of the patient.
3. It may be necessary to replace a portion of the prosthesis or the entire prosthesis every 18 months to 3 years for a body-powered prosthesis and every 2 to 4 years for a myoelectric device.

COMMON PROBLEMS

Neuroma Formation
1. Scar tissue forms around the severed nerve endings, resulting in a neuroma.
2. At the time of amputation, nerve endings should be buried in bone or deep tissues to prevent neuroma formation.
3. A painful neuroma is usually palpable on physical examination.
4. Initial treatment involves desensitization techniques and relief of direct pressures overlying the neuroma.
5. Injection with a mixture of local anesthetics and corticosteroid can be performed.
6. Surgical excision is reserved for patients refractory to conservative modalities who are severely symptomatic.

Dermatologic Problems
1. These include hyperhidrosis, folliculitis, allergic dermatitis, and even skin breakdown.
2. These are due to the problems with air circulation inside the prosthesis.
3. The patient should be trained in the proper washing maneuvers for the residual limb, socks, the socket, and its interface.
4. Prevention of these dermatologic conditions with frequent skin inspection cannot be overemphasized.

Pediatric Limb Deficiency and Amputation
(see Chapter 12)

1. The pediatric patient can have either an acquired or a congenital upper limb deficiency.
2. The child with a congenital limb deficiency usually has no sense of loss and does not have to go through the psychological adjustment process.
3. The incidence of congenital upper limb deficiency is approximately 4.1 per 10,000 live births.
4. Limb deficiencies can be classified as follows:
   a. Terminal: the limb has developed normally to a particular level, beyond which no skeletal elements exist.
   b. Intercalary: there is a reduction or absence of one or more elements within the long axis of the limb, and normal skeletal elements may be present distal to the affected segment.
5. The most common congenital limb deficiency is the *left terminal transverse radial* limb.

SPECIAL CONSIDERATIONS FOR THE PEDIATRIC PATIENT
1. Normal growth and development necessitate frequent prosthetic adjustments or change.

a. Multilayered sockets (i.e., onion sockets) can be used for body-powered devices, allowing removal of one layer at a time to accommodate increase in size.
   b. Length adjustment, although not as critical as with a lower limb prosthesis, is also important.
   c. Harnesses and cables need to be lengthened or replaced as the child grows.
2. Bone overgrowth calls for constant attention to the comfort of the socket and the condition of the soft tissue.
3. The vigorous use of the prosthetic device significantly shortens its life span compared with use in adult patients.
   a. It can be expected that all or part of a prosthesis will need to be replaced yearly in the first 5 years of life, every 18 months from 5 to 12 years of age, and every 2 years until age 21 years.
4. The need for frequent socket replacements, the cost of the prosthesis, and the weight and size of the components make myoelectric devices less practical for the pediatric patient. In addition, optimal electrode contact can be difficult to maintain in a growing child.
5. Timing
   a. Prosthesis fitting should be initiated at 6 to 9 months of age, which coincides with the beginning of bimanual activities. A passive prosthesis should be fitted at this stage so that a prosthesis can be incorporated into the child's body image.
   b. A body-powered prosthesis is often considered at 15 months to 2 years of age, and a terminal device can be activated at ages 18 to 24 months and at the elbow at ages 36 to 48 months.
6. The training period for a younger child is usually longer than that for an adult.

Spasticity Management

1. Spasticity is a motor disorder characterized by a velocity-dependent resistance to movement associated with exaggerated phasic stretch reflexes (e.g., tendon jerks).
2. Tone is the sensation of resistance the examiner feels within a muscle as it is stretched passively in a relaxed state.
3. Initial management should begin with a daily stretching program and avoidance of noxious stimuli.

PHARMACOLOGIC TREATMENT
Pharmacologic treatments are most effective in patients with mild to moderate tones. For severe cases, the drugs may not work or the cognitive side effects may be prohibitive. Commonly used agents include the following.

Diazepam (Valium)
1. Mechanism of action involves the facilitation of the postsynaptic effects of γ-aminobutyric acid (GABA).
2. GABA suppresses release of excitatory neurotransmitters.

3. Diazepam has been shown to be a successful treatment modality for spastic hypertonia in spinal cord injury.
4. It is unsuitable for patients with brain injury because of its sedative effect.

Baclofen (Lioresal)
1. Baclofen is a GABA analogue.
2. It is less sedating than diazepam and therefore is the drug of choice for spinal forms of spasticity or in patients with head injury.
3. Intrathecal delivery through a subdermal pump largely avoids the central nervous system side effects associated with oral intake.

Dantrolene Sodium (Dantrium)
1. Mechanism of action involves the reduction of calcium release into the sarcoplasmic reticulum of skeletal muscle induced by muscle action potentials.
2. It is the drug of choice for cerebral forms of spasticity.

Clonidine
1. This is an α_2-adrenergic agonist that is traditionally used as an antihypertensive agent.
2. It can be effective in controlling spasticity for patients with spinal cord injury.
3. It is not suitable for patients with autonomic nervous system instability.

SURGICAL MANAGEMENT
1. Surgical treatment of spasticity can involve lengthening of the musculotendinous unit by either Z-lengthening of the tendon or functional lengthening at the musculotendinous junction.
2. Motor nerve ablation can result in permanent elimination of spasticity.
3. Tendon transfers can also decrease spasticity.
   a. Superficialis to profundus (STP) transfers are indicated in patients with severe spasticity of finger flexion.
      i. It is contraindicated in patients with volitional control of the finger flexors.

ii. It can help with hygiene and skin care in the palm of the hand.

FOCAL SPASMS
Focal spasms can be managed by chemical neurolysis, paralysis, or surgical neurectomy. Commonly used agents for chemical neurolysis include phenol and botulinum toxin. If chemical blocks are not successful, surgical neurectomy of the affected site can lead to symptom improvement.

Phenol (2% to 6% Aqueous Solution)
1. Phenol is used to chemically disrupt a peripheral nerve at the neuromuscular junction or in the nerve parenchyma.
2. Denervation can last up to 6 months.
3. Disruption of sensory fibers may result in dysesthesias or causalgia.
4. For example, musculocutaneous blocks may be useful in the hemiplegic patient with upper extremity elbow flexion synergy or in the C5 quadriplegic patient who has elbow flexion unopposed by a paretic triceps muscle.
5. Patients with intrinsic spasticity can be treated with a phenol block of the ulnar motor branch at Guyon's canal. A surgical neurectomy can result in permanent nerve ablation.

Botulinum Toxin
1. This is a neurotoxin derived from *Clostridium botulinum* serotype A bacteria.
2. Mechanism of action involves the limitation of neuromuscular transmission by inhibition of the presynaptic release of acetylcholine, but not its synthesis or storage.
3. Intramuscular injection produces results similar to those of partial denervation.
4. Clinical effects are seen 24 to 72 hours after administration and peak 4 to 6 weeks later.
5. Because of the site of action, this agent is contraindicated in disorders of neuromuscular junctions, such as myasthenia gravis.
6. Dosing more frequently than every 3 months is not recommended to avoid the formation of antibodies.

◆ Table 13-4

RECONSTRUCTIVE OPTIONS FOR PATIENTS WITH UPPER CERVICAL INJURIES

Functioning Muscles Below Elbow	Procedure	Reconstructive Goal
None	Deltoid to triceps transfer or biceps to triceps transfer	Elbow extension
Brachioradialis (Br) [C5-6]	Moberg procedure (FPL tenodesis to distal radius + thumb IP fusion)	Simple hand grip (key pinch)
	Br to wrist extensor transfer (wrist extension), Moberg procedure	Wrist extension
ECRL [C6-7]	Moberg procedure (FPL tenodesis to distal radius + thumb IP fusion) or Br to FPL transfer + Thumb IP fusion	Simple hand grip (key pinch)
ECRB [C6-8]	Br to FPL transfer + thumb IP fusion	Simple hand grip (key pinch)
	ECRL to FDP	Finger flexion
	EDC tenodesis to distal radius	Finger extension
Pronator teres (PT) [C6-8]	PT to FCR transfer	Wrist flexion
	Br to FPL transfer + thumb IP fusion	Simple hand grip (key pinch)
	ECRL to FDP	Finger flexion
	Moberg procedure (FPL tenodesis to distal radius + thumb IP fusion)	Simple hand grip (key pinch)

7. The use of botulinum toxin has recently been expanded to reduce focal dystonia (co-contraction of agonist and antagonist muscles) (e.g., writer's cramp) in muscles by direct injection.

Tetraplegia

Reconstructive options for tetraplegia are outlined in Table 13-4.

Manual Dexterity Testing

Several objective tests have been developed to quantify dexterity.

1. Jebson-Taylor Hand Function Test evaluates manual dexterity and includes seven subtests. This test assesses gross coordination, is inexpensive, and is easy to administer.
2. The Minnesota Rate of Manipulation Test involves placing blocks into spaces on a board and assesses gross coordination.
3. The Purdue Pegboard Test evaluates finger coordination requiring prehension of small pins, washers, and collars.
4. The Moberg Pickup Test evaluates the sensory component of hand function and is not a test of manual dexterity. This is a timed test in which the patient must pick up an assortment of objects while the method of prehension is assessed.

Bibliography

Bowker JH, Michael JW, eds: Atlas of Limb Prosthetics: Surgical, Prosthetic, and Rehabilitation Principles, 2nd ed. Philadelphia, Mosby, 1992.

Challenor Y: Limb deficiencies in children. In Molnar G, ed: Pediatric Rehabilitation. Baltimore, Williams & Wilkins, 1992, pp 400-424.

Esquenazi A: Upper limb amputee rehabilitation and prosthetic restoration. In Braddom RL, ed: Physical Medicine and Rehabilitation. Philadelphia, WB Saunders, 1996, pp 275-288.

Esquenazi A, Leonard JA, Meier RH, et al: Prosthetics. Arch Phys Med Rehabil 70(Suppl):207, 1989.

Irani KD: Upper limb orthoses. In Braddom RL, ed: Physical Medicine and Rehabilitation. Philadelphia, WB Saunders, 1996, pp 321-332.

Katz RT: Management of spastic hypertonia. Am J Phys Med Rehabil 67:108-116, 1988.

Kejlaa GH: The social and economic outcome after upper limb amputation. Prosthet Orthot Int 16:25-31, 1992.

Leonard JA Jr, Meier RH III: Upper and lower extremity prosthetics. In DeLisa JA, Gans BM, eds: Rehabilitation Medicine: Principles and Practice, 3rd ed. Philadelphia, Lippincott-Raven, 1998, pp 669-680.

Mackin EJ, Callahan AD, Skirven TM, et al, eds: Rehabilitation of the Hand and Upper Extremity. Philadelphia, Mosby, 2002.

Malone JM, Fleming LL, Roberson J, et al: Immediate, early and late postsurgical management of upper limb amputation. J Rehabil Res Dev 21:33, 1984.

Schutt A: Upper extremity and hand orthotics. Phys Med Rehabil Clin North Am 3:223-240, 1992.

US Department of Health and Human Services: Current estimates from the National Health Interview Survey. Washington, DC, National Center for Health Statistics, 1990.

INDEX

Note: Page numbers followed by the letter f refer to figures and those followed by t refer to tables.